Prehospital Emergency Care

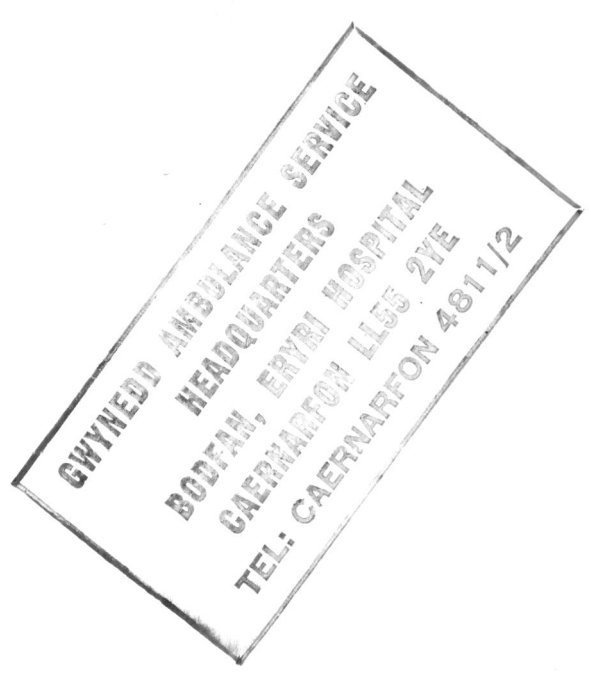

EMERGENCY CARE SERIES

Prehospital Emergency Care

S. James Mather MB BS LRCP MRCS DRCOG FFARCS
*Consultant Anaesthetist, Bristol Royal Infirmary and
The Royal Hospital for Sick Children, Bristol*
and
David L. Edbrooke LRCP MRCS FFARCS
Consultant Anaesthetist, Royal Hallamshire Hospital, Sheffield

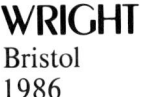
Bristol
1986

© **IOP Publishing Limited.** 1986

All Rights Reserved. No part of this publication may be reproduced, stored in a retrieval system, or transmitted in any form or by any means, electronic, mechanical, photocopying, recording or otherwise, without the prior permission of the Copyright owner.

Published under the Wright imprint by
IOP Publishing Limited, Techno House, Redcliffe Way
Bristol BS1 6NX, England

British Library Cataloguing in Publication Data

Mather, S. James
    Prehospital emergency care.—(Emergency care series)
    1. Emergency medicine
    I. Title   II. Edbrooke, David L.   III. Series
616'.025   RC86.7

ISBN 0 7236 0701 X

Typeset by
Severntype Repro Services Ltd, Market Street, Wotton-under-Edge, Glos.

Printed in Great Britain by
Henry Ling Ltd, Dorset Press, Dorchester

Preface

This book has been written to assist non-medically qualified personnel in the field of Emergency Medicine. In the past few years, research has established beyond reasonable doubt, that good training in specific skills in the field of resuscitation, can make considerable impact in morbidity and mortality outside the hospital environment. It is also clear that bystander-initiated resuscitation can have a similar impact in reducing morbidity and mortality 'in the street'.

It is the authors' opinion that substantial effort is worthwhile in both these areas and it is hoped that this book will go some way towards helping non-medically qualified personnel, working in the field of emergency medicine, attain the theoretical knowledge necessary for good patient treatment.

Finally, we would like to stress that this book is intended to complement practical training courses, as familiarity with practical procedures as well as theoretical knowledge is essential.

S.J.M.
D.L.E.

Contributors

M. L. Allen MBBS MRCP FRCS (Eng)
Senior Registrar in Accident and Emergency Medicine, Leeds Royal Infirmary

N. R. Bennett MBChB FFARCS
Consultant in Paediatric Anaesthesia and Intensive Care, The Children's Hospital, Sheffield and Honorary Clinical Lecturer, University of Sheffield

R. J. S. Birks MBChB FFARCS
Consultant Anaesthetist, Sheffield Health Authority and Honorary Clinical Lecturer, University of Sheffield

J. E. Butter SRN
Lecturer in Health and Community Studies, Highbury College of Technology, Cosham, Portsmouth

A. C. Crosby MBChB FRCS (Ed)
Senior Registrar in Accident and Emergency Medicine, The Royal Hallamshire Hospital, Sheffield

G. K. Davies MB FFARCS
Consultant Anaesthetist, Northern General Hospital and The Royal Hallamshire Hospital, Sheffield and Honorary Clinical Lecturer, University of Sheffield

D. L. Edbrooke LRCP MRCS FFARCS
Consultant in Anaesthesia and Intensive Care, The Royal Hallamshire Hospital, Sheffield and Honorary Clinical Lecturer, University of Sheffield

D. G. Ferguson MBBCh BAO FRCS
Consultant in Accident and Emergency Medicine, The Royal Hallamshire Hospital, Sheffield and Honorary Clinical Lecturer, University of Sheffield

J. C. Frankland BSc MBChB FRCGP DRCOG
General Practitioner, Lancaster; Medical Officer, Cave Rescue Organization; in charge of medical cover, Morecambe Bay Gas Field

M. J. Mangion SRN
Senior Sister, Intensive Care Unit, Rotherham District General Hospital, Rotherham

S. J. Mather MBBS LRCPMRCS DRCOG FFARCS
Consultant in Anaesthesia and Intensive Care, Sir Humphry Davy Department of Anaesthesia, Bristol Royal Infirmary and The Royal Hospital for Sick Children, Bristol and Honorary Clinical Teacher, University of Bristol

J. V. Mundy MBChB FFARCS
Senior Registrar in Anaesthesia, The Royal Hallamshire Hospital, Sheffield

J. R. Paskins MBBS FRCS
Consultant in Accident and Emergency Medicine, The Royal Infirmary, Doncaster

D. I. Rowley MBChB FRCS
Lecturer in Orthopaedic Surgery, Honorary Senior Registrar, The Royal Hallamshire Hospital, Sheffield

H. G. Schroeder MBChB FFARCS DA
Consultant in Anaesthesia and Intensive Care, The Royal Hallamshire Hospital, Sheffield; Lecturer in Clinical Anaesthesia, Resuscitation and Intensive Care, University of Sheffield

Claire M. Taylor SRN ARRC QARNNS
Superintending Nursing Officer, Royal Naval Medical Staff School, Gosport

P. C. Taylor MBChB MRCP
Senior Registrar (Haematology) South-West Regional Health Authority

R. A. Warren MBChB FRCS
Consultant Surgeon (Accident and Emergency), St Stephen's Hospital, London

M. J. Wolfe MBBS FFARCS
Consultant Anaesthetist, Chesterfield and North Derbyshire Royal Hospital, Calow, Chesterfield

Acknowledgements

The editors wish to acknowledge gratefully the help of Dr P. Baskett, Dr M. Bird, Dr A. Dixon and Mr K. Hoddy in the preparation of the manuscript, and Mrs M. Hunt for her secretarial assistance, and Mr J. Larder for help in preparing illustrations.

Contents

Chapter			
	1	Introduction	1
	2	Examination and Monitoring of the Patient *S. J. Mather, D. L. Edbrooke and M. J. Mangion*	4
	3	Nursing Care of the Injured *Claire M. Taylor*	22
	4	Fluid Balance and Therapy *D. L. Edbrooke and S. J. Mather*	25
	5	The Control of Pain *S. J. Mather and D. L. Edbrooke*	43
	6	Oxygen Therapy and Airway Management *D. L. Edbrooke and S. J. Mather*	48
	7	Cardiopulmonary Resuscitation *D. L. Edbrooke and S. J. Mather*	70
	8	The Respiratory System. I. Trauma *R. J. S. Birks*	82
	9	The Respiratory System. II. Non-trauma *P. C. Taylor*	91
	10	The Cardiovascular System. I. Trauma *G. K. Davies*	98
	11	The Cardiovascular System. II. Non-trauma *G. K. Davies*	105
	12	The Abdomen *R. A. Warren*	123
	13	The Musculoskeletal System *D. I. Rowley*	132
	14	The Nervous System. I. Trauma *A. C. Crosby and J. R. Paskins*	147
	15	The Nervous System. II. Non-trauma *S. J. Mather and D. L. Edbrooke*	152
	16	Damage to Special Senses *J. R. Paskins*	164
	17	Disorders of The Endocrine System *J. V. Mundy*	177
	18	Pregnancy and Related Problems *M. J. Wolfe*	190
	19	Shock and Thermal Injury *S. J. Mather and D. L. Edbrooke*	198

20	**Paediatric Emergencies** *N. R. Bennett*	210
21	**Toxicology and Common Poisoning** *H. G. Schroeder*	222
22	**The Trauma of Civil Disturbance** *D. G. Ferguson*	233
23	**Sports Injuries** *M. J. Allen*	244
24	**Cave and Mountain Rescue: Some Special Aspects of Prehospital Care** *J. C. Frankland*	258
25	**Aviation and Underwater Medicine** *J. E. Butter*	269
26	**Nuclear, Biological and Chemical Warfare** *J. E. Butter and S. J. Mather*	284
	Index	299

Chapter 1

Introduction

S. J. Mather and D. L. Edbrooke

When considering 'immediate care', road traffic accidents are the most obvious consideration, but industrial injury, accidents in the home, acute medical and surgical emergencies may also require early skilled intervention.

The wider concept of the care provided outside the hospital ('immediate' or 'prehospital' care), together with the continuing attention the patient receives in hospital, is embraced by the term 'critical care'. It is those aspects of critical care appropriate to emergency services personnel that we shall attempt to review in this book. In addition, some principles of early management in hospital are reviewed.

Often, the early treatment of sudden illness or injury can drastically influence the eventual outcome. This is particularly true in acute coronary ischaemia or myocardial infarction, poisoning and major trauma.

In recent years paramedical personnel have 'extended' the Accident and Emergency Department to the scene of the incident. This approach to critical care has been shown to have resulted in a statistically better outcome for patients. It is hard to quantify the benefit of prehospital care to any one individual and this has been one of the reasons for delay in the implementation of a nationwide paramedical ambulance service in the UK. The other main reason has, of course, been the cost. Training programmes are expensive and, once qualified, personnel are required to undertake regular periods of refresher training. The Department of Health seems to have developed a very cautious attitude towards advanced training. This attitude has brought a great deal of frustration to dedicated ambulance personnel and others in the field of prehospital care.

In certain other countries, but particularly in the USA, the 'paramedic' or Emergency Medical Technician has become a part of the structure of early medical care. Indeed, they have been welcomed and accepted by other professionals and the public alike. Today's public have a right to expect that their initial medical care will be provided by a highly trained person. This cannot always be a doctor and so an individual trained in the necessary skills to provide life support and pain relief, together with safe transport and monitoring, is the ultimate answer.

TRAINING OF CRITICAL CARE PERSONNEL

It should be the objective of all trainers to ensure that trainees are taught the skills necessary to care for the patient outside hospital. Training in these skills can be taught only to a limited extent in the classroom. Intubation models are useful but they are no substitute for the real life situation. Certain skills, notably airway care, endotracheal intubation and intravenous infusion, must be taught by an experienced clinician in hospital. Areas where useful experience is to be obtained include the intensive care and coronary care units, the Accident and Emergency Department, the operating theatre and, of course, experience 'on-site' at an actual incident where patients are receiving prehospital care.

It is, perhaps, important at this stage to clarify the nomenclature used throughout the book. *Prehospital care* will be used in preference to immediate care as the former term is completely self explanatory.

The term *paramedical personnel* will be used to describe highly trained but non-medically qualified individuals who have the expertise to treat patients either before qualified medical help is available or as part of a medical team.

Critical care personnel is a term which encompasses both medical and non-medically qualified personnel working in both the hospital and prehospital situations where the patient's life is at risk.

In some situations, prehospital care will inevitably have to be provided by, for example, soldiers, sailors, aircrew, mineworkers, mountain rescue teams, firemen or policemen. There are many other examples. Our aim is to provide an outline of the knowledge required of any person involved in the early care of patients from whatever 'service'.

All paramedical personnel should have some knowledge of the workings of their local hospital and should be familiar with the roles of medical, nursing and ancillary staff. This helps to achieve the liaison so vital to the provision of good medical care.

THE ORGANIZATION OF ON-SITE CARE

There is still much discussion regarding the most suitable personnel for attendance at road traffic accidents and emergencies in the home and factory. There is no doubt that if highly trained and experienced medical staff were available in large numbers then this would represent the ideal situation. This is, at the time of writing, unlikely to occur. At the other extreme, some doctors and ambulancemen firmly believe that a 'scoop and run' policy of getting the patient to hospital as quickly as possible is preferable. This is appropriate to a war situation, but is not accepted by most as ideal policy.

The authors believe that the best compromise is to train suitable paramedical personnel to a high level of competence and to discourage the involvement of doctors with no training in prehospital care.

MAJOR DISASTER PLANNING

We can define a major disaster as a situation which cannot be dealt with by the normal emergency procedure but requires mobilization of additional personnel and equipment.

It is often implicit in the organization of major accident teams that a medical practitioner with little experience of such situations is sent to organize the 'on-site' medical service.

We feel that, properly trained, paramedical personnel are more efficient in an organizational and therapeutic role at the scene than medical staff with no experience of on-site emergency care. Most doctors have never been to a major disaster, and most have never been taught even the rudiments of disaster planning. In the event, it is our view that medical staff who are to fulfil the role of 'site medical officer' should work with, and be familiar with the expertise of, their colleagues in the ambulance service. The same applies to doctors and nurses working with paramedical personnel on oil rigs or in the armed services.

Thus doctors who are involved in teaching these personnel will be best suited to liaise with them on-site. In many areas, such personnel do not exist and family practitioners, especially in rural areas, can provide the service of prehospital care. It must not be assumed, however, that all doctors are equally familiar with the skills required. Few family practitioners will be able to undertake advanced life support techniques without a period of further training. In urban environments, in the absence of advanced-trained ambulance personnel, hospital doctors and nurses may be better suited to this role.

Further reading
Zorab J. S. M. and Baskett P. J. F. (1977) *Immediate Care.* New York, Saunders.

Chapter 2

Examination and Monitoring of the Patient

S. J. Mather, D. L. Edbrooke and M. J. Mangion

EXAMINATION OF THE PATIENT

Assessment of the patient properly includes taking a history concerning the events which have led to the patient requiring care. It is important to elicit a history of any previous illnesses, hospitalization, drug therapy or allergy. Only then can we progress to *physical* examination of the patient. Specific questioning relating to particular injuries or pain may lead to better diagnosis and management.

One must not confine the history only to the patient. Any bystanders or witnesses to the event should be interviewed and any relevant information recorded. In the case of a road traffic accident such information might include speed of vehicles, direction of impact and the wearing of seatbelts.

It is useful to have a 'check-list' of points or 'scheme for history taking' such as that shown in *Fig.* 2.1 for the trauma patient.

We shall now describe in detail how to conduct the physical examination and its significance. A thorough examination can be performed quite easily in a few minutes.

1. General

If the skin or mucous membranes appears blue (cyanosed) there is a significant degree of hypoxaemia. In the peripheries this may be due to poor local blood flow but central cyanosis (i.e. blue lips) is always significant. Pale, sweating skin denotes increased activity of the sympathetic nervous system due, for example, to pain or low circulating volume (hypovolaemia), or indeed these signs can be produced by anxiety. Bleeding or leakage of cerebrospinal fluid from the nose or ear suggests a fracture of the base of the skull. Blood in the urine may

Fig. 2.1. 'Scheme for history taking'. Trauma patient.

History
Observed event e.g. head on collision. When?
Number of persons involved—in vehicles, pedestrian.
How many vehicles? Speed? Direction?
Any fuel or chemical spillage? Fire?
Any high-voltage cables? Gas or water mains damaged?

Injuries to each patient
Patient conscious or unconscious?
Predominant symptoms
Level of consciousness. Changing since accident?
Vomiting? Bloodstained vomit, urine?
Bleeding? (Don't forget per rectum)
Fitting?
History of alcohol or drugs?

Physical examination (proceeding down the body)
General appearance (pale, sweating, blue, etc.)
Surgical emphysema?   Loss of normal contours?
                     —deformity; malocclusion?
Heart rate—apex beat, carotid or femoral pulses.
Cardiac output—blood pressure
   a, by palpation
   b, by auscultation (Riva Rocci method)
Neck veins distended? Oedema
Any blood or CSF from nose or ears
Local trauma to neck or chest?
Spine—local tenderness? Lack of feeling or movement?
Respiratory rate and depth. Equal both sides?
Trachea—deviation?
Percussion of chest and vocal resonance?
Heart sounds, breath sounds
Abdomen—contour. Soft or tense? Bruising? Movement with respiration
Genitalia
Limbs—peripheral pulses
     —soft tissues
     —long bones
     —nerve or muscle damage

Write down the examination, preferably on a pro-forma, as follows:
General appearance
    pallor, cyanosis, sweating
    obvious deformities or lesions
    any CSF or blood from ear or nose?
    bleeding PR or in urine
Cardiovascular system
    pulse (heart rate at apex)
    distended neck veins?
    oedema
    heart sounds
    blood pressure

Fig. 2.1. (Cont.)

Respiratory system
    chest expansion; respiratory rate
    position of trachea
    percussion and vocal resonance
    auscultation
    presence of any cough or sputum
Abdomen
    shape, normal contour—
    distension? rigidity, tenderness?
    palpable swellings
    bowel sounds
Genitalia
Skull, spine, locomotor system
Nervous system
    any detectable deficit or abnormality
    (*See* Glasgow Coma Scale, p. 000)

indicate damage anywhere in the renal tract from the kidney to the urethra. A fractured pelvis may damage the bladder or urethra.

2. Cardiovascular system

A pulse can be felt in the left side of the chest (usually in the space between the 5th and 6th ribs) and is known as the apex beat. It can often be felt, or heard through the stethoscope, when no other pulses are palpable. Feeling (or palpation) and counting of this apex beat is the most accurate means of assessing the heart rate by manual means.

Rhythm

It is important to note whether the rhythm is regular or irregular. If it is irregular, is it so in time as well as in volume (strength)? Irregular pulses are common following myocardial infarction.

The pulse in atrial fibrillation is described as 'irregularly irregular', that is, irregular in both time and volume. If the pattern of irregularity recurs or occasionally a beat is 'missed' (in reality a premature beat) the cause is most likely to be extrasystoles. An extrasystole is merely a beat which occurs prematurely, and may be either atrial or ventricular. They occur when an ectopic focus in the heart depolarizes (initiates a wave of electrical activity) before the normal pacemaker (sino-atrial node). These extrasystoles are sometimes called 'ectopics'.

Venous pressure

An estimate of the venous pressure (and thus indirectly of the filling pressure of the right side of the heart) can be made by inspecting the jugular veins in the neck. In a healthy individual the veins should not stand out above the level of the manubrium (top of the breast bone) unless the patient is lying at an angle of less than 45° to the horizontal. In right heart failure, pulmonary embolus and circulatory overload, the neck veins may be engorged, even in a patient sitting upright.

Heart sounds

The modern stethoscope usually consists of a combined diaphragm/bell chestpiece connected by plastic tubing of high sound conductivity to two earpieces. The diaphragm and bell each best transmit different types of sound, the bell being better for low-pitched sounds.

Paramedical personnel would not be expected to use the stethoscope to detect the murmurs of cardiac valvular disease or the many different types of breath sounds found in lung disease. They will, however, need to be able to establish the presence of heart sounds and breath sounds since their presence or absence is most helpful in the diagnosis of certain conditions such as cardiac tamponade and pneumothorax.

Auscultation of the heart

Normally two heart sounds can be heard, the first and second sounds. The first corresponds to contraction of the ventricles (systole), the second to the beginning of ventricular relaxation (diastole). The first sound is due to closure of the atrioventricular valves. The second sound may be 'split', the aortic valve being heard to close a fraction of a second before the pulmonary valve.

There are certain 'areas' of the chest wall (e.g. aortic and pulmonary areas) where their respective sounds are supposedly best heard (*Fig.* 2.2).

3. Respiratory system

The colour of the patient is one of the first assessments to be made. The trachea should be felt in the neck and any deviation from the midline noted. Deviation occurs to the opposite side in pneumo- or haemothorax. In addition, air under the skin (surgical emphysema) should be sought as this may indicate injury to the lung, pleura or tracheobronchial tree. Note the shape of the chest and whether there is full and equal expansion on both sides when the patient breathes in.

Percussion

An appreciation of the resonant qualities of each side of the chest may be gained by striking the chest firmly with one finger (a finger of the opposite hand is used as a 'sounding board').

The chest can be likened to a drum. In pneumothorax, the air-filled cavity makes the chest more resonant on the affected side (hyperresonant). In contrast, when the lung is collapsed or consolidated (Chapter 8) the percussion note is dull. When fluid is present, as in a pleural effusion, the note is 'stony dull'.

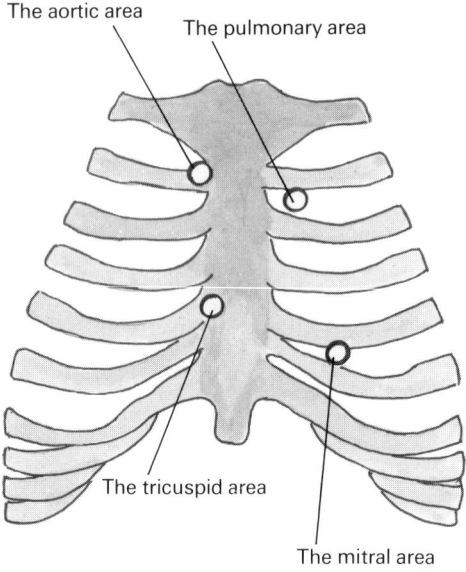

Fig. 2.2. The positions of the auscultatory areas.

Vocal resonance

If the patient can speak one should listen over the lung fields from above downward, comparing one side with the other whilst the patient says 'ninety-nine'. Any change in the perceived sound should be noted. This may yield valuable information as to the condition of the lungs (e.g. it will be diminished over collapsed lung or when there is a pleural effusion, and increased over consolidated lung).

Auscultation of the breath sounds

The character of normal breath sounds can only be appreciated by listening to the chest of a normal individual. The diaphragm of the stethoscope is most useful for this. Normal breath sounds are termed 'vesicular' sounds. One cannot really differentiate a distinct gap between the end of inspiration and the beginning of expiration.

Breath sounds are absent when the lung is collapsed or there is a pleural effusion. In lung disease the normal vesicular breath sounds may change. Over a lung affected by pneumonia (consolidated) the sounds heard resemble those audible over the trachea. There is a distinct pause between inspiration and expiration and the sound is harsher. This is known as *bronchial breathing*.

Added sounds

When fluid is present in the lungs a sound reminiscent of that made by rubbing one's hair together is often heard. It is due to changes in the opening characteristics of the smallest airways and is called *'crepitation'*. Crepitation is most usually associated with pulmonary oedema but occurs also in chest infection and certain other conditions.

Wheezes

Wheezes are termed rhonchi (rhonchus) by the medical profession. They are most often heard in obstructive airways disease such as chronic bronchitis and asthma.

4. The abdomen

When examining the patient look for changes in the normal contours. Does the abdomen move with respiration? Normally the abdominal wall bulges outwards when the patient breathes in. The *opposite* effect is seen when diaphragmatic function is lost. The presence of fluid within the abdominal cavity may splint movement of the walls. The abdomen may not move because there is muscle spasm due to underlying peritonitis.

Following the introduction of seat belts it is becoming more common to see clear marks of the seat belts on the abdomen. This is indicative of severe deceleration and damage to the abdomen must be assumed. At operation ruptured organs are very commonly found following seat belt injuries.

Palpation

This can only adequately be performed with the patient on his back. The whole abdomen is felt gently with the flat of the hand in a systematic fashion, e.g. beginning in the left lower quadrant and palpating each quadrant in turn. The liver and spleen are palpated whilst the patient takes a large inspiration.

Palpation (with a warm hand) should produce no discomfort. Look for local tenderness or rigidity of the abdominal muscles. In peritonitis maximum tenderness may occur when one lets go after pressing over the painful area. The liver and spleen are not normally palpable but may become so if swollen by haemorrhage or disease (e.g. the enlarged liver of right heart failure).

Paramedical personnel would not normally be expected to examine any other structures within the abdomen.

Auscultation

When auscultating the abdomen, one is listening principally for bowel sounds. Normal bowel sounds may be heard over any healthy abdomen, if one listens for a minute or two. The sounds are absent when there is peritonitis or ileus (a condition in which normal peristalsis has ceased) and increased in intestinal obstruction.

The genitalia

These should be examined when the abdominal examination has been carried out. Look for swelling, bruising (after trauma) and particularly examine any urine passed for blood. (Save this urine for later analysis in hospital.)

5. Nervous system

One cannot expect to perform an exhaustive neurological examination at the roadside but certain factors must be excluded or elicited particularly following trauma to the head or spine.

One should look for any facial asymmetry, drooling of saliva or inability to close the eyes and clench the teeth. Do the pupils react equally to light when a torch is shone onto each in turn; are they of equal size? Is the patient's hearing and sight intact? Can he protrude his tongue and does he gag when the back of his throat is touched with a blunt instrument? Can he shrug his shoulders? Abnormalities in these functions may indicate damage to the cranial nerves.

One should then examine each pair of limbs for muscle power and range of movement. Also note whether the muscle *tone* is increased (is the muscle floppy or stiff?) Next coarsely test sensation to light touch, moderate pressure and pinching the skin. Abnormalities can be elicited by comparing one side with the other. Great care must be taken in cases of spinal injury since the clue to the level or any cord lesion is dependent upon this clinical examination. Ask the patient, if conscious, if he can feel all his limbs and whether he has pain in his neck or back.

Before proceeding further a Glasgow Coma Scale should be instituted to produce a baseline of the patient's level of consciousness. This is described in detail in Chapter 14.

6. Locomotor system

The muscles, tendons, bones and joints collectively constitute the locomotor system.

Abnormal muscle movements or spasm may be important physical signs. They may be localized or generalized. Note that muscle pain may be the result of a protective reflex, for example in reducing the movements of the fragments of a fractured bone.

Bones and joints

One should look first for any change from the normal outline or shape, especially of limb bones, and for localized swellings or tenderness. Tenderness is also particularly important in the case of a suspected spinal injury. The joints should be examined carefully, first by

EXAMINATION AND MONITORING OF THE PATIENT

inspection, then by palpation (in an attempt to elicit tenderness or effusion, that is, fluid present around the joint). Finally the range of movement should be assessed *with reference to the opposite side*.

Caution

Extreme gentleness is required where a fracture is suspected. This is particularly so in the case of spinal injuries. Allow the patient to move for himself and never passively move the part further. Passive joint movement should never be performed by paramedical personnel on unconscious patients.

It is mandatory to remember that a cervical spine fracture may be present. It is, therefore, necessary to assume that one *is* present and not allow any degree of neck movement during examination or transport. It is best to apply a soft cervical collar or 'Hines' cervical splint to all patients who *could* have a neck or spine injury *before* moving them.

MONITORING

After careful examination, the patient must be monitored closely up to the time of arrival in hospital. This may be a matter of only a few minutes or may be considerably longer depending on the circumstances.

The most important facet of this is the documentation of such monitoring. By simply charting the progress of the patient before arrival in hospital, a much clearer impression can be gleaned in comparison to a quick resume in the resuscitation room. This should be standard practice for paramedical personnel.

A time-honoured method is to monitor progress by systems and this is still an excellent method.

1. General

By merely looking at a patient it is possible to glean quite a lot of information. In addition, the measurement of temperature classically does not fit into any of the systems and is so included in the general section. These general points can be subdivided as follows:

a. Temperature

The commonest method is by using the clinical mercury thermometer. This is quite accurate but is not really suitable for use in the field as it is extremely fragile. It is more practicable to use a modern thermistor thermometer (*see* Vol. 1, Chapter 22). These types of thermometers have the advantage of being portable, fairly cheap and very robust.

The site of measurement is also important. The axilla is a traditional site, is convenient but not very accurate. The other possible sites for use with the thermistor thermometer are the oesophagus, the mouth or the rectum. The oesophagus or rectum should be the sites of choice.

The use of temperature measurement in the prehospital environment is not yet accepted. To support the case for its use an example will be given. If a small child is seen and is convulsing then it is possible that these are febrile convulsions and this is one of the commonest causes in the small child. If this is the case then the standard policy of wrapping the patient in blankets will produce a rise in the central temperature. This is obviously not desirable.

In conclusion, it must be said that to monitor all patients' temperatures is obviously absurd. If, however, the journey to hospital is to be longer than 15 minutes, then the measurement of axillary temperature can be justified. If this is found to be more than $2°$ above or below normal then it is justifiable to insert a rectal thermistor thermometer. Patients with possible pelvic injury, especially if there is rectal bleeding, may be monitored by the oral thermistor probe.

b. Assessment of pain

This can be assessed by asking the patient whether there is any pain. This is very inaccurate but is the only indication available to the paramedic in the field. It is also important to locate the precise site of the pain and chart this. The character of the pain can also be assessed (e.g. sharp or dull).

c. Sweating

This is a non-specific sign but it is important to document it.

2. The cardiovascular system

This includes monitoring of the heart and peripheral circulation.

a. The heart rate

The rate and character of the heart rate should be monitored continuously. It must be stressed that monitoring of the heart itself is much more accurate than measuring the pulse at a peripheral site.

In addition to the rate of the heart, a note should be kept of the rhythm and rhythm changes throughout the monitoring period. There are two pieces of equipment which are useful in this respect. The first is a pulse monitor and the second an electrocardiographic monitor.

The pulse monitor

This is a device which measures the peripheral pulse rate and to some extent gives an indication of the peripheral blood flow.

The electrical activity of the heart can be monitored simply using portable monitoring apparatus. In the field it is not often feasible to make a full electrocardiogram which is printed on paper. It is possible to obtain a display of the electrical activity of the heart using an oscilloscope. It is

EXAMINATION AND MONITORING OF THE PATIENT

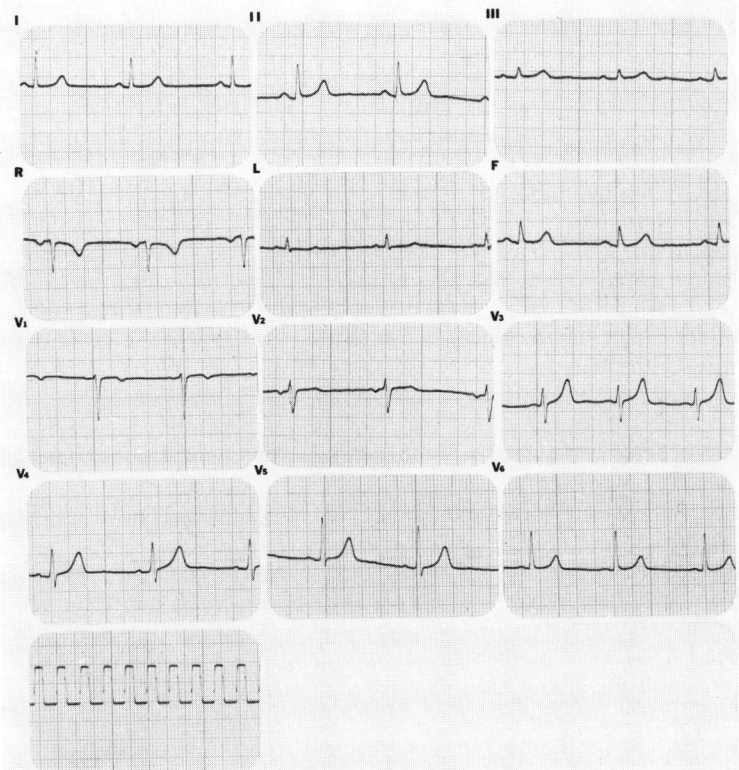

Fig. 2.3. The normal electrocardiogram.

necessary to understand the principles of electrocardiography and so a brief explanation of these is given below.

The electrocardiogram (Fig. 2.3)

The electrocardiogram (ECG) is a graphic representation of the electrical potentials produced by the heart. Electrodes are applied to the body surface and connected to an ECG machine which picks up the weak electrical current, amplifies it and reproduces it either on graph paper or on a cardiac monitor (oscilloscope). In a 12-lead electrocardiogram the heart is viewed from 12 different directions in two planes—frontal and horizontal.

The first six leads are known as limb leads. Leads I, II and III are bipolar leads, i.e. they have two poles, negative and positive. The bipolar leads compare the electrical potential between the two poles.

The arms and legs are extensions of the electrical field around the heart. Therefore, impulses sensed by an electrode on the right arm are the same that would be sensed by one on the right shoulder. The same applies to the left arm and shoulder and the right and left feet. Leads I, II and III form a triangle surrounding the heart, known as Einthoven's triangle (see Vol. 1, Chapter 24).

The axis of lead I extends from the right shoulder, (negative electrode) to the left shoulder (positive electrode). Lead I 'looks at' the lateral surface of the heart. The axis of lead II extends from the right shoulder (negative electrode) to the left leg (positive electrode) and views the inferior surface of the heart. The axis of lead III extends from the left shoulder (negative electrode) to the left leg, again viewing the inferior surface of the heart.

The next three limb leads, AVR, AVL, AVF, are unipolar, that is, they have one (positive) pole. The unipolar leads compare the electrical potential at the site of the lead with the negative potential at the centre of the heart.

The initials 'A' means augmented, 'V' vector and 'R, L and F' refer to the right, left and foot.

It was found that by eliminating the negative electrode that the amplitude of the tracing was increased by 50 per cent, hence the term augmented.

Lead AVR 'looks at' the right cavities of the heart, lead AVL at the left cavities and the lateral area, AVF at the inferior surface.

The other six leads are known as chest or precordial leads (V1–V6); they, too, are positioned on the chest wall with the negative potential pointing at the centre of the heart.

Precordial leads occupy the following positions on the chest wall:

V1—situated between the third and fourth intercostal spaces at the right sternal border. It views the right cavities and basal area of the heart.

V2—situated between the third and fourth intercostal spaces at the left sternal border. It views the basal area.

V3—between V2 and V4, views the interventricular septal area.

V4—in the fourth and fifth intercostal spaces at the left midclavicular line, again views the septal area.

V5—over the fourth and fifth intercostal spaces at the anterior axillary line, views the left cavities and the lateral area.

V6—situated between the fourth and fifth intercostal spaces in the left mid-axillary line, again views the left side of the heart and the lateral area.

The ECG paper is printed with 1-mm squares. Heavier lines running horizontally and vertically divide the squares into blocks of five. The horizontal lines represent time, each small square being 0·04 sec in duration, the larger square which is defined by a heavier line represents 0·2 sec in time.

EXAMINATION AND MONITORING OF THE PATIENT

The vertical plane measures amptitude (voltage). All twelve lead ECGs are standardized so that 1 millivolt (mV) is equal to 10 mm (two large squares).

Each cardiac depolarization is represented by the PQRST complex. On a 12-lead ECG, because the heart is observed from 12 directions, the configuration of the PQRST complex differs in each lead.

If an electrical current flows towards an electrode a positive deflection is seen, if it flows away a negative deflection is seen.

Lead II is commonly shown to illustrate the complex, but all the leads are looked at together in a diagnostic context.

The cardiac cycle

The heart has a specialized conducting system which accomplishes self-excitation and rapid conduction throughout the myocardium at regular intervals (see Vol. 1, Chapter 5). Under normal circumstances, at a rate of 70–90 times per minute an electrical impulse automatically arises in the sino-atrial (SA) node. This is an area of specialized conducting tissue situated in the right atrium. The atria are then depolarized and the impulse passes into the atrioventricular (AV) node.

Within the AV node the electrical stimulus is delayed before passing on to the bundle of His. This allows adequate ventricular filling time and also prevents the ventricles being bombarded by inappropriately high atrial rates (as seen in atrial flutter or fibrillation).

The electrical impulse then passes in to the common bundle of His and into the right bundle branch and the left anterior and posterior fascicles of the left bundle branch. It then passes into the ventricular myocardium and the ventricles are rapidly and efficiently depolarized.

The P wave represents atrial depolarization (the P-R interval is the length of time the impulse is being held in the AV node (normally 0·12–0·20 sec). The QRS complex is the graphic representation of ventricular depolarization. The interventricular septum is depolarized initially, then the right and left ventricles. The normal QRS duration is 0·6–0·10 sec. The T wave represents ventricular repolarization.

The normal PQRST is known as sinus rhythm.

The electrochemical activity of the heart

Each myocardial cell in its resting state carries a membrane potential of -90 mV.

Along the inner surface of each resting cell there are many negatively charged ions (anions). Conversely, on the outside of the cell membrane there are many positively charged ions (cations) of which sodium (Na^+ is in the highest concentration. The resting membrane potential prevents passage of sodium into the cell.

When an electrical stimulus arises in the SA node, it alters the membrane potential from -90 mV to $+40$ mV and also alters the permeability of the cell wall. This allows Na^+ to flood into the cell and the cation potassium (K^+) to leak out. The cell is then depolarized and mechanical contraction occurs.

The electrical impulse passes across the cell wall and the neighbouring cell is affected. This results in a wave of depolarization across the whole atria and through the conducting system into the ventricles.

A fraction of a second after depolarization there is another reversal of potential, the cations returning to the outside of the cell and the membrane potential falling from its active phase of $+40$ mV back to its resting state. This is known as repolarization.

A description of the commoner dysrhythmias which can affect the myocardium is contained in Chapter 11 of this volume.

b. *The blood pressure*

This is a basic and well tried measurement and should be measured as often as possible in the field. This means at least every 15 min, more frequently if conditions permit.

The measurement of blood pressure

Blood pressure can be measured in a variety of different ways.

The sphygmomanometer is the most usual method of measurement. The technicalities of the mode of use of this instrument are fully described in Vol. 1, Chapter 22.

The other methods include the oscillotonometer and direct methods such as intra-arterial pressure monitoring. The basic principles are similarly described in Vol. 1, Chapter 22.

There are problems with the measurement of blood pressure by these indirect techniques.

1. The radial or brachial artery can be impalpable in patients who are shocked and this can make measurement impossible. This is most commonly due to the fact that the blood pressure is so low that an adequate flow to the periphery is not being achieved. Less commonly, the central blood pressure can be adequate but peripheral blood flow cannot be detected.

2. In patients with extremely obese limbs, the blood pressure taken with a normal width of cuff will read falsely high. The correct procedure in these cases is to use a wider cuff. This may be impractical, and if a normal cuff is used a small allowance for this must be made. The reverse situation (i.e. very thin arms), produces the opposite effect.

3. It is quite impossible to measure blood pressure with any degree of accuracy in arms which are encumbered with articles of clothing.

To conclude, the measurement of blood pressure is an important indication of the physical state of the patient. It is, in the authors' opinion, quite feasible to measure this in the field and should be part of the normal techniques employed by skilled paramedical personnel.

EXAMINATION AND MONITORING OF THE PATIENT

c. *The peripheral circulation*
This can be assessed by using the capillary refill time. The principle of this is to press the skin at a suitable site (usually the ear lobe or the nail of the finger). The time of refill (when the colour returns) is under 2 sec in the normal person. In a patient with serious circulatory problems this time may be considerably extended.

d. *Blood loss*
An attempt should be made to monitor the blood loss. It will not be possible for the medical staff in the hospital to have any idea of how much blood has been lost at the site of the incident or during transportation to the hospital. An approximation of this as part of the documentation given to the doctor upon arrival in hospital will be invaluable.

3. The respiratory system
This includes monitoring of respiration and colour.

a. *The rate of respiration*
It is very important to measure the respiratory rate at regular intervals. As a general rule a sustained increase in the rate of respiration is a poor prognostic sign. The respiratory rate should be measured at least every 5 min.

b. *The 'depth' of respiration*
This is a measure of the tidal volume. An experienced observer can have an idea of the depth of respiration by observation.

It is possible to quantify the depth of respiration by using a face mask and spirometer (*see* Vol. 1, Chapter 23).

c. *Other respiratory signs*
Any other respiratory signs such as irregularities in the rate of respiration, coughing up of blood (haemoptysis), abnormal lung sounds or signs of a flail chest (*see* Chapter 8) should also be documented.

d. *Colour*
It is of vital importance to monitor the colour of the patient at all times. The onset of cyanosis can be extremely quick. The patient's colour must be observed centrally. It is no use to observe the fingers, for example, as the circulation at the periphery is influenced a great deal by the circulatory state. The most reliable site for observation is the lips (provided they are not obscured by cosmetics).

The two classic exceptions to the rule that a good pink colour means a well oxygenated patient are carbon monoxide and cyanide poisoning.

4. The central nervous system

The importance of monitoring the central nervous system is to document the level of consciousness and to watch for the onset of localizing signs.

a. The level of consciousness

The best simple and practical monitoring system is the Glasgow Coma Scale. This will be described in detail in Chapter 14. It is necessary to document the coma scale every 5 min.

b. Monitoring localizing signs

The purpose of this is to ascertain whether there are signs that bleeding is occurring inside the skull. If the brain is completely destroyed there will be no change in the conscious level or responses to reflexes. If, however, there is a blood vessel bleeding inside the skull on one side then one side of the brain will be slowly compressed and thus function will be lost. This will give physical signs on one side of the body. This change in physical signs should be looked for as early intervention may be lifesaving.

The most practical sign is the pupil's response to light. A strong light must be used, especially in daylight. The pupillary response should be brisk, and equal on both sides.

There are, of course, many pitfalls in this observation. For example, a glass artificial eye is (not surprisingly) completely unresponsive to light. Alternatively, it is possible that the patient may be receiving eye drops which enlarge the pupil.

It is also possible to detect a change in tone in the limbs. To elicit this it is merely necessary to gently move the limb. This may be flaccid or have varying degrees of rigidity. Again the same principle applies that a change in tone or a difference in response on both sides is important.

If the patient is conscious then he may be moving one side of the body and not the other, or one side of the body more than the other. If this is being monitored then a change will be detected early and so the chances of early alleviation of the problem will also, hopefully, be increased.

5. The abdomen

A note should be kept of the tenderness of the abdomen to touch and the presence or absence of bowel sounds but this will usually suffice in the prehospital phase of treatment.

6. The urinary system

This is difficult to monitor in detail without the presence of a urinary catheter. If a urinary catheter has been inserted it is important to monitor the urinary flow on an hourly basis.

Bloodstained urine may indicate damage at any point in the urinary tract.

7. Blood chemistry measurement in the field

In the field it is difficult to measure any chemical parameter other than blood sugar. This can be measured by a variety of commercially available sticks.

The technique depends upon obtaining a drop of blood and then carefully placing it upon the chemically impregnated end of the stick. After a short interval (which must be accurately timed) the blood is washed or wiped off and the colour of the chemically impregnated paper is compared against reference colours which are available on the side of the bottle in which the sticks are stored. It is vitally important to keep the bottle closed and the sticks dry or the test will be completely invalidated.

Indications for use

The most obvious indication for use is in the diabetic patient. Whilst this method is not as accurate as a blood sugar estimation in the laboratory, it is of sufficient accuracy (properly used) to initiate treatment in a patient who has severe hypoglycaemia.

It is good practice to estimate the blood sugar in the field in any patient with an altered conscious level as it is not impossible for a diabetic to be involved in a road traffic accident or to collapse for a variety of unrelated reasons.

Treatment

In the field it may be necessary to treat the hypoglycaemic patient. The simplest way of raising the blood sugar is by putting some sugar under the tongue. This has two disadvantages, the first being that the absorption is slower than the intravenous route but is still acceptably quick enough for all but the direst of emergencies. The second is that if this method is used in an unconscious patient it is possible for the sugar to be inhaled.

The most efficient way of getting sugar into the bloodstream is by a direct injection of dextrose. A 50 per cent solution is used for this purpose.

Further techniques used in the hospital environment

It is obviously possible to measure a great many haematological and biochemical parameters in the hospital. It is outside the scope of this book to review the whole range of these. Consequently, a few of the most commonly used and most important will be briefly discussed.

1. Haemoglobin

This is a measure of the oxygen-carrying pigment in the blood. If this is low then the ability of the body to transport oxygen to the cells is reduced.

In hypovolaemic shock blood is lost from the circulation and so the ability of the body to transport oxygen to the cells is severely reduced.

2. Platelets and clotting factors

The platelet count is used as one indicator of the ability of the blood to clot. Platelets are essential to the clotting process and if for any reason their number is depleted then the ability of the clotting mechanism is impaired.

3. Sodium

The sodium in the plasma is a major contributor to the maintenance of the osmotic pressure gradients in the vascular compartment. If the serum sodium is drastically reduced then the osmotic balance of the vascular compartment can be impaired and fluid will be 'sucked' out of the vascular compartment into the interstitial fluid.

On the other hand, if the serum sodium is raised, then fluid can be 'sucked' into the vascular compartment. In congestive heart failure one of the primary 'malfunctions' is sodium retention in the vascular compartment with consequent overloading of the circulation.

4. Potassium

Unlike sodium, potassium is mainly an intracellular ion and so tends to have only a 'token presence' in the plasma. As a direct consequence of this it should be realized that changes in the intracellular potassium may not be reflected by similar changes in the plasma potassium. Both sodium and potassium are necessary for the passage of impulses down a nerve fibre. If the level of potassium in the plasma is abnormal then conduction can be seriously affected.

5. Blood sugar

This has already been discussed. The laboratory is able to give more accurate results but the principles on which measurement is indicated are the same.

6. The partial pressure of oxygen (Po_2)

This is a measure of the amount of oxygen actually dissolved in the *plasma* at the time of sampling. It is not a measure of the oxygen combined with haemoglobin. It is used as a guide to the oxygenation of the patient, but many factors can influence this.

7. The partial pressure of carbon dioxide (Pco_2)

Carbon dioxide is excreted through the lungs. It is formed as a waste product and the level measured in the blood will give a rough guide as to the efficiency of this excretion. One of the commonest reasons for the carbon dioxide level building up is damage to the lung tissue itself. Perhaps the most well known example of this is chronic bronchitis. These patients due to the lung damage, have difficulty in excreting carbon dioxide and so the level will build up over the course of some years. The partial pressure of oxygen will then become a major factor in the control of respiration. (This is contrary to the normal patient when the partial pressure of carbon dioxide in the bloodstream controls respiration). Such patients are said to exist on 'hypoxic drive'.

8. The pH of the blood

This is a measure of the acidity of the blood. It is now measured as hydrogen ion concentration which is merely a different way of expressing the degree of acidity.

Further reading

Swash M. and Mason S. (1984) *Hutchison's Clinical Methods*, 18th ed. London, Bailliere Tindall.

Chapter 3

Nursing Care of the Injured

Claire M. Taylor

Having resuscitated the patient, the quality of life, however long or short it may be, depends to a large extent upon the nursing care the patient receives. This care commences at the scene of the incident and continues until the patient is able to care for himself again, or until he dies. Paramedical personnel must, therefore, be aware of, and provide for, the nursing needs of the patient from the time of their arrival at the incident until the patient is transferred to the care of a trained nurse.

Modern nursing is based upon the Nursing Process concept of individualized patient care. This is:

Assessment of the patient's needs
Planning of care to meet those needs
Implementation of the care required
Evaluation of the care given

The patient's needs are physical, mental, spiritual and social, any of which may take priority is any given situation. The Nursing Process approach to care, provides flexibility and an infinite variety of care to cope with any situation. As soon as the immediate life-threatening problems have been contained the patient should be covered, to avoid unnecessary exposure. At the same time the patient should be told what has happened and what the emergency services are going to do for him. Talking to the patient is extremely important, even if he appears unconscious, as hearing is the last sense the patient loses and the first he regains. A calm, reassuring voice will comfort the patient, even if he cannot understand or appreciate what is being said.

Any unforeseen incident tends to draw a crowd of onlookers, some eager to assist, others merely out of curiosity, and it may be necessary to organize the control of a crowd in order to avoid embarrassment to the patient and delay in any care required.

Most patients are part of a family or a group of friends and if these are present, the paramedic may have to deal firmly but tactfully with these shocked and often distraught people. Giving relatives something to do, perhaps writing down the patient's name, date of birth, address, any known medical history etc. will often help. Relatives or friends should be told the destination of the patient, if they have their own transport.

Records are a most important part of patient care. As soon as practicable, relevant details of the patient, the incident and the care given, must be recorded, as well as all subsequent observations and any drugs or treatment given. Where more than one patient is involved, it is often useful to tie the records to the patient. It is important not to attach the records to the patient's clothes as these will be removed. This will avoid confusion, especially if the patient's name is unknown.

Handling and transportation of the patient can also influence the extent of the patient's disease or injuries and possibly affect the rate or extent of recovery.

Paramedics must familiarize themselves with the area in which they work, as well as with their equipment. The needs of a golfer who has suffered from myocardial infarction on the golf course are very different from a seaman badly scalded in the engine room of a ship, or a family involved in a motorway accident in fog. Further trauma to any patient must be avoided if at all possible. Transportation should be by the smoothest, rather than the fastest route in most instances. During the journey the patient must be protected from not only excessive movement but from noise, lights and bright sunlight as well.

Positioning of the patient before and during travel is crucial and obviously depends upon the patient's condition and injuries. Adequate support for spine, head and limbs must be ensured whilst maintaining the comfort of the patient. If the journey is over two hours duration, or if the patient complains of discomfort, his position should be changed. Change of position will help to prevent pressure necrosis, especially over the bony prominences, and should be noted on the patient's record card or documents. Should the patient's condition, or injuries, preclude a change of position, then very gentle massage of the affected areas may be performed, always ensuring the patient is not lying on a wrinkled blanket, groundsheet or clothing.

If facilities are available and the patient's condition allows, washing of the face and hands to remove blood, dirt, perspiration etc. is very refreshing and comforting. Moistening of the lips with water, or a lanolin type of cream, prevents soreness or cracking when fluids must be withheld and especially if an oral airway is in situ. Hair falling over the patient's face is particularly irritating if the patient is unable to move or communicate. In order to prevent corneal abrasions the unconscious patient's eyes should be gently closed after pupil reactions have been checked. If the patient is positioned on his side, the ears should be flattened against the head to prevent folding and possible injury. Some dental prostheses may have to be removed and retained with the patient's personal effects and again a note made in the patient's records. The 'nurse' must decide, in the circumstances, whether there is a potential problem or not.

Restlessness in a patient may indicate pain or discomfort, haemorrhage or a full bladder. The cause should be elicited and the appropriate action taken.

Limbs and digits should be placed in as near a 'normal' position as possible and the patient should be kept warm but not overheated. It must not be forgotten that the lightest of covers may cause excessive pressure on an injury and any covers may need to be supported.

Injuries, infusion sites and dressings, must be easily accessible for observation without unduly disturbing the patient.

Touch is comforting to both the semiconscious and the conscious patient. Simply holding a hand, or touching the shoulder to indicate empathy is a reassuring gesture. Always tell the patient what is going to happen before carrying out any procedure, however small, as it is extremely frightening to be suddenly roused, particularly if the patient is recovering consciousness.

At all times, the patient must be cared for as a whole human being, not just a collection of signs and symptoms or a mass of injuries requiring attention. If conscious, the patient may ask questions and the appropriate reply must be given and not an evasive answer. A note of the question and reply given should be recorded in the patient's notes to ensure continuity of approach to what can be a changing situation. It is futile to be over-optimistic and cheerful but the patient must always be left with some hope, however disastrous the situation may be. The patient often has more trust in an honest 'I don't know' answer than one which is patently untrue.

At all times the paramedic should care for his patient in the professional way he would like himself or his dearest relative to be treated.

Further reading

Roper N., Logan W. W. and Tierney A. J. (1980) *The Elements of Nursing*. Edinburgh, Churchill Livingstone.
Skeet M. (ed.) (1981) *Emergency Procedures and First Aid for Nurses*. Oxford, Blackwell Scientific Publications.

Chapter 4

Fluid Balance and Therapy

D. L. Edbrooke and S. J. Mather

The body normally gains water from two sources: from drinking and, less obviously, from metabolism. In illness absorption from the gut is frequently impaired and it becomes necessary to administer fluids by other routes. By far the commonest, nowadays, is the intravenous route. Consequently the administration of intravenous fluids has become a vital part of modern medical management.

Before giving intravenous fluids it is essential to consider three basic questions:
 1. What type of fluid is required?
 2. What volume of fluid is appropriate?
 3. At what rate should the fluid be administered?

These questions can best be answered by considering the physiology of fluid balance (*see also* Vol. 1, Chapter 3).

As can be seen in *Fig.* 4.1 there are three compartments separated by semipermeable membranes, thus allowing fluid transfer between the compartments.

It is very important to clarify the terminology used in *Fig.* 4.1 as confusion often arises. All that portion of the body water which is contained outside the cells is called the extracellular fluid. This is made up of the intravascular compartment and the interstitial fluid. The remainder is contained within the cells and is termed the intracellular fluid. The extravascular fluid compartment is synonymous, for our purposes, with the interstitial fluid.

It is mandatory to assess the quantity and constituents of the fluid in both the vascular compartment and the extravascular compartment before any fluid is given. It is at the present time not feasible to assess the state of the intracellular fluid compartment.

ASSESSMENT OF THE VASCULAR COMPARTMENT

It is possible to divide the assessment into two parts:
 1. Present status
 2. Ongoing loss

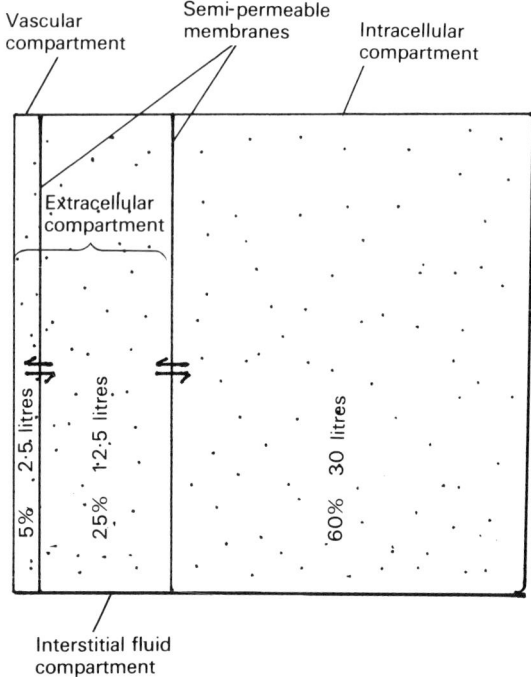

Fig. 4.1. The body fluid compartments. (The figures are very approximate.)

1. Assessing the present status

The vascular compartment may be underfilled, normal or overfilled. Conceptually, it is important to visualize the vascular compartment as a pump (the heart), pumping fluid around a series of pipes (the blood vessels). The number and diameter of the pipes through which the fluid is flowing can be varied, thus altering the volume of the system and the ease with which the fluid flows (resistance).

i. The underfilled vascular compartment

If insufficient blood is available in the vascular compartment, the venous return to the heart will fall. This will result in less stretch being exerted on the muscle fibres of the heart and the blood available for the heart to pump will be reduced. This will cause a decrease in cardiac output (Starling's Law. See Vol. 1, Chapter 5). The cardiovascular system will try to compensate for this lack of blood flow by an increase in heart rate and by reducing the flow to certain areas (selective vasoconstriction) which are not so vital e.g. the skin and gastrointestinal tract. This, of course, gives rise to the classic clinical signs of cold, pale extremities.

If the loss from the vascular compartment is extremely severe, the increase in heart rate and selective reduction in blood flow will not be sufficient to maintain a normal blood pressure and so the blood pressure will fall. In practice the compensatory mechanisms in young patients are much more efficient and this can lead (in extensive loss from the vascular compartment) to sudden severe reductions in blood pressure when the compensatory mechanisms suddenly fail. In older people the compensatory mechanisms are less efficient which tends to lead to earlier reduction in blood pressure.

It is possible to gain some impression of the vasoconstriction in the skin by measuring the peripheral temperature. This will gradually decrease with increasing peripheral vasoconstriction. It is, however, easy to be misled using this measurement as the peripheral temperature can be altered by other disease processes. The measurement of temperature is described in Chapter 2.

It is important to note that this explanation of vasoconstriction is of necessity oversimplified, but serves to give an indication of fairly complex physiological changes. The terms 'blood pressure' and 'blood flow' have been used in this discussion (see Vol. 1), but the two are not synonymous. Blood flow is of greater significance, as it is only by adequate blood flow that oxygen can be carried to the tissues. However, in a clinical situation blood pressure is much more easily measured and gives some indication of blood flow.

Urine output also tends to fall. This may not be obvious in the uncatheterized patient. In order to quantify this sign it is necessary to catheterize the patient. If the urine output falls to less than 0·5 ml/kg/h for more than 2 hours this constitutes an unacceptable urine output and may indicate underfill. As with all these signs each sign is only a guide to under- or overfilling of each compartment. However, taken in combination with other signs the sum total usually gives a good indication of underfill or overfill.

Another clinical indication of an underfilled vascular compartment is the capillary refill time. By depressing an easily visible area such as the lobe of an ear, and noting the time taken for the pale area to become pink again, it is possible to get a crude assessment of the peripheral blood flow. In cases where the flow is reduced, the capillary refill time will be much longer than normal. Obviously this test is not an absolute indication of underfill, as extraneous factors such as cold can slow capillary refill.

It is possible to obtain a direct measurement of how much blood is being returned to the ventricles by measuring the pressure directly via a catheter placed in the left or right atria.

In addition to the measurement of the volume of fluid in the intravascular compartment, it is also necessary to monitor the constituents of the fluid.

The haemoglobin level is important as the haemoglobin in the red cells is the main mechanism for oxygen carriage in the body. If the blood flow is severely reduced however, the oxygen will not find its way to the tissues.

The blood flow will be modified by the ratio of the volume of red blood cells to plasma (the haematocrit or packed cell volume). The normal value is approximately 0·45. This means that 45 per cent of the space in the vascular compartment consists of red blood cells and 55 per cent plasma (including white blood cells and other constituents).

ii. The overfilled vascular compartment

The vascular compartment may be overloaded (e.g. simply as a result of too much fluid being introduced too quickly during intravenous therapy) or may appear to be overloaded by virtue of the heart's pumping action being compromised.

In clinical practice the term 'heart failure' is loosely used and can cover a wide variety of conditions. Heart failure is commonly insidious in onset and may involve both sides of the heart. It is then termed 'congestive cardiac failure'. This is associated with a retention of sodium ions thus producing, by osmosis, a retention of water in both the extracellular vascular compartment and the vascular compartment. This fluid retention becomes apparent clinically at such sites as the lung where (using a stethoscope) it is possible to hear 'wet sounds' or the liver, which becomes enlarged with fluid, or by noting the presence of fluid at such sites as the ankle and sacrum where it tends to accumulate due to gravity. It is not uncommon for this failing of the circulation to cause a diminution in kidney blood flow which can lead to less fluid being removed by the kidneys and a consequent further build up of fluid.

Heart failure can occur on either side of the heart without involving the other side. Right heart failure leads to overfilling of the right atrium, which leads to an increase in the central venous pressure and this is characterized clinically by engorged neck veins. In addition, the systemic circulation is overfilled and this leads to engorgement of the liver, which is consequently enlarged, and to the development of peripheral oedema which is usually first seen at the ankles.

Left heart failure leads to overfilling in the left atrium. This in turn leads to an increase in the pulmonary capillary pressure and consequently fluid is forced into the lung tissue. This is detected clinically by the 'wet sounds', described above, and can be seen on X-ray as an increase in vascular markings in the lung fields.

Although congestive cardiac failure has been discussed in this section on the overfilled vascular compartment, it is important to stress that it cannot be simply described as a vascular compartment problem as it involves the extracellular fluid compartment as well.

Summary of methods of assessment of present status of the vascular compartment
1. Heart rate
2. The peripheral circulation
3. Ventricular filling
    a. Right side—observing the neck veins or measuring the central venous pressure
    b. Left side—measuring the pulmonary or 'wedge' pressure with a flotation catheter (this can only be done in hospital)
4. Blood pressure
5. Haemoglobin
6. Haematocrit
7. Urine output

2. Assessing the ongoing loss in the vascular compartment
Losses can occur from the vascular compartment in the form of plasma, blood or water. Plasma loss as such in any quantity only occurs in special situations such as severe burns, when the skin covering is lost from the body and the plasma can seep out. The measurement of this loss is very specialized and is beyond the scope of this book.

Assessment of blood loss can be divided into two distinct categories:

i. Assessing visible loss
Blood lost in the operating theatre or in the resuscitation room can be measured in various ways.

a. Clinical observation
With experience, it is feasible to assess with reasonable accuracy the blood lost at operation, by assessing the blood on swabs, or drapes around the patient, and the content of suction bottles. There are, however, two situations in which this is not practical. First if the volume lost is large, then it is very difficult to gauge and secondly in small babies when 10 per cent of the blood volume may only be 30 ml. Consequently more accurate methods of measuring this blood loss are essential.

b. Weighing swabs
This is the commonest way of estimating blood loss in clinical practice. The method assumes that 100 ml of blood weighs approximately 100 g. Swabs of a standard weight are used, and the swabs with blood on them are weighed. The weight of blood can then be calculated.

It is important to note that swabs must be weighed immediately, otherwise inaccuracies develop due to evaporation of water from the swabs.

c. Colorimetric method

This is a much more accurate method of assessing the loss. The principle is that the bloody swabs are washed in a solution which destroys the red cells releasing the haemoglobin. Thus the solution becomes red. The colorimeter is able to measure the colour density of this red solution and this is proportional to the haemoglobin concentration. Knowing the patient's haemoglobin level before commencement of surgery it is possible with some accuracy to estimate the blood loss.

ii. Assessing non-visible loss

Bleeding may not only be external to the body, but internal or both. For example, if the spleen is damaged bleeding will occur into the abdomen and it will be necessary to replace the loss as it is still outside the vascular compartment.

Similarly, in cases of fractured long bones it is possible to lose a considerable quantity of blood (up to 700 ml) into the soft tissues. Again this blood will be outside the vascular compartment. In these situations it is essential to realize that blood is being lost and assessment is carried out as described in 'assessing the present status'. For this reason careful and diligent monitoring of seriously ill patients is at all times essential.

ASSESSMENT OF THE EXTRAVASCULAR COMPARTMENT

Theoretically the vascular compartment is part of the extracellular fluid. However, for the sake of this discussion it is, perhaps, simpler to consider the vascular compartment as a separate entity. The extracellular fluid compartment bathes the cells of the body in fluid and it is not a discrete entity. Consequently, it is sometimes difficult to imagine the size of this space and its ability to 'soak up' fluid.

Vascular compartment + 'interstitial' fluid
= Extracellular fluid volume

b. Assessing the present status

This chapter attempts to consider the three spaces separately, in different sections. In reality, however, all three spaces are continuously being adjusted to keep the balance of the fluid volume and its constituents constant.

i. The underfilled extravascular compartment

If fluid depletion occurs, the fluid loss occurs uniformly throughout the compartment. It will only become noticeable clinically in certain areas. A fluid loss of less than 10 per cent will not be obvious. If a loss of greater than 10 per cent occurs this will be detectable clinically and laboratory tests will support this.

Underfilling can be assessed as follows:

a. Skin elasticity

In extravascular fluid loss the skin tends to lose its elasticity. Thus, in picking up a fold of skin, for example, on the front of the patient's neck, it will have less recoil than in a normally hydrated patient. This test is, however, unreliable in older patients as the skin loses its elasticity with age.

b. Eyeball tension

The eyeball in a patient with an underfilled extravascular compartment tends to have a sunken appearance, and if pressed (with the eyelid closed) will feel soft. The pressure in the normal eye is such as to make it feel hard.

c. The tongue

The tongue will appear quite dry. This is a very commonly used clinical sign.

ii. The overfilled extravascular compartment

Overfilling of the extravascular compartment has rather fewer clinical signs to aid detection.

a. Urine output

The kidneys will try to compensate for this fluid overload by increasing the urine output. This, however, is not a reliable sign as there are many other causes of an increased urine output.

b. Oedema

This is the term given to accumulation of fluid outside the cells. The fluid is distributed throughout the body, but tends to be more noticeable in areas where it accumulates with gravity. So it is commonly seen around the ankle region where it can be identified by pressing a thumb into the affected region for a few seconds. The fluid is pressed out of this area leaving a depression. This is classically known as 'pitting oedema'. Collection of fluid at the ankle can also occur in extremely hot weather and in old people.

In patients lying in bed the fluid will accumulate at the lowest points and consequently the fluid collects at the area around the sacrum rather than the ankles. Oedema also collects at sites which are not visible. For example, fluid can collect in the lungs, giving rise to pulmonary oedema. This is detectable clinically as shortness of breath and using a stethoscope 'wet sounds' can be heard at the bases of the lungs ('crepitations', *see* Chapter 3). Fluid may also collect in the liver and thus the liver will be palpable below the right costal margin (normally the liver lies above and behind the right costal margin).

Summary of methods of assessment of the extravascular compartment
1. Underfill
    i. Skin elasticity
    ii. Eyeball elasticity
    iii. The tongue
2. Overfill
    i. Urine output
    ii. Oedema

THE INTRACELLULAR COMPARTMENT

The compartment that contains the most fluid as previously described (*see also* Vol. 1, Chapter 3) is the intracellular fluid compartment. Unfortunately, it is impossible to assess the state of this compartment and as this accounts for the largest volume of fluid (*Fig.* 4.2) it will inevitably lead to inaccuracies in the assessment of the fluid requirements of the body as a whole.

FLUID THERAPY

Once it is established that the fluid status of a compartment is significantly abnormal it will then be necessary to either reduce the amount of fluid or increase it.

Fluids can be administered by different routes. These routes are summarized below.
1. Oral
2. Nasogastric
3. Rectal
4. Subcutaneous
5. Intravenous
6. Intraperitoneal

1. Oral administration
This is by far the most physiological route of administration. there is no doubt that this route should always be preferred. However, in some

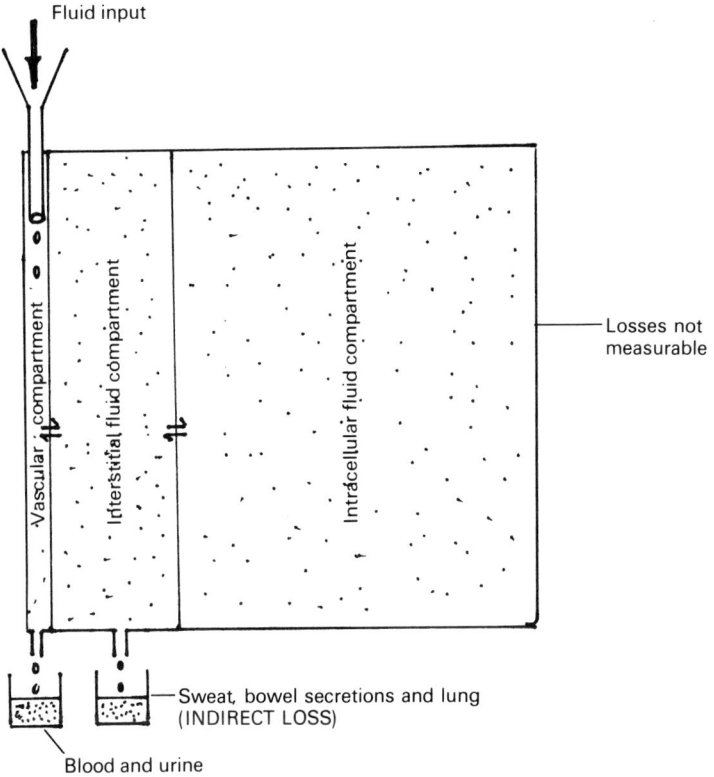

Fig. 4.2. Input and output in the body fluid compartments.

circumstances it may not be possible to do this. In patients who are in hospital recovering from surgery in the abdominal region, the gastrointestinal tract will not necessarily be functioning, and so fluids will have to be administered by another route. In patients who are likely to be admitted to the Accident and Emergency Department it would not be advisable to give oral fluids as it may be necessary to give the patient a general anaesthetic after admission. Also, gastric stasis commonly occurs following trauma.

2. Nasogastric administration

In essence this route of administration is the same as the oral route. Fluid is being placed into the upper gastrointestinal tract. Consequently the advantages and disadvantages are the same.

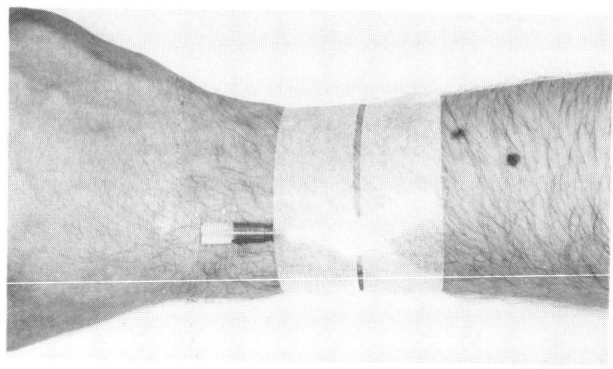

Fig. 4.3. Intravenous cannula in position in forearm vein.

3. Rectal administration

This is merely another route of access into the gastrointestinal tract. The risks of vomiting are minimized but absorption is less predictable.

4. Subcutaneous administration

This is really only included for the sake of completeness but has no real place in modern fluid therapy.

5. Intravenous administration

This will be considered in more detail as it is the most direct way of correcting fluid balance problems. Access is achieved by inserting a needle or preferably a plastic cannula into a vein. It is much safer to insert a plastic cannula as this is less likely to perforate the vein with movement.

The site of insertion will depend upon the ease of access to veins but it is a very important rule to choose the simplest available site. The commonest site in clinical practice is the arm and virtually any large vein on the arm is suitable. It is preferable, but not essential, to avoid siting the cannula over a joint as this will minimize movements of the cannula. *Fig.* 4.3 shows a cannula inserted into a forearm vein.

It is possible that a vein in the arm is not accessible or that the patient is sufficiently shocked for the veins to be collapsed and an alternative site has to be found. Another suitable site is shown in *Fig.* 4.4.

If these veins are not accessible then certain other sites are possible. It is *not* recommended that these sites be utilized in the field and they are only used in hospital by doctors with specific expertise in this field, but if no suitable peripheral veins are available then it is possible to cannulate the external or internal jugular veins, the subclavian vein or the femoral vein.

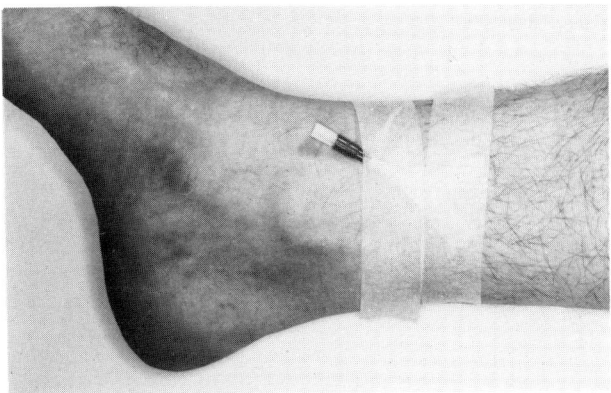

Fig. 4.4. Intravenous cannula in ankle vein.

Once a cannula has been inserted under sterile conditions it will then be necessary to decide what type of intravenous fluid is suitable for the patient.

Different fluids tend to migrate to the three compartments at different rates. Consequently, it is mandatory to look first in some detail at the range of fluids available for intravenous infusion.

6. Peritoneal fluid administration

Theoretically this is a suitable route for the administration of crystalloids, particularly as they are rapidly absorbed into the circulation from the peritoneal cavity. In most cases, however, the intravenous route is more practical.

Crystalloids and colloids

It is possible to divide intravenous fluids into two basic categories.

Crystalloids

These solutions are usually colourless and are made up of small molecules that can pass through semipermeable membranes rapidly. Consequently, they do not stay in the plasma for a long time and most of the fluid has left the vascular compartment in less than one hour.

Not all crystalloid solutions in clinical use are iso-osmotic with plasma. An iso-osmotic solution has the same osmotic pressure as that of plasma (*see* Vol. 1, Chapter 18). If the osmotic pressure was the same as that of tap water then the osmotic balance in the plasma would be disturbed and fluid would be drawn into the red cells and they would swell and ultimately burst. If the osmotic pressure was greater than that of the plasma then the reverse would apply.

There are many different types of crystalloid solutions in clinical use and it is beyond the scope of this book to describe them all. However, a few of the more commonly used ones are described below. The following shows the constituents of 1 litre of some of the commonly used crystalloids. All are iso-osmotic with plasma.

Isotonic Saline

pH	5·0	
Sodium	154	mmol
Potassium	0	mmol
Chloride	154	mmol
Calories	0	

This is misleadingly called 'normal' saline by some. 'Normal' saline is not the same as a normal solution in chemistry which contains 1 gram molecular weight of sodium chloride in 1 litre. As can be seen it does contain a lot of sodium. As has already been described, the basic pathology in congestive cardiac failure is sodium retention and so it is not advisable to choose this particular crystalloid in patients who may have this condition.

4% Dextrose–0·18% Saline

pH	4·5	
Sodium	31	mmol
Potassium	0	mmol
Chloride	31	mmol
Calories	180	

This crystalloid has much less sodium. The number of calories it contains is minimal and 1 litre contains the equivalent number of calories (approximately) as 24 grams (almost 1 oz) of cheddar cheese.

Dextrose 5%

pH	4·0	
Sodium	0	mmol
Potassium	0	mmol
Chloride	0	mmol
Calories	205	

As can be seen this fluid contains slightly more calories than dextrose-saline but no electrolytes.

Ringer Lactate (Hartmann's Solution)

pH	6·5	
Sodium	131	mmol
Potassium	5	mmol
Chloride	112	mmol
Calories	0	

FLUID BALANCE AND THERAPY 37

This particular crystalloid contains an electrolyte balance which is closest to that of plasma. It is, therefore, used commonly and is particularly noteworthy in that it is the only commonly used crystalloid that contains potassium. Potassium salts may be added to the others if required.

Colloids

These fluids are made up of larger molecules and spend a longer time in the vascular compartment. Those in clinical use persist in the circulation for up to 6 hours.

These fluids are usually used when it is necessary to 'expand' the plasma volume and are thus commonly used in the acute situation to replace blood loss.

When blood is unavailable commonly used colloid solutions include:

1. Polygeline (e.g. Haemaccel)
2. Dextran
3. Plasma protein preparations
4. Blood
5. Hydroxyethyl starch (e.g. Hespan)

1. Polygeline (Haemaccel)

This is made up as 3·5 per cent solution of a type of gelatin and has a molecular weight of 35 000. The volume of blood or plasma lost can be replaced by an equal volume of haemaccel. It is stable for 8 years at room temperature and only gels if the temperature falls below 3°C. It can, rarely, give rise to allergic reactions due to histamine release. If used in excess it may give rise to cardiac failure due to overloading of the circulation.

It can be used to replace up to about 25 per cent of the circulating volume and is now one of the commonest colloids in routine use. It does not result in difficulties with cross-matching of blood. However, citrated blood should not be mixed with haemaccel as the calcium in haemaccel can cause recalcification of the blood, which may clot.

2. Dextran

Dextran is formed by bacteria which chemically alter sucrose. There are three types: dextran 40, dextran 70 and dextran 110. Dextran 70 is the most commonly used because the average molecular weight of the molecules is 70 000. Dextran 70 is made up as 6 per cent dextran solution in either 0·9 per cent saline or 5 per cent dextrose. Dextran 70, like polygeline, can also cause allergic reactions but again this is rare.

The most important disadvantage of dextran 70 is that if administered before blood is taken for cross-matching it can invalidate the crossmatch. For this reason it is less suitable for use in the prehospital situation than haemaccel.

3. Plasma protein preparations

A great many preparations have been used over the years and it is probably unnecessary to consider these. Nowadays the preparation available from the Blood Transfusion Service is called Human Albumin Solution (HAS) (formerly plasma protein fraction, HPPF).

Human Albumin Solution is a 4 per cent albumin suspension made from pooled human plasma. It is stated that the risk of acquiring hepatitis B (type II hepatitis) is minimal. It can be kept at room temperature for a time not exceeding five years. The solution should be inspected before use to make sure that no cloudiness is present. It can be given to donors of any blood group.

The commercial equivalent is 4 per cent Buminate which is exactly the same and can be used in place of HAS.

4. Blood

Blood is obviously the most appropriate substance to give to a patient to replace loss of blood from whatever cause. It would be preferable to replace the losses with the patient's own blood (autotransfusion).

The alternative to this is to give stored blood and it is advantageous to use blood that is relatively fresh.

The technology of the storage of the blood has become extremely sophisticated. The modern trend is to separate the red blood cells from the plasma. The plasma is then refined and specialized products such as platelet concentrates and clotting factors are produced. Some plasma is frozen to be used in patients with bleeding problems but most is used to produce HAS.

The red cells are now resuspended in a mixture of saline, adenine, glucose and mannitol. This is termed SAGM blood. As yet, little clinical experience has been gained with this suspension as it has only been introduced in 1984. If up to 4 units of blood are to be transfused then no additional replacement therapy is necessary. However, if it becomes necessary to transfuse more blood, then fresh frozen plasma (FFP) should be added in the proportion of 1 unit of FFP to every unit of blood.

ACD and CPD blood have both been in use over the past decade. ACD blood is thus named as the blood is stored in acid citrate dextrose. CPD blood means citrate phosphate dextrose stored blood.

CPD blood is, perhaps, better as it has a higher pH and hence the red cell survival time is longer.

It is important to note that problems are likely to occur with haemostasis with all blood preparations (see below). Consequently, laboratory testing of clotting function must be undertaken with large transfusions (transfusions in excess of 4 units).

5. *Hydroxyethyl starch*

This high molecular weight colloid has recently been introduced into clinical practice. It persists in the circulation longer than either polygeline or dextran. At present clinical experience is limited but its use will probably become widespread in the field of prehospital care.

Artificial blood

It would be an attractive hypothesis to have a blood substitute which will both act as a volume replacement fluid and also have the ability to transport oxygen without the problems associated with the administration of stored blood.

Work in this field has been going on for a number of years, and the most promising blood substitutes at this time are the perfluorocarbon emulsions. At the moment the studies are confined to animal work and seem to indicate that these substances compromise the immune system. There is little doubt, however, that artificial blood will become a reality in the future.

Hazards associated with transfusion of stored blood and blood products

1. The transmission of infection

Although rare, blood may become infected and the organisms passed on to the patient. In the UK all donors are screened for venereal disease and type 2 hepatitis. Potential donors are refused if they have had malaria or brucellosis or recent immunization with certain live viruses. Transmission of infection is minimal in the UK but in certain other countries where paid donors are employed and the screening procedures are less rigorous, the risk of infection is much higher.

Recently screening of blood for the HTLV III (AIDS) virus has been introduced in the UK.

2. Pyrogens

Certain bacterial products called pyrogens may be present in the anticoagulant. These are less common following the introduction of disposable apparatus.

3. Transfusion reactions

Severe febrile or allergic reactions or haemolysis, occasionally occur. They may be due to mismatch or to incorrect storage of the blood. The routine crossmatch will not detect all incompatibilities and minor reactions lead to decreased red-cell survival which passes unnoticed clinically.

4. Coagulation problems

Stored blood more than 48 hours old contains few platelets. Further, clotting factors are severely depleted. Disseminated intravascular coagulation (DIC) occurs when the clotting process takes place within the circulation consuming both platelets and clotting factors. It may lead to platelet deficiency and clinical bleeding. The condition can be detected by various clotting studies and treated by the administration of FFP (to provide clotting factors) and platelet concentrate.

5. Hyperkalaemia

The amount of free potassium ion in stored blood increases with the age of the blood. Unless old blood is given very rapidly, hyperkalaemia is rarely a problem.

6. Temperature changes

Blood is stored at 4°C. Infusions of large amounts of cold blood may rapidly lead to hypothermia and even cardiac arrest, especially if, as in major vascular and cardiac surgery, the blood is given into a central vein.

7. Acidosis

The pH of stored blood (ACD or CPD) is approximately 6·7. This is obviously a disadvantage especially in a shocked patient who may already have a metabolic acidosis.

8. Mismatch transfusions

These are usually the result of infusion of incompatible donor cells. Occasionally, however, they are due to high levels of antibodies (agglutinins) in the recipient serum. The result of mismatch is haemolysis. Fever with rigors may occur after less than 50 ml of blood have been transfused. For this reason the patient must be carefully monitored and his temperature taken regularly throughout the transfusion. Headache, loin pain and tenderness (due to the deposition of free haemoglobin in the renal tubules), nausea, vomiting, shortness of breath, persistent capillary oozing and hypotension may also occur. However, in the unconscious or anaesthetized patient the only sign of incompatibility may be the rise in temperature and the fall in blood pressure with persistent venous oozing.

As soon as any mismatch is suspected the transfusion must be stopped and the remaining blood sent for detailed crossmatch.

9. Aggregates in old blood

It has been discovered in the past few years that cellular debris is present in old blood which, when transfused into the body, tends to block capillaries. This embolization is especially important in the lungs where these aggregates can impair gas exchange. As a result of this discovery, the filter in a normal infusion set is not considered to be adequate as the pore size is too large except to screen large clots. Special blood filters have been introduced which filter out aggregates of a size of 40 μm or greater (this is an approximation). They are of two basic types: screen filters and depth filters. The screen filters act by behaving simply as a physical screen to the passage of particles. Depth filters act by adsorbing particles onto their surface. Some commercial filters incorporate both actions into their design.

It is becoming more accepted that a blood filter should be employed if old blood is to be used at all especially if the volume to be transfused is unknown (several transfusions in succession may be required). The filter should be changed after some 6 units of old blood.

Blood filters should not be employed if 'fresh' blood (blood less than 48 hours old) or blood products are to be used as the platelets themselves have a physical size in excess of 50μm. SAGM blood consists of resuspended red cells in a modified saline solution. Micro-filtration of this product is not required.

The rate of infusion of fluids

The rate of administration of intravenous fluids is dependent on the situation. In the hospital environment it can be controlled using careful monitoring. This is obviously not available in the field.

It is therefore necessary to use 'rules of thumb' in this circumstance. In the first instance it is essential to divide the administration into two main groups.

1. If the patient is losing blood then a colloid solution must be administered. Polygeline, e.g. Haemaccel, is the colloid of choice. One unit should be administered as quickly as gravity will allow.

2. If there is no blood loss and fluid therapy is clinically indicated, then a crystalloid solution should be used in the first instance. The crystalloid of choice is dextrose saline. Again this should be given as quickly as gravity will allow. It is possible that if the patient is in heart failure, the administration of fluid will make this condition worse, but in the authors' opinion the underadministration of fluids is a much commoner problem.

Whilst this fluid is being administered the patient should be examined and an assessment of the fluid status ascertained as has been previously described.

In addition to clinical assessment it is important to realize in patients who have suffered trauma that fractures always indicate blood loss. In the long bones and pelvis this blood loss is significant. For example, a fracture of the femur is indicative of a blood loss over 2 hours of 2–3 units. A fractured tibia 1–2 units and a fractured pelvis can loose into the soft tissues 4 units of blood or more.

In this chapter the basics of fluid management have been discussed with reference to management of the patient outside the hospital environment. It must be stressed again that this chapter is meant to be used in parallel with in-hospital training as the skill necessary for paramedical personnel in this field requires a combination of theoretical knowledge and practical experience.

Further reading

Willatts S. M. (1982) *Lecture Notes on Fluid and Electrolyte Balance.* Oxford, Blackwell Scientific Publications.

Chapter 5

The Control of Pain

S. J. Mather and D. L. Edbrooke

Control of pain is often not uppermost in the clinician's mind when dealing with severely ill patients but it deserves high priority. Adequate analgesia (pain relief) reduces 'stress', thus lessening adverse effects upon the body. One must also consider the patient's mental well being. Severe pain may imprint itself indelibly on the patient's memory and pain increases anxiety with consequent adverse effects upon the cardiovascular system. In short, adequate control of pain will reduce stress and anxiety resulting in the best physiological and psychological state for the patient.

THE PREHOSPITAL PHASE

Whatever the cause, a patient in pain will almost certainly travel better if his pain is relieved. 'Shock' and autonomic nervous system stimulation will be minimized. Complete relief of pain may not be possible outside hospital but it should be possible to reduce it to a tolerable level.

1. Physical methods
a. Splintage (to minimize movement and thus further painful stimulation and trauma).
b. Traction of fractured limbs (traction splint).
c. Transport in the most comfortable position.

2. Analgesic drug therapy

a. Inhalational analgesia with nitrous oxide
Fifty per cent nitrous oxide in oxygen provides very effective analgesia, equivalent in most subjects to that provided by standard doses of morphine. In the UK it is available premixed in cylinders (Entonox),

with a patient-operated demand valve. Administration by this method is considered very safe since the patient must achieve a good seal with the face mask or mouthpiece in order to operate the valve. Should the patient become very drowsy the mask will fall away and no more gas will be delivered. Care must be exercised when using Entonox under freezing conditions since the liquid nitrous oxide may separate out (see Vol. 1, p. 274). There is then a risk that the patient may receive 100 per cent oxygen followed by 100 per cent nitrous oxide. For this reason some regard the use of separate cylinders with a mixing valve as more appropriate. Entonox is available for use by UK ambulance crews at their discretion following special training in its use. It is without doubt the safest effective analgesic for use outside hospital but care must be exercised when a pneumothorax is suspected since diffusion of the nitrous oxide into the air-filled space may dramatically increase the size of the pneumothorax.

Table 5.1. Strong analgesics. Doses for intermittent administration

Drug	TOTAL dose in fit adults (mg)
Diamorphine (heroin)	5–10
Morphine	10–15
Pethidine	100–150
Papaveretum	10–20
Levorphanol	1–2
Piritramide	10–20
Nalbuphine	10–20
Buprenorphine	0·3–0·6
Pentazocine	30–60

In 'shocked' patients approximately one-fifth of the dose for a fit adult is usually adequate if given intravenously. The dose is repeated when discomfort returns.

Each increment should be about one-tenth of the total dose listed above.

b. Parenteral analgesics

This means drugs given by subcutaneous, intramuscular or intravenous injection. Strong analgesics (Table 5.1) may be administered, usually by medical practitioners but also by others (for example cave or mountain rescue teams) in the prehospital care situation. It is our view that intramuscular administration of such analgesics should be avoided unless the intravenous route is not available. The reason for this is that muscle blood flow may be very poor in a traumatized or shocked patient and absorption of the drug is unreliable. Further, a subsequent dose given because the first proved apparently ineffective may lead to respiratory depression if rapid absorption occurs following resuscitation and restoration of muscle blood flow.

The drug is best administered incrementally through an indwelling intravenous plastic cannula, allowing at least 5 min between increments for the full effect of each dose to be evaluated. Analgesia can then be titrated to the individual patient's requirement. Confusion has arisen over the use of the term 'narcotic analgesic' following the introduction of the partial agonist drugs (pentazocine, buprenorphine, nalbuphine). For this reason we have avoided the use of the term in this discussion. Suffice it to say that some 'strong' analgesics are better able to control pain than others and some produce marked euphoria.

However, such 'strong' analgesics can cause severe respiratory depression in 'shocked' patients. Nausea and vomiting may also be a problem. The partial agonist drugs appear to cause respiratory depression less readily but the relief of the patient's distress may be inferior to that of morphine or diamorphine due to lack of any associated euphoriant effect.

It is essential to dilute the drug to ten times its volume with isotonic saline to enable accurate incremental administration.

3. Sublingual administration

In patients who are able to co-operate, buprenorphine may be given as a tablet. Held under the tongue, this is rapidly absorbed. Each tablet contains 200 µg (0·2 mg).

4. Ketamine

Although not ordinarily considered an analgesic, in subanaesthetic doses (0·5 mg/kg) ketamine provides excellent analgesia with very few side-effects. Hallucinations and unpleasant dreams tend not to occur with such doses and the catecholamine release associated with its administration helps to maintain cardiac output. It has proved to be particularly useful in cases of severe partial thickness burns which could not be controlled by intravenous morphine in full dosage. Ketamine should only be administered by doctors experienced in its use.

5. Local analgesics

It is rare for local analgesics to be used in the prehospital phase of treatment because such procedures are time-consuming, require special skills and are often ineffective unless carried out under ideal conditions. Local analgesics may, however, be used for the insertion of chest drains or large bore intravenous cannulae and bladder catheters.

IN THE ACCIDENT DEPARTMENT

Following his arrival at hospital, the patient may wait for a variable period in the accident department pending radiography and assessment. Intravenous analgesia is most appropriate here as the patient should be under constant supervision, but if the patient is not 'shocked' the intramuscular route may be justifiable. However, it must be remembered that 30–45 min may be required for adequate analgesia to develop following intramuscular injection of a 'strong' analgesic. Nerve blocks with local analgesic drugs may occasionally be used for such injuries as fractured shafts of femur, fractured ankles, forearm bones and digits. If good analgesia is achieved it may even be possible to manipulate the fracture without resort to general anaesthesia.

POSTOPERATIVE ANALGESIA

Following a minor operation of manipulation, strong analgesia is rarely required. However, major operations result in a great deal of pain and discomfort which must be adequately treated. Parenteral analgesia is the usual method of pain relief, the drugs being given by intramuscular or intravenous injection together with a drug to control nausea (an antiemetic). Nowadays, continuous intravenous infusions of strong analgesics are gaining in popularity. Intramuscular injection, although widely practised, is less than satisfactory because 'peaks and troughs' of analgesia occur between doses. The result is that the patient alternates between painful and pain-free periods. This method continues to be used because it is the most practical, the majority of nurses on general wards not being allowed, at present, to administer drugs intravenously.

Sublingual administration of buprenorphine is a useful alternative where the pain is of moderate degree and the patient is able to co-operate, but again peaks and troughs occur because the administration of the analgesic is intermittent. Continuous intravenous infusion is ideal from the patient's point of view because once a steady state has been achieved, and the correct dose found, continuous infusion avoids the 'troughs' which precipitate him into pain. Furthermore, the onset of analgesia is rapid following an intravenous dose. The drawbacks of such a method, however, mean that it is far from universally practised at present, mainly because staff need to constantly supervise the patient to avoid respiratory depression, but also because each patient receiving an analgesic infusion requires a mechanised pump or syringe to control accurately the infusion rate and these are expensive.

IN THE INTENSIVE CARE UNIT

It is widely agreed that almost all intensive care patients require some form of analgesia. In this environment the intravenous infusion of analgesics is a real possibility since both the patients and the apparatus can be closely supervised at all times. Furthermore, intensive care nurses are trained in the administration of intravenous drugs.

A relatively short-acting drug (when compared to morphine) is most appropriate for intravenous infusion as the degree of analgesia can be rapidly altered simply by adjusting the infusion rate. Fentanyl, a drug related to pethidine, is the drug of choice and is administered at the rate of about 0·030–0·045 µg/kg/min. If the infusion is stopped, analgesia wears off in about 15–20 min.

'MILD' ANALGESICS

We consider that 'mild' analgesics, such as aspirin and paracetamol, have no place in the management of the emergency patient. Their use should be restricted to the rehabilitation phase of treatment when pain is minimal and only discomfort persists (*see also* Vol. 1, p. 238).

Further reading

Bullingham R. E. S. (1985) Synthetic analgesics. In: Atkinson R. S. and Adams A. P. (ed.) *Recent Advances in Anaesthesia and Analgesia* No. 15. Edinburgh, Churchill Livingstone.

Chapter 6

Oxygen Therapy and Airway Management

D. L. Edbrooke and S. J. Mather

Oxygen is a necessary requirement for all the cells in the body. The lungs and circulation merely act as transport mechanisms to allow the passage of oxygen molecules to their eventual destination in the cells. Without oxygen cells die; some, however, are more at risk than others. Fat cells, for example, are quite tolerant of lack of oxygen, whereas cells in the brain are extremely intolerant and cannot survive for more than 3 min without adequate oxygenation.

Lack of oxygen is termed hypoxia and the total absence of oxygen, anoxia. Classically hypoxia can be subdivided thus:
A. Hypoxic hypoxia
B. Anaemic hypoxia
C. Stagnant hypoxia
D. Histotoxic hypoxia

This classification indicates the precise site where the 'blockage' of the oxygen passage to the tissues has occurred.

Oxygen in the air ⟶ Lungs ⟶ Circulation ⟶ Cells
(A)   (B, C)   (D)

A. HYPOXIC HYPOXIA

This implies that the oxygen pathway is blocked at some point up to its distribution to the circulation. Consequently the hypoxia may be due to insufficient oxygen in the atmosphere. Examples of this include the oxygen availability at the top of Mount Everest or in an unpressurized aircraft flying at, say, 20 000 feet.

Alternatively, it may be due to damage to the lung tissue itself, through disease processes such as chronic bronchitis. It can also be due to trauma, an example of which would include pneumothorax.

B. ANAEMIC HYPOXIA

This term indicates that oxygen is not being transported efficiently by the red blood cells. This can occur for a number of reasons. The commonest cause is the lack of haemoglobin due to anaemia. This can be a chronic condition and can be due to malnutrition, chronic renal disease, leukaemia, women having severe blood loss during menstruation and a variety of other causes.

Alternatively, the blood loss can be acute. This often occurs following trauma. As the blood is lost the amount of blood reaching vital organs will diminish and it is thus extremely important to minimize the bleeding.

Anaemic hypoxia can occur in other rare circumstances when the haemoglobin level remains within normal limits. The best example is, perhaps, carbon monoxide poisoning when the carbon monoxide replaces oxygen attached to haemoglobin. This occurs because the affinity of the haemoglobin for carbon monoxide is far greater than its affinity for oxygen. It results in the classic clinical presentation of a patient with a cherry red complexion.

C. STAGNANT HYPOXIA

Here the blood is oxygenated by the lungs in a normal fashion, but its transport to the tissues is slowed or even stopped.

This can occur generally throughout the whole body or, alternatively, in a localized area. There are many causes for the diminution of blood flow in a localized area. A good example is an embolus becoming impacted in a coronary artery. Blood is unable to flow past this obstruction and consequently the heart tissue distal to the embolus will die. This is known as a myocardial infarction. Cerebral or pulmonary emboli will produce tissue death in the same manner. Stagnant hypoxia can also be generalized throughout the body. This is caused by the inability of the heart to act as an efficient pump. The most florid example is cardiogenic shock which is described in more detail in Chapter 11.

D. HISTOTOXIC HYPOXIA

This variety of hypoxia occurs at the receptor site where oxygen is to be utilized, but due to a malfunction at cellular level it is unable to be utilized. A good example of this is cyanide poisoning when the cyanide interferes with an enzyme system stopping the oxygen molecules being available for use by the cell.

THE CLINICAL FEATURES OF HYPOXIA

1. The cardiovascular effects

As a general rule the heart rate rises with hypoxia and continues to rise until the hypoxia becomes extremely severe. At this point it falls producing a bradycardia and eventually asystole. Depending upon the state of the myocardium, atrial or ventricular arrhythmias can occur at any stage.

The blood pressure follows the same pattern with rises in the systolic and diastolic pressures until the hypoxia becomes very severe. At this point a catastrophic fall can ensue.

Cyanosis may be observed when the saturation of oxygen in combination with the haemoglobin falls below 75 per cent. This, however, can be misleading as the patient could be suffering from chronic anaemia. These patients do not display cyanosis until the oxygen saturation is much lower. This is due to the fact that the low level of haemoglobin is balanced by a very high level of 2,3-diphosphoglycerate (*see* Vol. 1, Chapter 6).

2. The respiratory effects

The most consistent finding is hyperpnoea (increased rate of respiration). Again, however, this is a non-specific feature as the increased respiratory rate may be due to a chronic disease.

3. The central nervous system effects

The effects of hypoxia on the central nervous system can be extremely variable, but by far the commonest and most important clinical sign is confusion. Generalized epileptic fits can occur in severe cases. Conversely, generalized fits are an extremely potent method of producing hypoxia. The oxygen consumption of the body will be increased vastly. It is, therefore, of vital importance to reduce the oxygen consumption as a matter of urgency by controlling the fits.

WHEN IS TREATMENT NECESSARY?

The previous section has described the clinical features of hypoxia and highlights the problem that these features are in themselves non-specific. The most obvious clinical feature is cyanosis but it is beyond doubt that the treatment of hypoxia should be initiated at a much earlier stage.

It is of dubious value to give a list of indications for the administration of oxygen but it is undoubtedly true that 'too little, too late' is often the case.

A list of indications for the administration of oxygen can be found in many books, but it is the authors' opinion that all patients who are being treated as emergencies should be given oxygen. It can be argued that this will result in many patients being given oxygen who do not need it, but it is the authors' contention that too many patients who do need it do not receive it. The percentage of oxygen to be given and how it should be administered will be reviewed below.

Most people with normal physiological function depend on the level of carbon dioxide in the blood to regulate the respiratory pattern. This phenomenon is termed the respiratory 'drive'. However, in some patients with severe chronic obstructive airways disease in which the carbon dioxide level in the blood is very high (hypercarbia), the respiratory centre in the brain becomes insensitive to the level of carbon dioxide. In this way the carbon dioxide 'drive' to stimulate respiration is removed. In contrast to the high level of carbon dioxide, these patients also have a low level of oxygen in the blood (hypoxia) due to the poor respiratory function. As a result the respiratory centre in the brain uses this hypoxia as a stimulus to respiratory drive and tends to ignore the hypercarbia. These patients are said to exhibit 'hypoxic drive'.

Thus it is clear that if high percentages of oxygen were given to these patients, the oxygen levels in the bloodstream would swiftly rise and equally swiftly the drive to support respiration would diminish. This is the most important contraindication to oxygen administration. It is, however, not an absolute contraindication and this will be discussed in the next section.

HOW IS THE OXYGEN TO BE ADMINISTERED AND HOW MUCH SHOULD BE GIVEN?

Oxygen is administered to the patient via the respiratory tract and thus circulates via the bloodstream to the tissues. It is 'sucked in' as air into the lungs by respiratory movements. If these movements are judged to be inadequate (in the hospital environment usually with the aid of laboratory testing of the blood to ascertain the level of oxygen and carbon dioxide) a state of respiratory failure is diagnosed. It is then likely that the patient's inadequate respiratory movements will be suppressed with the aid of drugs and air with oxygen added will be pumped into the patient's lungs under positive pressure. This is called intermittent positive-pressure ventilation (IPPV) and usually a machine (ventilator) is used for this purpose.

1. Oxygen treatment without respiratory failure

In the absence of respiratory failure, oxygen can be given by one of the following methods.
  a. Oxygen masks
  b. Nasal cannulae
  c. Oxygen tents

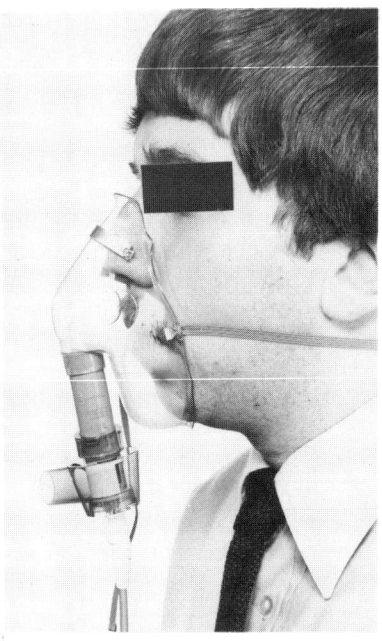

Fig. 6.1. Present-day oxygen mask, with adjustable oxygen flow rates.

a. Oxygen masks

A great many oxygen masks are available (*Fig.* 6.1). Some, however, suffer from the disadvantage that a precise percentage of oxgen in air is not administered to the patient. Nowadays, oxygen masks are designed to administer accurately precise concentrations of oxygen in air. The preset percentages include 24, 28, 40 and 50. The flow rate of oxygen necessary to achieve this percentage will be indicated on the mask. This is of paramount importance as if the patient does rely on hypoxic drive then a maximum of 28 per cent oxygen should be administered. All other patients should be given a minimum of 40 per cent oxygen.

The problem lies in the identification of those patients who rely on hypoxic drive. This is not easy in the absence of a laboratory. If relatives

or close friends are in attendance then a brief history should be sought. Any longstanding history of shortness of breath may be an indication of the patient relying on hypoxic drive.
If a history is not available then assessment is more difficult. However, it is extremely unlikely that patients under the age of 40 years will be dependent on hypoxic drive. Outside the hospital environment it is impossible to identify this group of patients more clearly. It must be stressed that this group of patients forms a very small percentage of the general population and so in the authors' opinion the following schedule should be adhered to:
  i. If the patient is under 40 years of age then an oxygen concentration of 40 per cent or greater should be administered.
  ii. If the patient has a history of severe shortness of breath then he should be given 28 per cent oxygen.
  iii. If the patient is over 40 years of age and no history is available then a concentration of 40 per cent or more of oxygen should be given.
In the last group, there will undoubtedly be a very small percentage of patients who do depend on hypoxic drive. If a concentration of oxygen in excess of 28 per cent is given then the respiratory effort will diminish and may cease entirely. At this stage intervention will be necessary and the patient will require some form of respiratory assistance (described below). It must be emphasized that this scheme for treatment must only be followed if personnel have undertaken full training and are qualified and competent to treat a patient with respiratory failure.

b. Nasal cannulae
This is a method of administering oxygen without enclosing the patient's face in a mask (Fig. 6.2). This device depends upon the effectiveness of the breathing of the patient through the nose, and is particularly effective if the patient is confused and will not tolerate an oxygen mask.

c. Oxygen tents
These consist of plastic canopies which fit over the patient's head and upper trunk and thus form a loose seal around the bed. They are not much used nowadays as they render observation of the patient difficult.

2. Oxygen treatment with respiratory failure
If, despite the use of an oxygen mask to increase the percentage of oxygen available to the patient, the respiratory rate and frequency deteriorate and cyanosis ensues, then a state of respiratory failure is said to exist. This simply means that the body's tissues are receiving inadequate oxygen for their needs. If this occurs the following steps should be taken:
  i. The airway should be checked to establish that no obstruction to the airway exists.

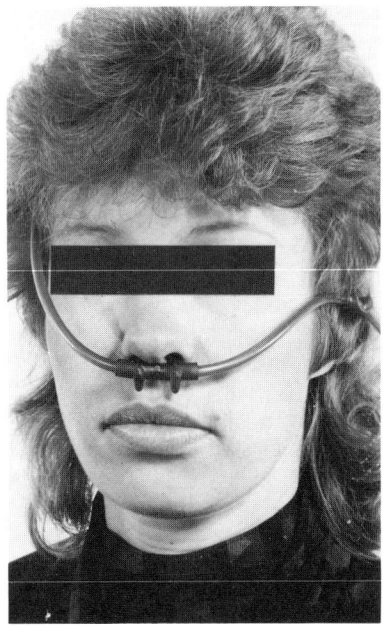

Fig. 6.2. A nasal oxygen cannula.

ii. Intermittent positive-pressure ventilation should be instituted. This may or may not be accompanied by intubation of the trachea.

CHECKING THE AIRWAY
1. Removal of foreign bodies

It is important to remove any large foreign bodies that could be causing an obstruction. Depending on the circumstances these could include loose teeth, large pieces of vomit or, in the case of children, almost any object could be the cause of an obstruction.

The most efficient way of finding and removing large objects is to use a finger to sweep around briefly inside the mouth. In small children a different technique can be employed. The child can be turned upside down and a few slaps on the back administered. This can be a life-saving manoeuvre. Another useful technique for removing foreign bodies trapped in the oropharynx or trachea is the Heimlich manoeuvre (*Fig.* 6.3). To do this the operator places himself behind the patient and places his arms around the patient under his ribs. The operator then administers

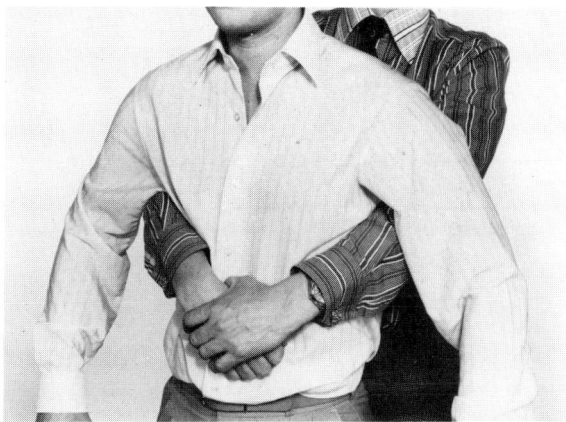

Fig. 6.3. The Heimlich manoeuvre for removing foreign body from oropharynx or trachea.

a sharp squeeze which expels air at some force out of the trachea. This can dislodge foreign bodies from the airway.

Dentures or dental appliances of different shapes and sizes may be discovered upon examination of the airway. Any dentures or dental bridges that do not constitute the entire dentition of the upper or lower jaw should be removed. If full sets of dentures are found in the mouth then they should be retained. As they are large it is not possible for them to be inhaled and if they are in position they provide a great deal of support for the lips and thus the airway. When they are removed the lips collapse on to the gums and make artificial or mechanical ventilation a great deal more difficult.

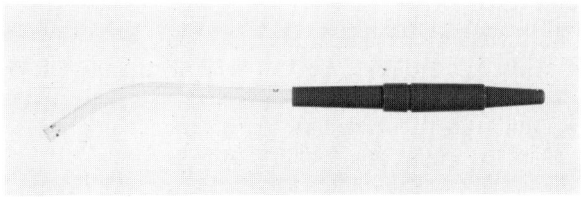

Fig. 6.4. A rigid sucker for removal of liquid debris.

2. Removal of liquid debris

Once large foreign bodies have been removed liquid debris can be removed with the aid of a specially designed sucker (*Fig.* 6.4).

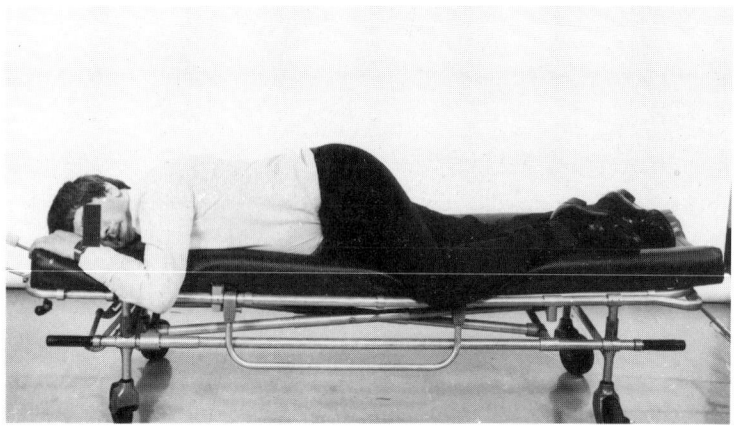

Fig. 6.5. The recovery position.

3. Positioning the patient

In order to achieve optimal air exchange it is vital to position the patient in the correct manner. The standard first aid manuals recommend the use of the recovery position for patients who may not be able to protect their own airways (*Fig.* 6.5).

This has the advantage of allowing free drainage of liquid debris from the mouth and nose and prevents the soft tissues in the oropharynx from obstructing the airway. It does, however, present significant disadvantages. First of all it is very difficult to observe the rate and depth of respiration and to observe the colour for the onset of cyanosis. It is also difficult to apply an oxygen mask successfully. Transporting the patient usually requires this position to be modified or abandoned, patients often being carried supine.

The authors wish to propose a position for transport of the patient which has many advantages. We will refer to this as the emergency position (*Fig.* 6.6).

The 'emergency position' consists of the patient being placed with the right side raised to form an angle of 30° to the horizontal. In addition the body should be tilted so that the feet are approximately 25 cm above the head. This position has the following advantages:
  i. It allows access to the upper airway.
  ii. Observation of the patient's pattern of respiration are simplified.
  iii. If vomiting occurs, the risks to the airway are diminished (compared to the supine position) as the head-down and lateral tilt allows the patient to be rapidly moved on to the side.

OXYGEN THERAPY AND AIRWAY MANAGEMENT

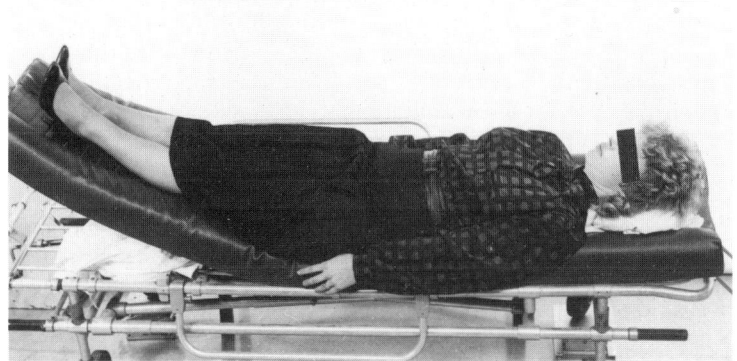

Fig. 6.6. 'Emergency position' for transporting patient.

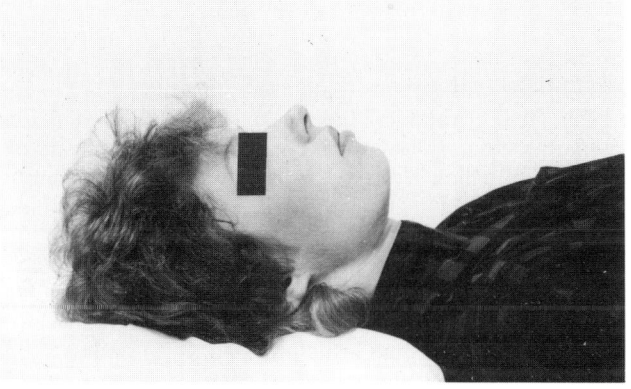

Fig. 6.7. 'Sniffing the morning air' position, with a small firm pillow.

iv. The head-down tilt improves the venous return to the heart.
v. Cardiac massage can be effectively undertaken in this position.
vi. Soft-tissue obstruction of the airway is less of a problem than it would be if the patient was in the supine position.

It is the authors' contention that ambulance stretchers should be redesigned to allow the patients to be transported in the emergency position. At present this position can be achieved by the judicious use of pillows.

In addition to the use of this position it is mandatory to use a small but firm pillow to allow the head to adopt the 'sniffing the morning air' position (*Fig.* 6.7).

This is, anatomically, the position in which the trachea, the oropharynx and mouth approximate most closely to a straight line and thus allow free passage of air. It is important to note that this does not apply to children of 2 years or younger (this is an approximation), as the relationship of the trachea and oropharynx is different. To achieve the best airflow no pillow should be used in these patients.

4. Improving the airway mechanically

After cleaning the mouth and oropharynx and positioning the patient, significant improvement should have been made to the airway. The tongue falling back or the presence of soft-tissue damage may still, however, cause significant airway obstruction. It is possible to improve the airway by the use of mechanical devices.

a. The oropharyngeal airway (Fig. 6.8)

This is the airway used most commonly. It is available as a disposable item in a variety of different sizes. Its shape is designed to fit the airway and it is strengthened near its exit point from the mouth (when in position) to stop the possibility of it being obstructed by biting.

It must only be utilized if the patient has lost the ability to control his own airway. If the patient 'objects' to its insertion then it must be withdrawn immediately as it can produce laryngospasm or induce vomiting, both of which are catastrophic. It is also important to choose the correct size as an incorrectly sized airway can produce airway obstruction in its own right.

b. The oesophageal obturator airway

The oesophageal obturator airway, is similar in construction to a cuffed endotracheal tube, connected at its proximal (top) end to a face mask. The inflated cuff occludes the oesophagus. Early versions were designed with a blind-ending tube having holes along the length of its upper, pharyngeal, portion to allow ventilation of the lungs via the holes in the tube. This design, however, did not allow decompression of the stomach. If vomiting occurred, the oesophagus might be ruptured, with fatal results. The later design, called the oesophageal gastric tube airway, allows drainage of gastric contents through the tube, the patient being ventilated via the face mask in the same manner as 'bag and mask' ventilation.

These devices have been widely used abroad, especially by the military. The device is passed 'blind' into the oesophagus and when correctly inserted functions reasonably well. However, in the civilian situation at least, it is the authors' opinion that endotracheal intubation, which is a technical skill most personnel can acquire in a reasonable time, is preferable. Ventilation is more effective via the endotracheal tube compared with either of the oesophageal airways.

OXYGEN THERAPY AND AIRWAY MANAGEMENT

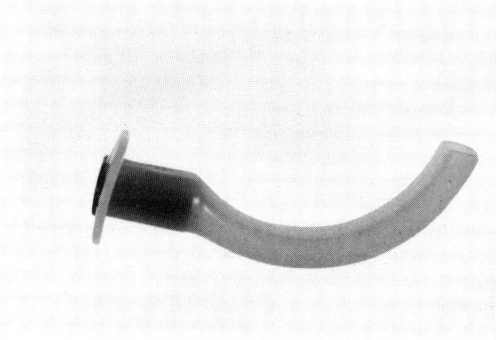

a

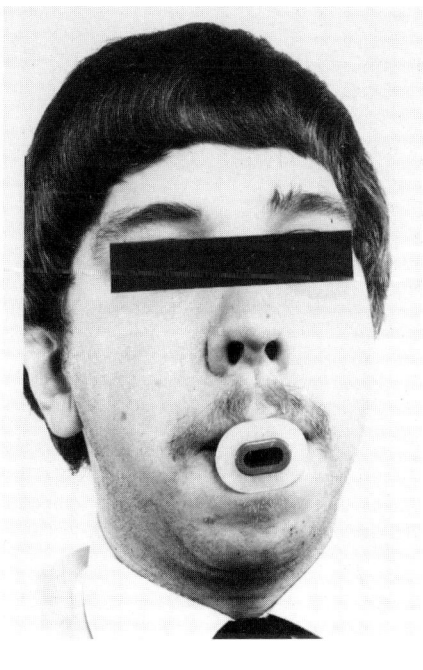

b

Fig. 6.8. *a,* The oropharyngeal airway. *b,* In use.

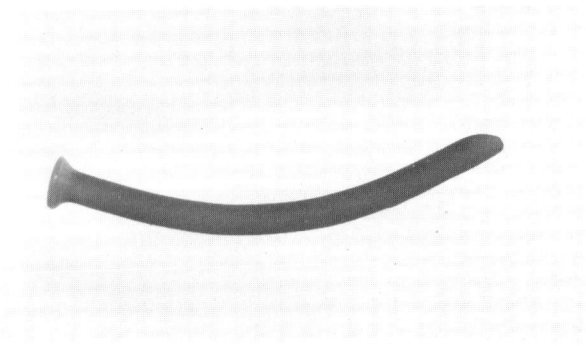

a

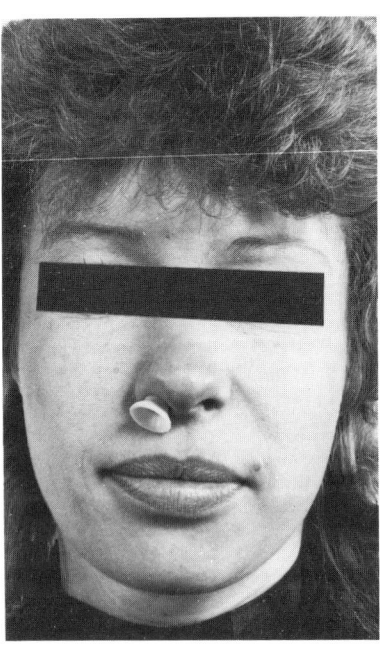

b

Fig. 6.9. *a,* The nasopharyngeal airway. *b,* In use.

c. The nasopharyngeal airway

This airway is positioned in one nostril and passes into the oropharynx (*Fig.* 6.9).

It is sometimes of value if it is difficult to maintain the patient's airway using the commoner oropharyngeal airway. A good example of its benefit would be if the mouth is badly lacerated following trauma. It should be standard equipment in an ambulance manned by emergency medical technicians.

INTERMITTENT POSITIVE-PRESSURE VENTILATION WITHOUT INTUBATION

It is a widely held but inaccurate belief that for intermittent positive-pressure ventilation to be undertaken an endotracheal tube must be inserted.

It is perfectly feasible and sometimes preferable to undertake intermittent positive-pressure ventilation without an endotracheal tube in position. To achieve this a source of oxygen is necessary together with a reservoir bag, valve and face mask. Two examples of this are shown in *Fig.* 6.10.

In a patient with respiratory failure, the airway is cleared, an airway inserted and the mask is fitted over the face. If respiration is present but inadequate, the patient's own respiratory efforts can be gently assisted by squeezing the bag. Synchrony with the patient's respiratory pattern is mandatory.

If the patient's respiratory efforts have ceased, then the operator can completely take over the ventilation of the patient using this technique.

It is the authors' opinion that this technique should be undertaken in the following circumstances:
  i. If the skill of the operator will allow it.
  ii. Before endotracheal intubation is undertaken to allow the body's oxygen store to be replenished.
  iii. If the endotracheal intubation is likely to be technically difficult.

It must be noted that the skill of ventilating a patient by this technique is complementary to the skill required for endotracheal intubation and both should be learned together in the practical environment.

ENDOTRACHEAL INTUBATION (*Fig.* 6.11)

This technique requires an endotracheal tube to be placed in the patient's trachea and this tube will then be connected to an anaesthetic circuit or self-inflating bag and the lungs insufflated manually.

This technique can only be learned successfully in a controlled environment, for example, the anaesthetic room of a theatre suite. In this environment, however, the doctor is at an enormous advantage as he can intervene before respiratory failure is very severe. This intervention

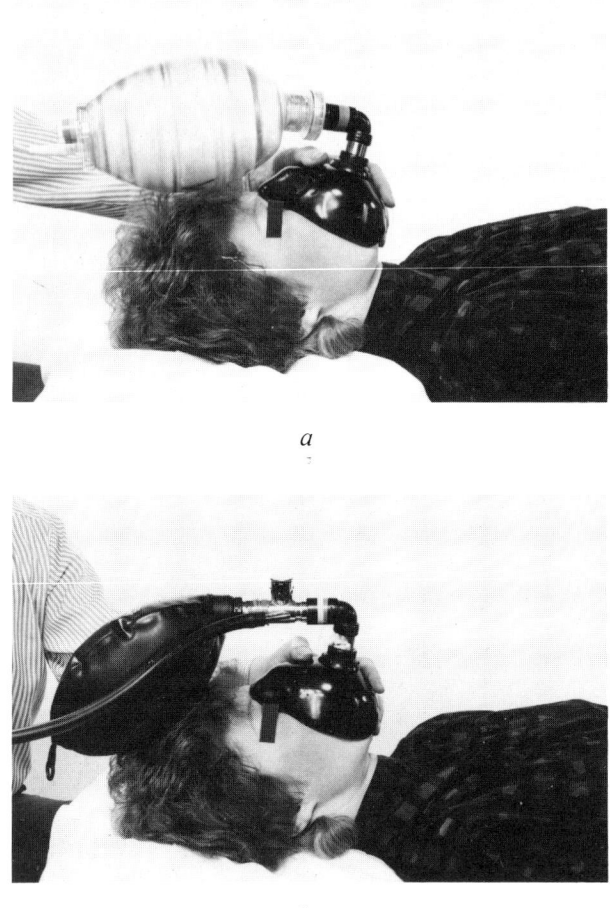

Fig. 6.10. a, b. Examples of reservoir bag, valve and face mask in use for intermittent positive-pressure ventilation.

takes the form of the administration of drugs which will sublimate the patient's efforts to respire allowing ease of access to the trachea and the placement of an endotracheal tube. In addition, he will be working in a well lit room with all the necessary equipment neatly laid out, the patient's respiratory and cardiovascular systems monitored and adequate assistance available.

OXYGEN THERAPY AND AIRWAY MANAGEMENT

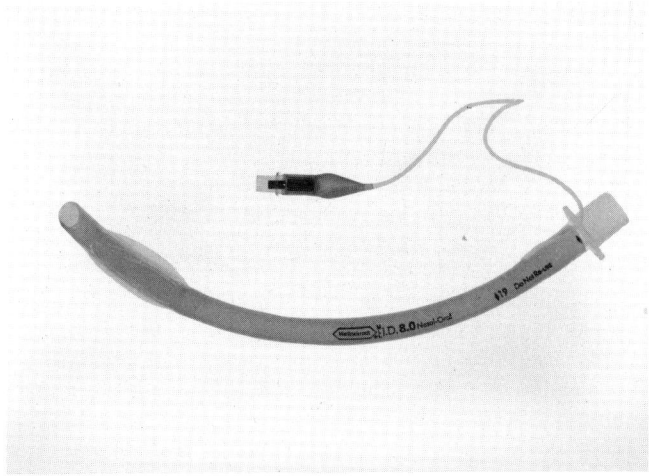

a

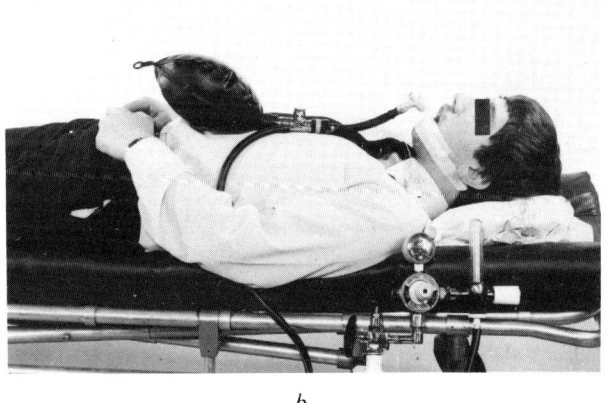

b

Fig. 6.11. *a, b,* Endotracheal intubation.

By contrast, the emergency medical technician is likely to be working in a very difficult environment with only basic equipment. This may involve working at night sometimes in appalling weather. Secondly, the anaesthetic and muscle-relaxant drugs do not form part of the armamentarium of the emergency medical technician. Consequently, he will have to intervene at a much later stage of respiratory failure, when the patient's protective reflexes guarding access to the larynx and trachea are obtunded by the onset of unconsciousness. It could be argued that these drugs should, therefore, be available to the emergency medical technician. The authors feel strongly, however, that the advantages of this argument are small as compared with the enormous risks of using these drugs. In fact a number of doctors specializing in emergency care believe that they should not even be employed by doctors skilled in intubation techniques working outside the hospital.

Indications for intubation

Intubation should, therefore, only be employed if it is impossible to maintain adequate oxygenation of the patient by the means described above. This could arise if, for example, the patient's facial tissues are severely distorted by trauma and consequently an adequate seal cannot be maintained around the face mask. It can be argued that an endotracheal tube should always be inserted if the patient develops respiratory failure as this will eliminate the risk of the patient inhaling saliva, foreign bodies or vomit. Against this, however, must be balanced the risks of a failed intubation and it is the authors' strong contention that these constitute the greater risk. Even the most skilled anaesthetist cannot guarantee intubating every patient successfully, let alone intubating a patient in a ditch, at night during heavy rain. Consequently, only if it is extremely difficult to maintain adequate oxygenation using a mask and airway should intubation be attempted.

The equipment necessary for intubation

A list of equipment necessary to undertake endotracheal intubation is given below:
 Two working laryngoscopes
 A selection of endotracheal tubes of different sizes
 A 20 ml syringe
 A sterile lubricant (e.g. KY gel)
 A self-inflating bag (e.g. Laerdal bag)
 A strong tie
 An introducer
 Suction equipment
 A stethoscope
 A catheter mount
 This is the minimum of equipment necessary to undertake intubation of the trachea.

The technique of intubation

Once again it must be stressed that the technique of intubation is a skill which can only be learnt by practical teaching in a controlled environment. It is not proposed to discuss the procedure in full. This

OXYGEN THERAPY AND AIRWAY MANAGEMENT

section is merely provided as an adjunct to the practical teaching. The points below are written in the chronological order in which they will occur during the actual procedure.

1. Before starting check twice that all the necessary equipment is present.
2. Check that all the connectors fit together.
3. Check that all the batteries in the laryngoscopes and the bulbs are working.
4. Check that the cuffs on the endotracheal tubes do not leak.
5. Try to ensure that you have an assistant who is familiar with the technique of intubation and that he is giving you his undivided attention.
6. Whilst checking the equipment preoxygenate the patient for 3 min with 100 per cent oxygen.
7. Optimize the patient's position as described earlier ('sniffing the morning air').
8. Ask the assistant to provide gentle cricoid pressure. This means that when the operator inserts the laryngoscope in to the patient's mouth, the assistant will gently press over the cricoid cartilage. This compresses the oesophagus and reduces the likelihood of the stomach contents being regurgitated to the mouth.
9. Instruct your assistant to keep a hand on the pulse at all times during the procedure and watch the patient constantly for signs of central cyanosis. He must inform you of any change in the patient's condition.
10. You are now ready to intubate. If you take longer than 20 sec, withdraw the laryngoscope and oxygenate the patient again. Repeat the process after 30 sec of oxygenation with a mask and manual ventilation. Allow yourself three attempts before reverting to a mask and airway, or if this is unsuccessful a tracheostomy may be necessary.
11. Once the endotracheal tube is in position, start to inflate the patient's lung whilst asking your assistant to inflate the cuff. Do not let go of the endotracheal tube at any time.
12. Tie the endotracheal tube in position with a strong tie. Make sure that it is impossible to pull the tube out.
13. Check with a stethoscope that both lungs are being equally inflated. If the endotracheal tube is placed too far down the trachea, it is possible that only the right lung will be inflated. This means that the endotracheal tube is situated in the right main bronchus. If this is the case, withdraw the endotracheal tube 2 cm, check again and then retie in position.
14. The safeguarding of the endotracheal tube will remain your responsibility, and your responsibility alone, until a formal handover takes place at the hospital. Do not hand over to anyone at any time other than this.

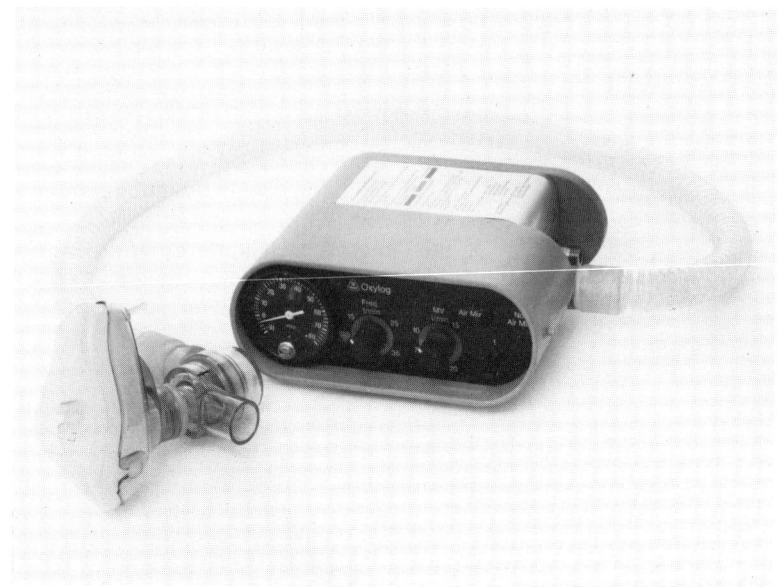

Fig. 6.12. Variety of portable oxygen apparatus. (By courtesy of Dragerwerk AG, Lubeck.)

15. If for any reason the circuit fails to work (for example if the self-inflating bag breaks) then it is always possible to blow down the endotracheal tube. In this way acceptable, if not optimal, oxygenation of the patient can be continued. If the pressure needed in insufflation is very great, then this may be due to some pathology in the patient's chest (e.g. severe asthma). However, it is important to ensure that this is not due to a physical blockage such as an overinflated endotracheal tube or a kink in the mouth.

It is also good practice to insert an oropharyngeal airway into the patient's mouth once the endotracheal tube is in position. This will stop any possibility of the patient biting the endotracheal tube, thus obstructing his own airway.

Continue the ventilation of the patient once endotracheal intubation has been successfully accomplished.

It is mandatory to insufflate the patient's lungs with oxygen until hospitalization. The best way of achieving good manual insufflation is by matching the patient's breathing pattern to your own. It is important to insufflate sufficient air to make the patient's chest wall visibly rise and fall. If this does not occur then the entire procedure must be rechecked.

It is, however, in the authors' opinion far superior to use one of the portable ventilators made specifically for this purpose (*Fig.* 6.12).

The use of this apparatus will reduce the risks of 'operator error' during manual ventilation and, of equal importance, free the operator's hands to check continuously the circuitry and the patient's condition.

TRACHEOSTOMY

This section is the last in the chapter and is so positioned as it represents the ultimate intervention to support the respiratory system. If it is found impossible to support the airway using the techniques described above then entrance to the trachea in the neck may have to be sought. It may also be necessary to intervene in this manner if no equipment at all is available.

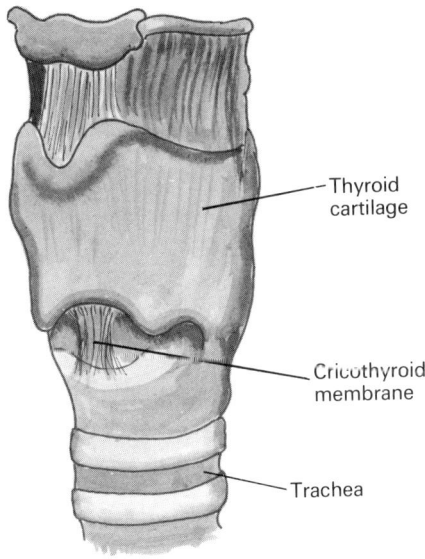

Fig. 6.13. The laryngeal cartilages showing the cricothyroid membrane.

It is important to remember that if the patient is in life-threatening respiratory distress due to the obstruction of an upper airway from trauma or inhalation of a foreign body, it is better to attempt a tracheostomy than do nothing at all; this may appear obvious but, sadly, the latter has happened too often in the past.

The type of tracheostomy described here is an emergency 'stab' tracheostomy and is a totally different technique to the tracheostomies

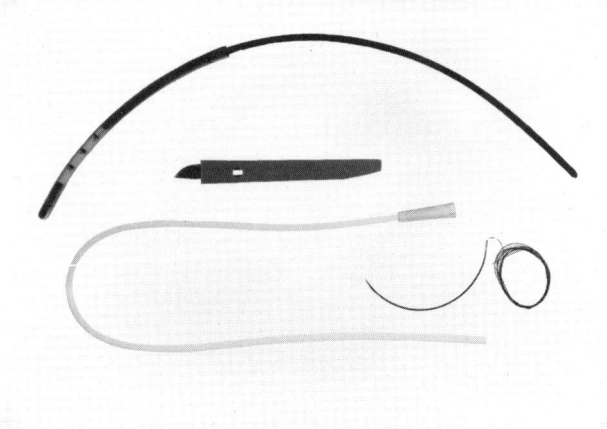

a

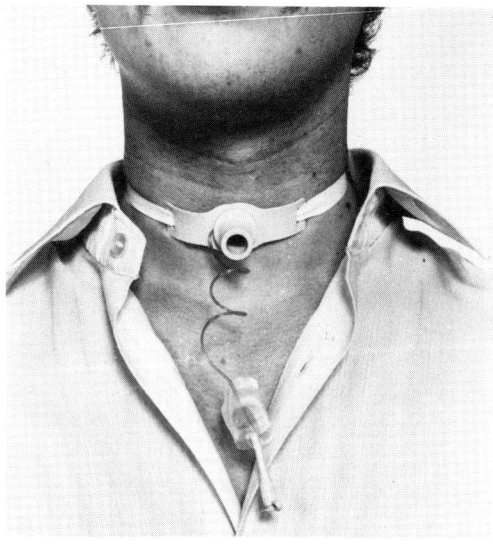

b

Fig. 6.14. *a,* Tracheostomy set. Mini-or 'stab'. *b,* A cuffed tracheostomy tube in situ.

done in the operating theatre. It is merely an emergency measure and in no way will it replace a more formal surgical approach.

The site for tracheostomy

The site for this 'stab' tracheostomy is the cricothyroid membrane. It is easily located using the thyroid cartilage (Adam's apple) as a guide. Feeling down from the uppermost border of the thyroid cartilage the cricothyroid membrane lies approximately 2 cm below this in the midline. It can be felt as an indentation in the cartilage (*Fig.* 6.13).

Tracheostomy technique

In the field the equipment necessary for this may be limited or non-existent. It is possible to make an incision at the site described above using a penknife and then supporting this opening in the airway using the outer casing of a Biro pen.

This is obviously only a temporary measure as the resistance of such a narrow tube is very great. Once the immediate threat to life is alleviated it is possible to enlarge the opening in the trachea and put a larger tube of some sort in position. An endotracheal tube is acceptable for this purpose.

Specially designed disposable 'stab' tracheostomy sets are now available on the market (*Fig.* 6.14 *a*) These are relatively cheap and incorporate a specially designed knife which is the correct width for insertion of the small tracheostomy tube in the same pack. In addition, it is short and consequently is unlikely to cause damage to the posterior wall of the trachea. This equipment should be carried in the emergency ambulance.

In conclusion, it can be said that with application and some specialized training the patients treated by emergency medical technicians should not die from the lack of airway support. Unfortunately, at the time of writing, this happens too often in the UK. It is hoped that with the acceptance of better training in the emergency services in these techniques deaths will not occur from this cause in the future.

Further reading

Shapiro B. A., Harrison R. A. and Walton J. R. (1977) Oxygen therapy. In: *Clinical Application of Blood Gases*, Chicago, Year Book.

Chapter 7

Cardiopulmonary Resuscitation

D. L. Edbrooke and S. J. Mather

(Cardiopulmonary resuscitation in infants and children is dealt with in Chapter 20)

INTRODUCTION

Any scheme of resuscitation must be committed to memory and must therefore contain didactic statements. We make no apology for this as we feel that to list minor deviations from generally agreed practice would serve to cloud rather than clarify the issue.

It must be remembered also that the scheme presented here represents current practice. This will change in years to come as techniques evolve, we have therefore included one blank page to enable the reader to update information as change occurs.

SCHEMES OF ACTION

Any resuscitation procedure must be pre-planned and executed according to a protocol well learnt and rehearsed. Familiarity with the procedure will make success more likely.

'CARDIAC ARREST'

Not all patients who require resuscitation have had a true cardiac arrest. Some suffer respiratory arrest only, e.g. the unconscious patient with airway obstruction. However, it is obvious that in a short space of time the ensuing hypoxia will lead to cardiac dysrhythmias, hypotension and eventual cardiac arrest. It must be borne in mind that successful management of an arrest will not necessarily have removed the initial cause. Vigilance must, therefore, be maintained for some time following restoration of the cardiac output.

'Cardiac arrest' is taken to mean the absence of an efficient cardiac output, i.e. impalpable major pulses.

An attempt should be made to feel a major pulse at two different sites (carotid and femoral) as occasionally the pulse in any one site may be impalpable.

In addition, one or all of the following signs may be present:
1. Respiratory arrest
2. Pallor or cyanosis
3. Absent heart sounds
4. Unconsciousness
5. Dilatation of the pupils
6. Cold and sweating

Successful cardiopulmonary resuscitation will achieve 'A B C':
1. An open *Airway*
2. Resumption of spontaneous *Breathing*
3. *Circulation* restored

Major causes of cardiac arrest

a. Cardiac
   i. Ventricular fibrillation
   ii. Asystole
   iii. Other cardiac dysrhythmias caused by, for example,
       heart block
       electric shock
       myocardial infarction
       myocardial depressant drugs

b. Non-cardiac
   i. Airway obstruction
   ii. Pulmonary embolus
   iii. Septic shock
   iv. Hypovolaemic shock
   v. Neurogenic shock
       spinal cord damage
       accidental total spinal anaesthesia
   vi. Hyperkalaemia
   vii. Hypocalcaemia
   viii. Vagal stimulation
   ix. Respiratory depressant drugs, including self-poisoning

There may be *no* preceding symptoms or signs but chest pain suggestive of myocardial ischaemia often precedes cardiac arrest. The patient is often nauseated and may vomit.

Management
Remember A B C—airway
   —breathing
   —circulation and conscious level

A—The Airway

Establish a patent (open) airway by lifting the jaw forward.
Relieve mechanical obstruction (i.e. dentures or other foreign body, blood, vomit) if possible with fingers or Magill's forceps and suction.

B—Breathing

Ventilate, initially by the expired air (mouth-to-mouth) method (*Fig. 7.1*) and then by self-inflating bag and mask with high concentrations of

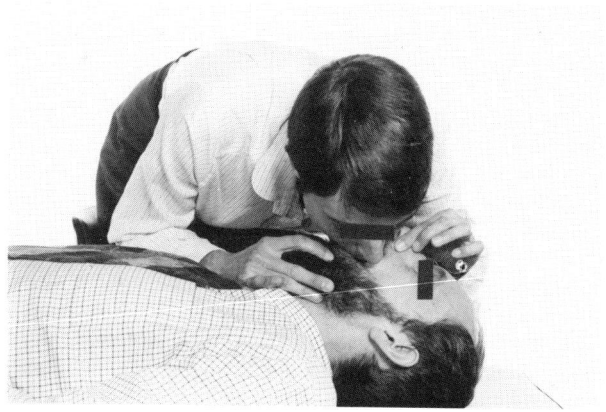

Fig. 7.1. Mouth-to-mouth resuscitation.

oxygen. The chest should be auscultated to confirm bilateral air entry. Adequate movement of the chest wall must be achieved.

If this is not seen, laryngoscopy may be necessary to remove a foreign body in order to allow adequate ventilation.

Effective ventilation should be established before intubation is attempted.

Intubation should only be performed by trained personnel. If ventilation by bag and mask is feasible and effective, intubation is not mandatory.

C—Circulation

Closed chest cardiac massage (CCCM) should be administered as soon as ventilation has been established.

The patient should be placed on a hard surface (floor or board) if possible. Massage is most effective if the resuscitator kneels beside the patient and provides downward movement of his hands by rocking forward. CCCM is achieved by placing the heel of one hand over the

CARDIOPULMONARY RESUSCITATION

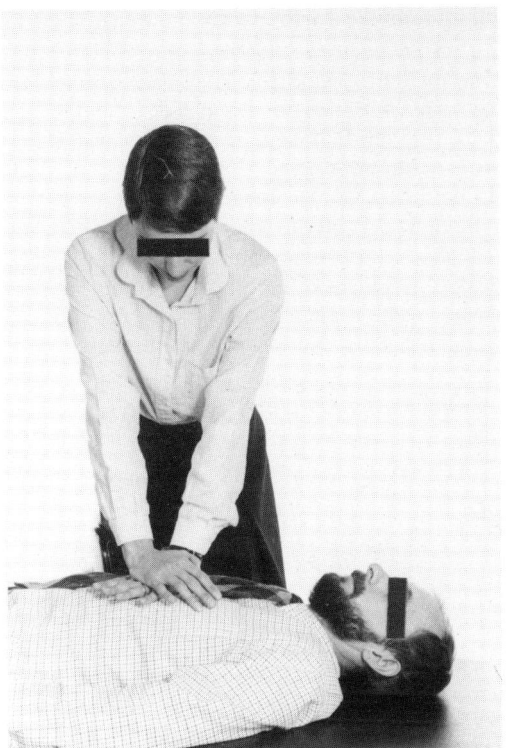

Fig. 7.2 Closed chest cardiac massage.

lower third of the sternum and the heel of the other hand upon the first. The arms must be kept straight (*Fig.* 7.2).

The patient's sternum should be depressed 4–5 cm (2·5–3 in) about sixty times per minute in the adult (rather more than one per second if working alone, to allow for ventilation). With two operators, it is not necessary to discontinue massage during ventilation. If a carotid or femoral pulse is not palpable the massage given is inadequate and the technique should be modified.

A ratio of fifteen compressions to two breaths is advised when working alone, one breath per five compressions when there are two operators. Effective cardiopulmonary resuscitation (CPR) can be maintained by trained operators for at least an hour. All medical and paramedical personnel should undergo regular refresher training in basic life support.

Points to consider in the further management of cardiac arrest
1. Cardiac rhythm *must* be ascertained by ECG monitoring, either via the defibrillator paddles or by monitoring leads. Adhesive electrodes may not stick to a sweating, shocked patient.
2. Access to the cardiovascular system should be provided by intravenous cannulation.
3. It should be noted that prolonged ventilation with a self-inflating bag may lead to carbon dioxide retention. Mechanical ventilation should therefore be considered and expert advice sought.
4. Correction of acidosis should be based upon the results of blood gas analysis. Sodium bicarbonate should not routinely be given on an *ad hoc* basis after the initial administration of 1 mmol/kg.

DYSRHYTHMIAS (*See* Chapter 11)

These may range in severity from a few ectopic beats to ventricular fibrillation. Protocols for the treatment of important dysrhythmias are given below:

1. Supraventricular dysrhythmias

Supraventricular tachycardia

a. Attempt vagal stimulation by carotid sinus massage (this is rarely successful)
b. If the patient is stable and not distressed, give:
    i. *Verapamil* 5 mg intravenously (which may be repeated after 15 min), *or*
    ii. *A beta blocker such as practolol* (2 mg increments to a total of 10 mg over 15 min).

Do not give verapamil and beta blockers together. Verapamil should not be given within 12 hours of any beta-blocking drug (significant risk of cardiac arrest).
If this is unsuccessful, give:
    iii. *Disopyramide* in a dose of 2 mg/kg intravenously over 5 min may be tried.

If these drugs are ineffective, or the patient's condition is deteriorating:
    administer synchronized DC shock starting with low energy (180 J).

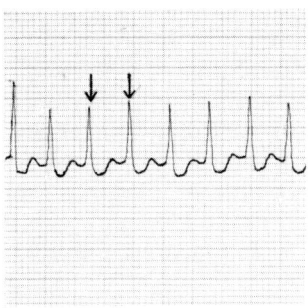

Supraventricular tachycardia.

2. Ventricular dysrhythmias
Ventricular tachycardia
This is a medical emergency as it may rapidly lead to ventricular fibrillation
If the patient is distressed:
   give DC shock
If the patient is stable and not distressed:
   give lignocaine 1 mg/kg over 2 min followed by an intravenous infusion (in 5 per cent dextrose) of 4 mg/min for 1 hour (this may need to be continued at a lower rate). If lignocaine is not effective, give DC shock as for ventricular fibrillation.

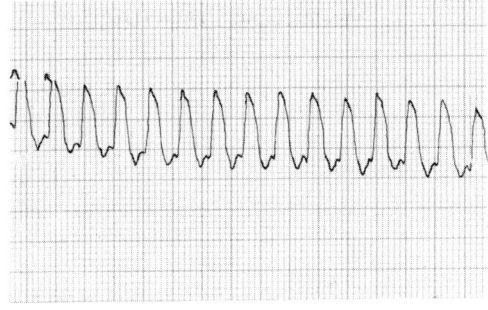

Ventricular tachycardia.

3. Ventricular fibrillation

Immediate action is required.
One DC shock may be effective. If not, follow the scheme outlined below.

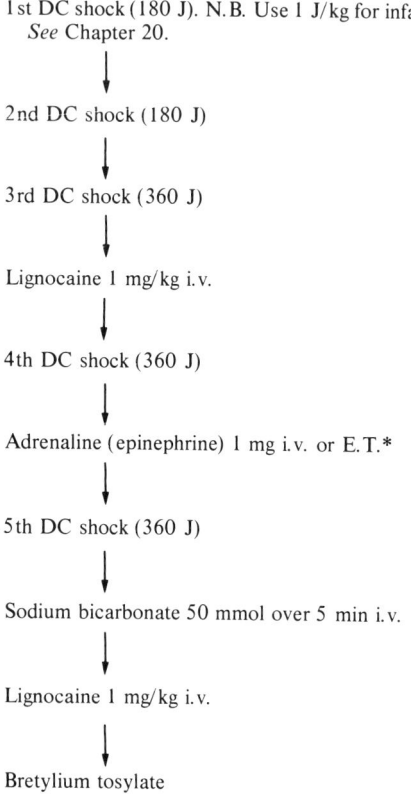

1st DC shock (180 J). N.B. Use 1 J/kg for infants and children. *See* Chapter 20.

↓

2nd DC shock (180 J)

↓

3rd DC shock (360 J)

↓

Lignocaine 1 mg/kg i.v.

↓

4th DC shock (360 J)

↓

Adrenaline (epinephrine) 1 mg i.v. or E.T.*

↓

5th DC shock (360 J)

↓

Sodium bicarbonate 50 mmol over 5 min i.v.

↓

Lignocaine 1 mg/kg i.v.

↓

Bretylium tosylate

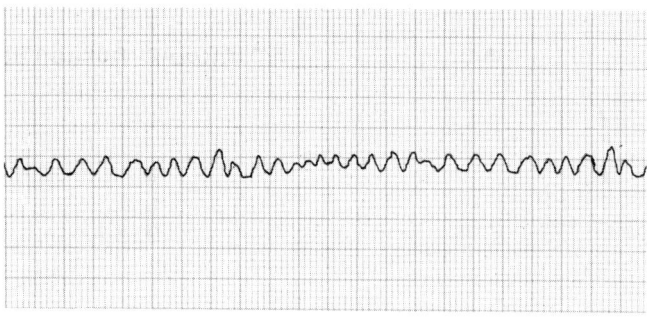

Ventricular fibrillation.

CARDIOPULMONARY RESUSCITATION

4. Asystole
The object of treatment is to restore a rhythm which can ultimately be converted to normal sinus beats.

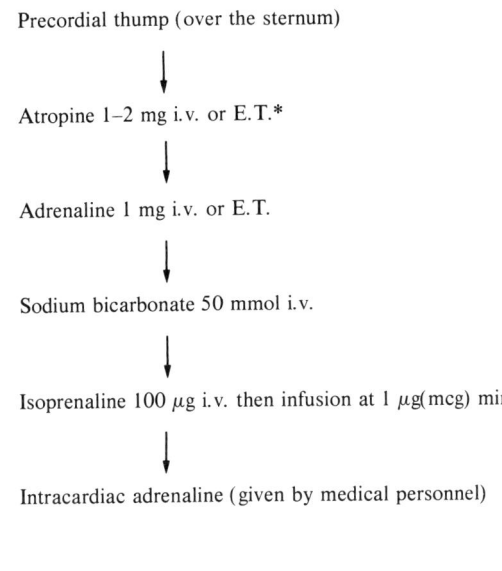

Precordial thump (over the sternum)
↓
Atropine 1–2 mg i.v. or E.T.*
↓
Adrenaline 1 mg i.v. or E.T.
↓
Sodium bicarbonate 50 mmol i.v.
↓
Isoprenaline 100 μg i.v. then infusion at 1 μg(mcg) min

If unsuccessful it may be necessary to resort to
↓
Intracardiac adrenaline (given by medical personnel)

or

Electrical pacing

*E.T. = endotracheal route
 i.v. = intravenous route

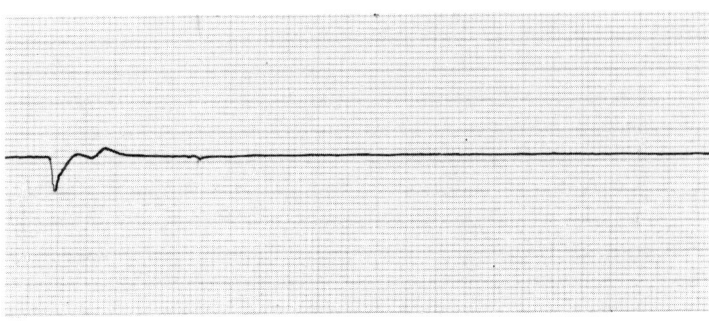

Asystole.

5. Heart block and electromechanical dissociation
Heart block
Only second or third degree heart block is likely to be a problem. Treatment is required for slow ventricular rates (less than 40 per minute).

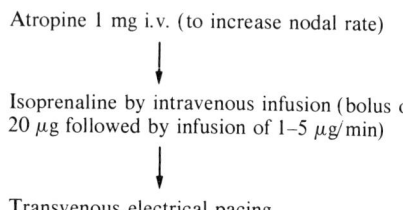

When available   Transvenous electrical pacing

Electromechanical dissociation
This implies that there are ECG complexes, showing electrical activity in the heart, but without cardiac output.

N.B. *Cardiac tamponade and tension pneumothorax must be excluded.*

Calcium gluconate 1 g i.v. (10 ml of 10 per cent solution)*
↓
Adrenaline 0·1–1 mg i.v. or E.T.
↓
Isoprenaline (bolus of 100 μg, then i.v. infusion at 1 μg/min)

*Must not be given concurrently with sodium bicarbonate through the same needle due to physical incompatibility.

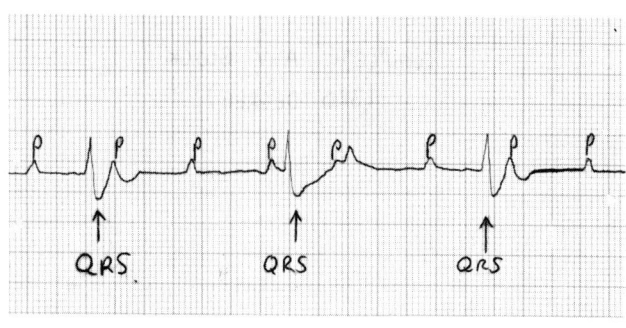

Complete heart block. (*See also* Chapter 11.)

CARDIOPULMONARY RESUSCITATION

ASSOCIATED PROBLEMS

These will require immediate treatment to maximize the chances of success.
1. Cardiogenic shock—*see* Chapter 11
2. Pulmonary oedema due to left ventricular failure
   This may be life-threatening and requires prompt treatment. The patient is classically in a state of extreme agitation, apparently

   Treatment
   The patient should be given:
   a. High concentrations of oxygen.
   b. Morphine or diamorphine by intravenous increments to achieve analgesia, sedation and tranquillity. The associated vasodilatation is also advantageous.
   c. Intravenous 'loop' diuretics such as frusemide 40 mg or bumetanide 4 mg.
   d. If life-threatening bronchospasm is present, aminophylline 250 mg slowly intravenously. *Caution.* Extreme care must be exercised in the administration of aminophylline in the hypoxic patient as serious dysrhythmias may be precipitated by rapid injection of the drug. It should be given under ECG control.
   e. Digitalization may be considered.
   f. Refractory cases should be managed in an intensive care unit where positive pressure ventilation may be employed.
3. Hypoglycaemia
   This *must* be excluded (*see* Chapter 17).

COMPLICATIONS OF CARDIOPULMONARY RESUSCITATION

1. Fractured ribs or sternum
2. Trauma to heart and lungs: cardiac tamponade; ruptured heart; ruptured diaphragm; pneumothorax; haemothorax.
3. Trauma to other viscera: liver; stomach; spleen.
4. Metabolic acidosis
5. Renal failure
6. Cerebral oedema
7. Resuscitation to the point of brainstem viability with cortical death. Other, less severe, neurological sequelae are common.

Often the patient will suffer several of these complications which may lead to prolonged cardiorespiratory instability necessitating mechanical ventilation and circulatory support for several days or weeks. There may be permanent neurological damage resulting in severe handicap.

USE OF THE DEFIBRILLATOR

The types of defibrillator available for use locally should be familiar to all personnel involved. A cardiac arrest situation is no time to begin reading the instructions!

DEFIBRILLATORS

Defibrillators are not used solely to treat ventricular fibrillation (*see above*); 'DC shock' or 'cardioversion' are therefore preferable terms.

A defibrillator is a device which is designed to depolarize a large mass of cardiac muscle fibres in unison. The pulse waveform and energy are important with respect to myocardial damage and the development of further (post-shock) dysrhythmias.

Crudely speaking, the DC defibrillator (which is superior to the previously used AC type) consists of a large capacitor (*see* Vol.1, p. 149) discharging through an inductor (which lengthens the current pulse). The discharge time is of the order of 12 msec. The skin resistance (about 1 megohm when dry) and that of the thorax (about 50 ohm) also affects the waveform and the amount of energy delivered. Skin resistance is minimized by using conductive electrode jelly on the electrodes ('paddles').

Modern defibrillators are capable of storing up to 400 joules (watt.sec) of energy. Experimentally, most defibrillators will deliver around three-quarters of this energy through a resistance of 50 ohm at the paddles. Skin resistance, however, is about 1000 ohms even with electrode jelly. The pulse is delivered by manually pressing a button (usually on the 'paddles' or by synchronization with the 'R' wave of the ECG. Most modern defibrillators have the facility of recording the ECG through the 'paddles'. When electrodes are applied directly to the heart, much smaller energies are required.

Defibrillators currently in use are about the size of a small attache case though research is at present being carried out into pocket-sized and even implantable defibrillators.

Dangers associated with the use of defibrillators

1. Up to 35 amperes may flow for a few milliseconds during the discharge. If there is any air gap or poor contact, significant sparking and burning may occur to the patient's *or even the operator's skin.*
2. The operator must be well insulated to avoid a potentially lethal shock.
3. Repeated defibrillation, especially at high energies, may cause myocardial damage.

UPDATE INFORMATION

Chapter 8

The Respiratory System.
I. Trauma

R. J. S. Birks

The bony skeleton and soft tissues can be affected by direct external insults but, peculiar to the lung, soft-tissue damage may occur from insults within the respiratory tract itself, e.g. from smoke and fumes inhalation.

TRAUMA TO THE BONY SKELETON

The main airways and lungs are protected within a bony skeleton. Posteriorly (behind) lie the 12 thoracic vertebrae. The ribs are attached behind to these vertebrae and surround the thoracic cage, being attached anteriorly (at the front) to the sternum (*Fig.* 8.1).

Damaging forces may act upon the thoracic spine from above, e.g. when a victim is buried in a rock fall, or from below as in a heavy fall onto the feet or buttocks, In either event such forces tend to flex the spine.

In the main, three types of damage to the spine may follow such a flexion injury. First, the body of the vertebra may 'explode' into the two intervertebral discs above and below it, the so-called 'burst' fracture.

Secondly, one or more of the vertebral bodies may collapse at the front. This is known as a 'wedge compression fracture'.

Thirdly, especially when the flexion injury is accompanied by some twisting of the spine, a fracture-dislocation occurs. This is the most dangerous of fractures in this region as it is unstable and may lead to damage of the spinal cord or damage to the intercostal nerves themselves (*Fig.* 8.2).

It is sound policy to treat all back injuries initially as having an unstable fracture until proved otherwise. The immediate care of patients with spinal injuries is discussed in Chapter 13.

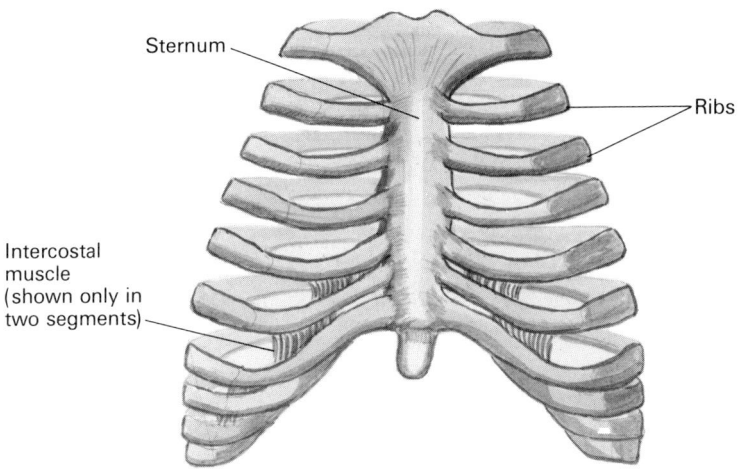

Fig. 8.1. The rib cage from the front.

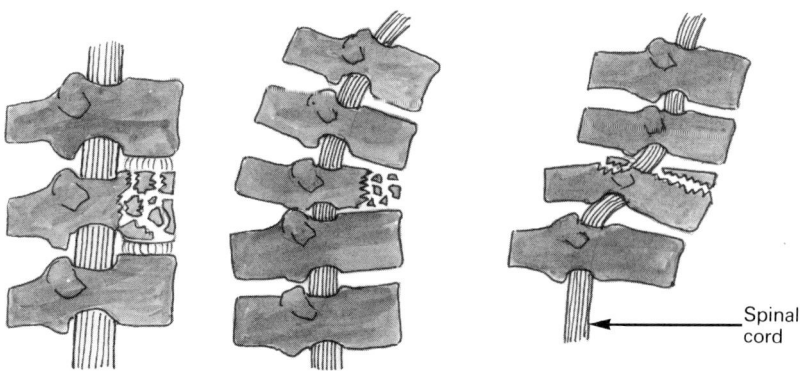

Fig. 8.2. Fracture of a vertebra leading to spinal cord injury.

Fracture of the thoracic spine may be associated with fracture of the breast bone or sternum. A fracture of the sternum may also occur on its own after direct injury. Sternal fracture rarely causes major problems.

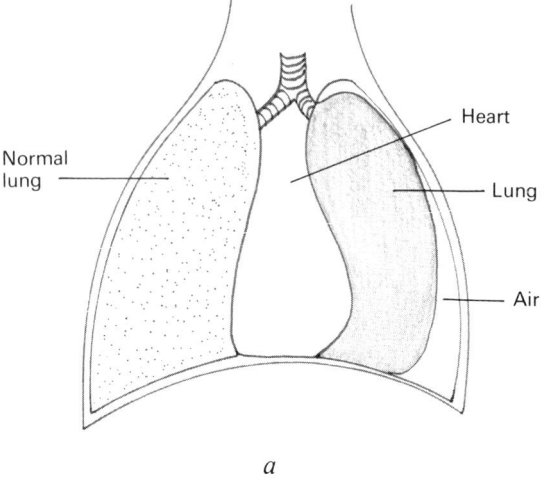

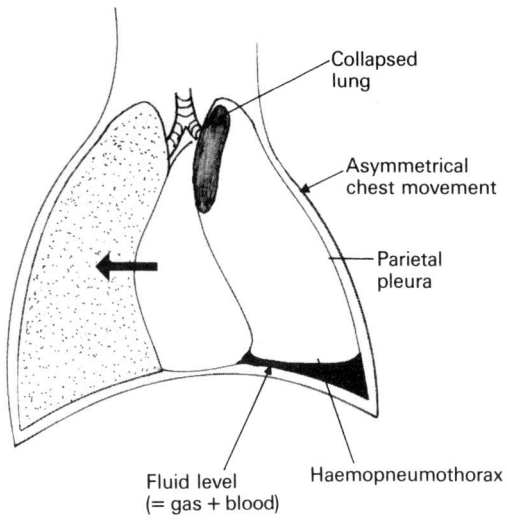

Fig. 8.3. *a*, Pneumothorax without tension. *b*, 'Tension' pneumothorax—heart displaced by air under pressure.

FRACTURED RIBS

Most fractures of the ribs are caused by direct injury, but rarely a rib may be fractured by laughing or coughing. Fractures usually occur at the angle of the rib and are held together well by the surrounding muscles without severe displacement. If marked displacement does occur then a fragment of the rib may pierce the lung or pleura leading to bleeding within the pleural space (haemothorax) or an air leak into the pleural space (pneumothorax). A combination of these two conditions is not infrequent (haemopneumothorax) (*Fig.* 8.3).

Clinically there is marked local tenderness over the site of a rib fracture. The fractures themselves unite spontaneously and treatment is designed to reduce pain, particularly when breathing deeply (which should be encouraged to prevent pulmonary collapse and the development of chest infections). Usually adequate analgesia can be given by mouth for one or two uncomplicated fractures. A patient with several fractured ribs, however, may require strong analgesics to be given by injection or a local anaesthetic 'block' of the intercostal nerves in the affected segments.

Rarely, the ribs are fractured in two places producing a mobile segment of chest wall. This is known as a 'flail' segment and is recognized by the segment being indrawn when the patient breathes in, the normal chest wall, by contrast, expanding (paradoxical respiration) (*Fig.* 8.4). Such patients may require mechanical ventilation to splint the chest wall as well as to improve respiratory function.

Treatment of the complications of haemo- and pneumothorax may require drainage of the pleural cavity as outlined below.

TRAUMA TO THE THORACIC CONTENTS

Damage to the thoracic contents, i.e. the heart and lungs and their respective coverings, together with the major thoracic blood vessels, may occur following trauma with or without damage to the overlying thoracic cage. Blunt trauma, e.g. a crush injury or steering wheel impact in a road traffic accident, may lead to lung contusion. In this condition there is disruption of the small blood vessels within the lung. Bleeding and extravasation of fluid into the interstitial tissues of the lung occurs with encroachment on and bleeding into the alveoli themselves. Small amounts of blood may be coughed up by the patient (haemoptysis).

On examination there are decreased breath sounds over the affected area and a chest radiograph shows a picture similar to that of pneumonia.

The degree to which the patient is compromised by lung contusion depends upon how widespread the contused (bruised) area is and the presence or absence of other injuries. Small areas of contusion with no

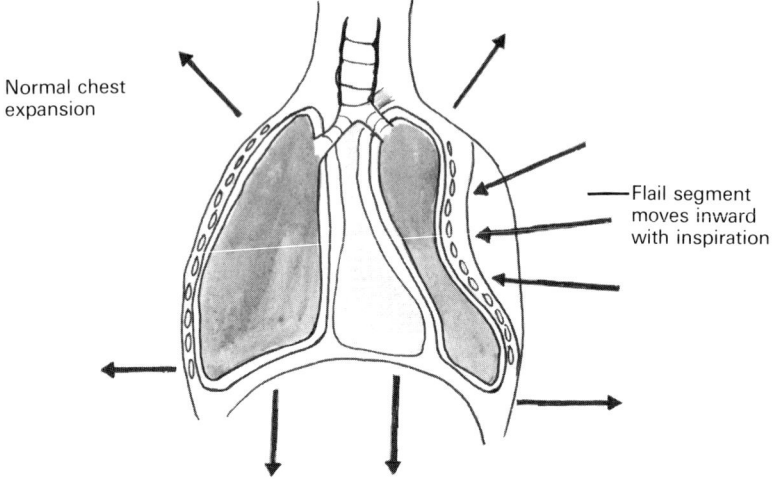

Fig. 8.4. The flail segment.

other damage will heal spontaneously with little upset to the patient. Antibiotics are often given to prevent infection of the damaged area.

More severe wounds may lead to laceration of the lung. Laceration is in effect 'traumatic cutting'. This permits leakage of blood and air into the pleural cavity. Minor lacerations heal spontaneously. Major lacerations with large haemopneumothoraces may need urgent drainage of the pleural space and resuscitation followed by surgical intervention.

Secondary infection of the damaged lung is again an important complication prevented by antibiotics, bronchial aspiration and physiotherapy.

Severe chest trauma may be associated with rupture of a major thoracic blood vessel. Aortic or main pulmonary artery rupture may be instantly fatal. Rupture of a major branch of the pulmonary artery will require an attempt at resuscitation and immediate thoracotomy. Insertion of a special double-lumen endobronchial tube may be required to isolate the damaged lung and allow ventilation of the undamaged side. Furthermore, this procedure prevents 'spillover' of blood from one lung into the other.

SMOKE AND FUMES INHALATION

In the event of fire in an enclosed space, damage to the lungs can occur from the inhalation of smoke or other products of combustion. Damage to the respiratory tract may have occurred to a much greater degree than any external burns might suggest. Indeed, the patient may have little or no evidence of superficial burning.

Experiments in dogs have shown that when air at 270°C is blown into the larynx, the temperature has fallen to 50° by the time the trachea is reached. Thermal injury, therefore, only occurs to the larynx and pharynx. Damage, however, is not only related to the amount of heat but also to the nature of the toxic fumes or smoke.

Smoke variously contains carbon monoxide, oxides of nitrogen and sulphurous compounds, depending upon the nature of the burning material, together with solid particles. Various aldehydes and hydrochloric acid are usually present which, together with the other compounds, cause direct damage to lung tissue.

Polyurethene foam, present in many articles of modern furniture, is particularly hazardous. Different products are given off at different temperatures, with increasing toxicity, until at 1000°C hydrogen cyanide predominates.

Laryngeal oedema may ensue following smoke inhalation and eventually laryngotracheobronchitis occurs with the formation of slough in the airways. These may become detached causing complete airway obstruction.

It is imperative that any patient who has inhaled smoke should be well oxygenated while being transported to hospital and on arrival should be closely observed, preferably in an intensive care unit. Respiratory support, with intubation and mechanical ventilation may be urgently required. The patient should breathe humidified oxygen-enriched air. Antibiotics should be administered as the damaged lung may quickly become infected.

BLAST INJURIES

Blast injuries are caused by explosions of one form or another. They may be due to a terrorist bomb or an explosion of gas in a confined space. When an explosion occurs, energy is dissipated outwards with a spherical pressure wavefront (*see* Chapter 22). Many people may be injured in a single explosion and their management involves well rehearsed disaster planning as well as individual clinical management.

Injuries from an explosion may be direct or indirect (*Fig.* 8.5). Indirect injuries are caused by large or multiple small foreign bodies, e.g. glass, pieces of metal, wood or stones flying through the environment as a result of the blast. These may cause a variety of injuries to the respiratory system, e.g. fractured ribs, laceration or contusion of the lung, pneumothorax, haemothorax and combinations of all of these.

In the lungs, damage consists of alveolar disruption and haemorrhage causing hypoxia. The degree of damage is very variable. Small home-

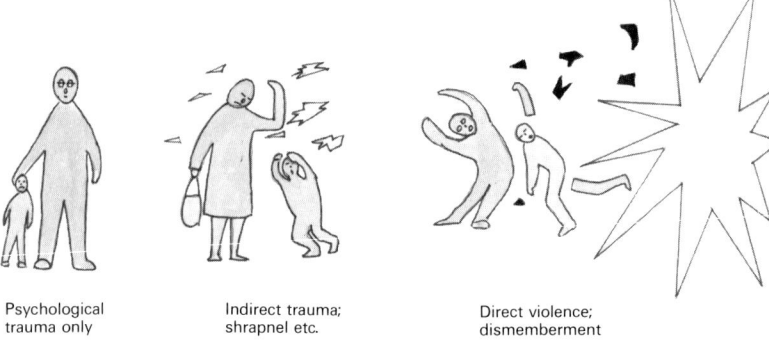

Psychological trauma only   Indirect trauma; shrapnel etc.   Direct violence; dismemberment

Fig. 8.5. Blast injury

made bombs have limited blast pressures and blast injuries are uncommon, injury largely being the result of flying missiles.

Both massive haemorrhage into the lung and oedema are common findings in those killed by more sophisticated devices.

Blast-injured patients require the administration of oxygen during transport. Where facilities allow, the more severely injured may require intubation and positive-pressure ventilation before evacuation to hospital. One must also be aware, of course, that other related respiratory damage may have occured such as haemo- or pneumothorax which may require on-site insertion of a chest drain before the casualty is moved.

FOREIGN BODY

Foreign bodies in the thorax may occur due to direct penetration of the thoracic wall by missiles which include bullets, bomb fragments, etc., or stabbing by knives or other sharp implements. Foreign bodies are also commonly inhaled and frequently cause partial or complete respiratory obstruction.

As a general rule, foreign bodies should not be removed unless facilities for resuscitation and immediate surgical intervention are available.

Inhalation of a foreign body is a common occurrence, especially among children. The foreign body may lodge anywhere in the respiratory tract depending upon its size. A large foreign body may cause sudden respiratory obstruction and if not treated with the greatest urgency the patient will rapidly succumb to hypoxia. Foreign bodies may also cause vagal stimulation and cardiac arrest.

Heimlich described a manoeuvre designed to forcefully expel foreign bodies from the respiratory tract (see Chapter 6, Fig. 6.3).

If the Heimlich manoeuvre fails, the use of back blows must be considered. In an adult, short, sharp slaps between the shoulder blades will provoke coughing. An infant may be held upside down and similar treatment applied.

If these methods are unsuccessful, and the patient is suffering from hypoxia, artificial respiration by the expired air method or ventilation with a bag and mask must be commenced without delay. Such therapy may, in fact, move the foreign body into one or other main bronchus, thus relieving the hypoxia by allowing ventilation of one lung. The foreign body may then be removed at operation when the patient has been properly prepared.

A cricothyroid puncture may be undertaken (see Chapter 6). This technique is only suitable for cases where the foreign body is lodged above the cricothyroid membrane, i.e., in the larynx.

If facilities are available, rapid recourse to a tracheostomy may become necessary. This should ideally be performed by someone skilled in the technique.

PNEUMOTHORAX

This condition has been mentioned already. One must always consider the possibility of a pneumothorax when dealing with any thoracic injury. It may be caused by apparently minor injury. For example a small spicule of bone from a single fractured rib may tear the pleura overlying the lung, causing air to escape into the pleural cavity. There may be associated bleeding resulting in haemopneumothorax.

A small pneumothorax may occur asymptomatically, that is the patient feels no symptoms and may not realize anything is wrong with his lungs. The diagnosis is made radiologically (on a chest X-ray).

Most serious, however, is the development of a 'tension pneumothorax'. In this condition, air can enter the pleural cavity but, because the pleural tear is valvular in nature, cannot then escape. Air gradually accumulates and compresses the lung. The heart may be deviated into the opposite side of the chest (see Fig. 8.3 b). The condition will be made worse if the patient is subjected to positive-pressure ventilation.

Treatment must be given quickly and effectively as such a tension pneumothorax is life-threatening. The patient should be inclined toward the affected side to allow the uninjured side of the chest to expand.

A needle inserted into the pleural space will bring immediate relief of the problem; there is little risk of damage to the underlying lung when so much air is present. Of course, the pneumothorax will still be present but no longer under tension. The needle (or preferably a plastic intravenous

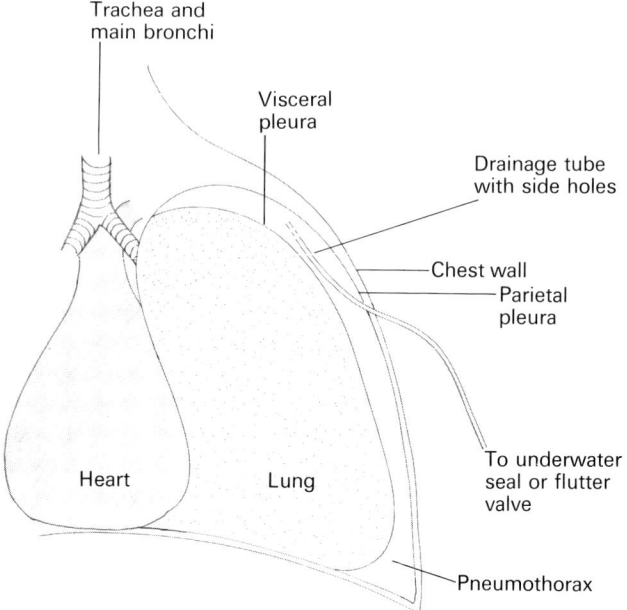

Fig. 8.6. Diagram showing chest drain in situ.

cannula) can then be connected to a flutter valve (Heimlich valve) or underwater seal (Fig. 8.6). When conditions allow, a formal chest drainage procedure can be performed in hospital when the patient has stabilized.

Sometimes air escapes also into the subcutaneous tissues producing surgical emphysema.

Pneumothorax may also result from penetrating wounds of the chest, such as from a knife or bullet. The lips of the wound may have a valvular effect and air may be sucked into the chest ('sucking wound').

Penetrating wounds of the chest require immediate application of a dressing in order to minimize the entry of air into the pleural space. Small wounds with an underlying pneumothorax will require wound toilet and the placement of a chest drain in hospital. Larger wounds will require formal surgical exploration and repair of any underlying damage. A thoracotomy (opening of the chest) may be necessary and, if the diaphragm has been breached, a laparotomy (opening of the abdomen) as well.

Further reading

May, Harold L. (ed.) (1984) *Emergency Medicine.* New York, Wiley.

Chapter 9

Respiratory System.
II. Non-Trauma

P. C. Taylor

STRIDOR

This is a condition caused by partial obstruction of the airway resulting in a severe and usually acute respiratory distress.

The condition most commonly occurs following upper respiratory tract infection in infants. The infection may in fact affect the epiglottis (the flap which covers the airway on swallowing). (*Fig.* 9.1.)

Adults, having larger airways are less likely to develop stridor although this can be a consequence of inhaled foreign bodies, toxic chemicals or injury.

The sound of stridor is caused by air being drawn through a narrow orifice, in this case the patient's upper airway. There may also be coughing and respiratory difficulty.

Stridor may precede acute and fatal respiratory obstruction. Infants are particularly prone to rapid deterioration, especially if laying flat. They should always be observed in hospital.

QUINSY

Quinsy is an abscess involving the tonsil causing swelling in and around the tonsil which can compromise the airway. It is caused by repeated infections of the tonsils.

The infection is almost always unilateral and begins during an attack of tonsillitis. The patient complains of severe pain, his temperature rises and he may well have difficulty opening his mouth. With rupture of the abscess there is immediate relief of symptoms.

In the first instance treatment with antibiotics is indicated. An abscess may well form despite such treatment and will require incision after 2–3 days.

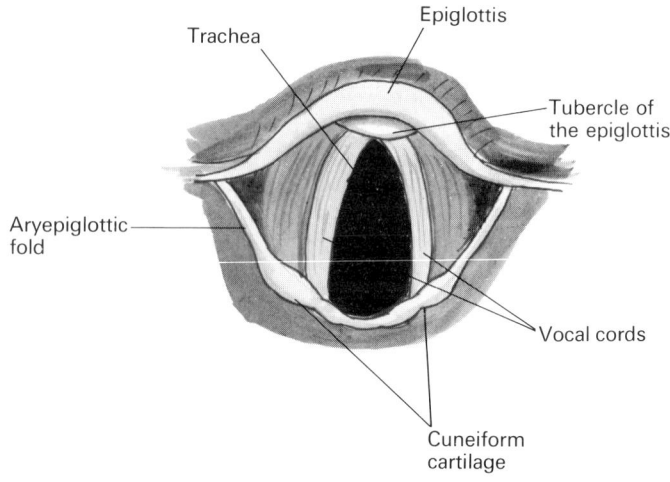

Fig. 9.1. The larynx.

PNEUMONIA

This is an infection of the lung, when the products of infection (pus cells, exudate) fill the air spaces of the lung which is then said to be consolidated.

Pneumonia is due to viral or bacterial infection. Aspiration of caustic substances, particularly vomitus, inhaled after a vomiting episode, will directly damage the lung tissue, thereby reducing resistance to infection.

In practice pneumonia is commonest in patients with chronic bronchitis and emphysema (usually secondary to smoking) when recurrent episodes of infection are the rule.

Young, apparently fit people can, however, develop pneumonia. The organism usually responsible is the pneumococcus (*Streptococcus pneumoniae*).

The symptoms are fever and cough, dry at first but later productive of thick green or occasionally bloodstained sputum. Breathlessness is almost always a feature as is a feeling of marked general malaise. Pain is present if the lung infection spreads to the surface, when the lining membranes (pleura) become inflamed and rub together on breathing. The typical pain is sharp, worse on deep breathing and is called pleuritic.

The patient should be put to bed, his temperature reduced either by tepid sponging or aspirin and treatment with antibiotics commenced. Viral infections, although in themselves not amenable to treatment with antibiotics, are usually complicated by secondary bacterial infection. In addition to the above measures, oxygen by face mask is required for severe infections when lung function is seriously impaired. Pain relief may be necessary and also physiotherapy to encourage the patient to cough up any secretions, thereby clearing as much as possible of the infected material.

The outcome in patients with normal lungs is almost invariably completely satisfactory. However, the risks are undeniably greater in patients with underlying lung disease.

BRONCHITIS

Bronchitis is a condition characterized by repeated chest infections with increased production of sputum. This leads to recurrent infections and is then referred to as 'chronic' bronchitis.

The most significant cause is tobacco smoking although atmospheric pollution and exposure to dust and fumes are also important.

The development of chronic bronchitis is very slow and to many people the earlier stages pass completely unnoticed. Subsequently, however, the increased sputum production leads to infections with prolonged bouts of coughing. Recurrent infection is common. The disease may end in respiratory failure.

Cigarette smoking should be strictly prohibited. Prompt treatment of all infective episodes is advised and regular physiotherapy given to help clear the chest of sputum.

The outcome depends on the severity of the disease and the ability to stop smoking. There is no doubt that life expectancy is significantly reduced in severe cases.

EMPHYSEMA

This is a condition characterized by destruction and dilatation of the terminal air spaces.

The underlying cause is unknown. A rare type is due to an enzyme deficiency but this accounts for less than 1 per cent of all cases.

The predominant symptom is breathlessness which usually develops slowly over several years to leave the sufferer incapacitated after the most minimal of exertion. There is little in the way of cough and the chest is over expanded due to air trapping in the enlarged air spaces. Occasionally one of the terminal air spaces (bullae) ruptures and produces a pneumothorax with its accompanying symptoms (*see below*).

The disease is irreversible and there is no treatment available for the underlying condition, only antibiotics for the inevitable complicating infective episode.

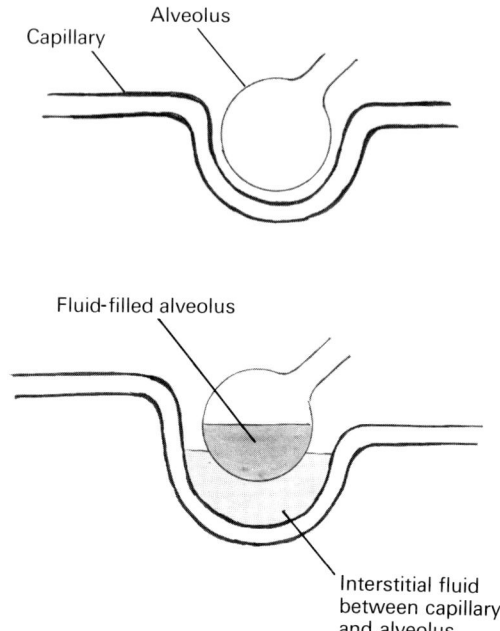

Fig. 9.2. Diagrammatic representation of alveolus and capillary.

For established cases presenting to hospital for the first time, only 50 per cent will survive the following five years.

PULMONARY OEDEMA

This is a condition characterized by widespread leaking of fluid from the circulation into the air spaces of the lungs (*Fig.* 9.2).

The most common cause of pulmonary oedema is blood 'damming back' into the lungs when the left side of the heart fails to pump adequately ('heart failure').

The outstanding symptom is breathlessness which can be very severe. A cough can be present but is usually mild though irritating and is classically productive of pink frothy sputum.

The mainstay of treatment is diuretic therapy (*see* Vol. 1, Chapter 32). This therapy aims to remove water from the body, and therefore from the lungs. Also oxygen by face mask is given.

The outcome relates to the underlying cause, and in the case of heart failure, which is progressive, repeated episodes are the rule.

PULMONARY INFARCTION

This is a condition caused by a blockage in the main artery to the lung (or one of its branches)—usually with a clot of blood—which results in death of the lung supplied by the affected artery, and subsequent bleeding into the area of lung supplied by that vessel.

The blood clot responsible may form in the venous system, commonly in the leg or pelvis.

The variety of presentation which may bring the patient to medical attention reflects the sizes of the blood clots responsible and the response of the arteries in the lung to this insult. The symptoms can vary from mild chronic progressive breathlessness to sudden shortness of breath with pain on deep breathing and coughing up of blood (haemoptysis). Occasionally the patient may just collapse.

The mainstay of treatment in the initial phase, apart from cardiopulmonary resuscitation if required, is heparin (see Vol.1, Chapter 34), which when injected intravenously stops the blood clotting and reduces the likelihood of further blood clots hitting the lung. Unfortunately it does not dissolve clots which are already formed. After several days of such treatment the patient is gradually changed over to oral anticoagulant therapy (e.g. warfarin). Anticoagulant treatment is usually continued for 6–12 months depending upon the severity of the pulmonary embolism.

ASTHMA

Asthma is a condition in which a variable degree of breathlessness is caused by narrowing of the airways, this narrowing is reversible either with or without treatment.

There are three possible mechanisms:
1. Contraction of the muscular wall of the airway.
2. Swelling of the lining of the airway.
3. Sputum blocking the airway.

Typical precipitating factors are exercise, chest infections, emotion and drugs (aspirin and drugs which cause beta-adrenergic blockade). (see Vol. 1, Chapters 8 and 28).

During the attack the patient may experience severe breathlessness with and accompanying tightness of the chest, and audible wheezing. Attacks may be of very variable severity and duration, some resolving spontaneously.

Status asthmaticus is a life-threatening form of asthma, when continued symptoms are unassisted by treatment. In this condition plugging of the smaller airways is a major problem.

The mainstay of treatment are drugs which reverse the constriction of the airways. Beta-adrenergic stimulating drugs relax smooth muscle and bring about relief, salbutamol being the most widely used. Aminophylline has a similar relaxing activity and is commonly used in the acute situation (*see* Vol. 1, Chapter 43).

Further treatment consists of oxygen by face mask, treatment of possible infection and reassurance as this can be a particularly frightening episode. In the worst cases artificial ventilation may be required.

For long-term treatment use of drugs such as disodium cromoglycate which prevent release of the agents responsible for the airway narrowing are very effective. As a last resort, steroids may be necessary for the more protracted attacks. Steroids work by decreasing the swelling of the lining of the airways. Finally, avoidance of, or desensitization to, a specific allergic stimulus can be attempted if one is found. However, more commonly, several such stimuli are present and this therapy, therefore, is impractical.

SPONTANEOUS PNEUMOTHORAX

This is a collection of air occurring between the lung and the chest wall, thereby restricting expansion of that lung. This type of pneumothorax is unrelated to injury.

The condition usually occurs in tall, thin, fit young adult males for no apparent reason and rarely with any past history of previous lung disease. However, once it has occurred there is a marked tendency to recurrence.

There is usually a sudden onset of sharp stabbing pain at the site of rupture made worse by breathing and accompanied by breathlessness. The pain disappears after a few hours, the degree and duration of breathlessness depending on the size of the pneumothorax. A chest X-ray confirms the diagnosis in case of doubt.

In rare instances air will continue to escape, the lung is increasingly compressed, and eventually the other lung is also affected. This is called a tension pneumothorax, and constitutes a medical emergency (*see* Chapter 8).

If left alone 70 per cent of cases reinflate on their own. These are the smaller pneumothoraces, constituting less than a quarter of the lung area on the affected side.

ADULT RESPIRATORY DISTRESS SYNDROME (ARDS)

This is a condition with many possible causes, often complicating trauma or other major illness. The syndrome has attracted attention recently because of its very high mortality rate. This increases dramatically when other organ involvement is present.

The immediate cause is a leak of haemorrhagic and proteinaceous fluid into the air spaces of the lung. The syndrome occurs in a variety of conditions including infections, thrombosis, major trauma, aspiration into the lungs of vomit or seawater, shock states and immunological diseases. In many (50 per cent) evidence of major or small vessel thrombosis in the lungs occurs and in all, abnormalities of blood coagulation are likely to lead to thrombosis and release of agents which damage the alveoli.

There are four major symptoms which characterize this condition: progressive respiratory distress, increased stiffness of the lungs and hence increased work of breathing, acute lowering of the oxygen tension in the blood (despite breathing oxygen) and diffuse shadowing of both lungs on the X-ray.

Treatment is aimed at maintaining the oxygen tension in the blood, by keeping the airways open using a ventilator. Those with extensive X-ray changes requiring ventilation for prolonged periods with high levels of oxygenation are a particularly poor risk group, having a high mortality rate. Moderate degrees of ARDS produce widespread though not complete changes on the X-ray but still require ventilation. In a mildly affected group there are only faint X-ray changes and the patients fare much better. They require only oxygen by face mask and usually do not need to be ventilated. There are only faint X-ray changes.

Further reading

Harvey A. McG., Johns R. J., McKusick V. A. et al. (1984) *The Principles and Practice of Medicine*, 21st ed. New York, Appleton-Century-Crofts.

Houston J. C., Joiner C. L. and Trounce J. R. (1982) *A Short Textbook of Medicine*, 7th ed. London, Hodder & Stoughton.

Chapter 10

The Cardiovascular System. I. Trauma

G. K. Davies

TRAUMATIC HAEMORRHAGE

Bleeding following road traffic accidents and other forms of trauma is still a frequent cause of death. Haemorrhage can arise from three sources:

Arterial
Pulsating
Bright red in colour
Large volumes
Often the most serious type of bleeding

Venous
Flows rather than spurts
Darker red
It, too, can be serious, especially if a major vein is involved

Capillary
Slow ooze
Rarely serious unless the patient has a clotting defect

Bleeding can be internal or external. In the former case large volumes of blood may be lost within the body cavities and tissues. Whatever and wherever the cause of bleeding, the blood loss may range from trivial to severe or fatal. When blood loss becomes significant then the patient will become *shocked* (*see* Chapter 19).

In untreated haemorrhagic 'shock' the body brings into play several compensatory mechanisms.

10 per cent Blood Loss: Receptors in the low-pressure venous system

THE CARDIOVASCULAR SYSTEM. I. TRAUMA

Table **10.1.** Blood loss

	10–20%	25–30%	50%
Central Nervous System	Normal	Restless, confused complaining of thirst	Impaired consciousness coma
Respiratory System			
a. Respiratory distress	Normal	Rapid and shallow	Severe respiratory distress
b. Blood gases	Normal	*Pao_2 ↓ † $Paco_2$ ↓	Pao_2 ↓↓ $Paco_2$ ↓ or ↑
Cardiovascular System			
a. Blood pressure ↓	often only in upright position	↓ Mild ↑ ↓	Not measurable ↑↑ ↓↓ ↓↓
b. Heart rate ↑			
c. Central venous pressure ?			
d. Peripheral blood flow	Slight	Skin cold and clammy	
Urinary System			
Urine output	Normal	↓	Absent

* Arterial partial pressure of oxygen.
† Arterial partial pressure of carbon dioxide.

cause an increase in sympathetic tone which reduces the size of the vascular bed and restores normal heart rate and blood pressure.

10–20 per cent Blood Loss: Pressure receptors on the arterial side bring about a release of catecholamines. This increases the heart rate. Blood pressure is maintained. Blood flow to the brain and heart is maintained in preference to other organs such as the skin, gut and kidneys.

30 per cent Blood Loss: Reflex mechanisms are maximal at this time. Kidney blood flow is reduced further and the urine output falls. There is a reflex increase in breathing because of hypoxia and metabolic acidosis.

50 per cent Blood Loss: Blood flow to the heart and brain is now impaired. Blood pressure falls and is often unrecordable.

CLINICAL SIGNS AND SYMPTOMS IN HAEMORRHAGIC SHOCK

The normal circulatory blood volume of an adult is said to be in the order of 65 ml/kg.

Patients with minimal blood loss will be conscious, alert, a good colour and with a normal heart rate and blood pressure. As blood loss increases then the signs and symptoms of shock will develop (*Table* 10.1).

TREATMENT OF HAEMORRHAGIC SHOCK
(*see also* Chapter 19)

When treating any injured patient one must establish an order of priorities which includes:
Establishment of an airway
Administration of oxygen and maintenance of respiration
Pain relief
Obtaining a history from patient, relative or passer-by
Assessment of other injuries
Establishing priorities of management when there are multiple injuries

Specifically when dealing with a haemorrhaging patient one must:
Control haemorrhage
Establish an intravenous line for blood and fluid replacement
Monitor the efficacy of treatment

Control of haemorrhage
There are three methods available:
Pressure
Elevation
Tourniquet

Pressure
Direct pressure over a bleeding site, preferably with a sterile dressing. If this is not available a clean article of clothing will be acceptable.

Arterial pressure points
Knowledge of arterial pressure points can be extremely useful when direct pressure is not possible or applicable.
 Useful pressure points are the brachial artery in the arm (felt at the crease of the elbow) and the femoral artery in the leg (felt over the groin). Clots should not be dislodged for fear of re-starting significant bleeding.

Elevation
Elevation will reduce the pressure in the vessels on the low-pressure venous side. One must use caution when there are associated injuries to that limb, e.g. a fracture.

Tourniquet
The use of a tourniquet is controversial and should only be considered if the bleeding cannot be controlled by any other means. A tourniquet can be extremely useful when applied properly.

The tourniquet must be:
1. A pneumatic type so as to apply uniform pressure.
2. Wide enough to exert even pressure, thereby reducing local tissue damage.
3. Always inflated above systolic blood pressure. Failure to do so will result in blood continuing to flow into the venous system thereby increasing venous pressure and leading to further venous blood loss.
4. Placed on the upper part of the extremity thereby exerting maximum pressure on a major artery. It should be applied in the upper limb between shoulder and elbow and in the lower limb between groin and knee.

Note the time of application (maximum 1 hour). Dangerous release of metabolites may occur on deflation with marked falls in blood pressure. This should be anticipated by pre-loading with intravenous fluids.

Fluid replacement

In response to trauma, oedema develops in the injured area. This oedema forms at the expense of intravascular volume, interstitial fluid and intracellular fluid (ICF).

Fluid replacement is given in the form of crystalloids, colloids and blood (*see* Chapter 4).

Afterwards the oedema is lost from the body via the kidney.

General guidelines of fluid replacement

1. Two large bore intravenous lines should be inserted in the arms, particularly when abdominal injuries are suspected so that the fluid replacement is not lost into the tissues from rupture of large abdominal veins.
2. Blood for cross-matching should be taken at the time of venous cannulation.
3. Suitable intravenous fluid replacement should be given whilst waiting for blood to be cross-matched.
4. Vital signs should be evaluated.

Usually if the patient has responded to a fluid infusion of 2 litres then blood loss is not critical. However, if the patient remains hypotensive then blood loss is continuing and whole blood can be used.

There is controversy regarding the use of crystalloids alone for resuscitation of trauma patients. The criticisms include:
1. Weight gain after resuscitation
2. Dilution of plasma proteins which may decrease osmotic pressure and may lead to pulmonary oedema
3. Reduction of clotting factors and platelets

However, there are distinct advantages to the use of crystalloids for field work:
1. Easily stored
2. Do not cause reactions
3. Inexpensive

Colloids in common use
Whole blood
Packed cells
Plasma protein fractions
Vegetable colloids (Dextran and Haemaccel)

A wider discussion regarding the relative merits of the various intravenous fluids is dealt with in Chapter 4.

INJURIES TO HEART AND GREAT VESSELS
Injuries to the heart
These can be classified into: Blunt trauma; Penetrating trauma.

Blunt trauma
This occurs in accidents involving a sharp blow to the chest, e.g. steering wheel injuries. The resulting injury can be cardiac contusion and/or rupture of the heart valves.

The signs and symptoms of *cardiac contusion* vary and may even be absent, depending upon the severity of injury. The following should alert one to the possible diagnosis:
1. History of blunt trauma to the chest
2. Pain in the chest mimicking that of myocardial infarction
3. Tachycardia or other dysrhythmias
4. ECG evidence of myocardial damage
   Q waves in Leads I, II and III
5. Raised cardiac enzymes

The treatment is symptomatic and should include:
1. Bed rest
2. Continuous cardiac monitoring
3. Treatment of dysrhythmias
4. Serial ECG tracings

Major surgery should be avoided if at all possible.

Valvular damage is an extremely rare injury, but rupture of the aortic and mitral valves has been reported. Signs and symptoms will include:
1. Shortness of breath
2. Dysrhythmias
3. Chest pain
4. Heart murmurs

The treatment of this condition is emergency open heart surgery to replace the damaged valve.

Penetrating injuries to the heart

Many of these injuries are immediately fatal, particularly wounds of the left ventricle where the entry wound is sufficiently large to cause the patient to exsanguinate in a matter of seconds. There may also be penetration of more than one chamber of the heart, laceration of the coronary vessels or laceration of the pericardium. The bleeding that follows can exit:
1. Into the chest cavity to produce a haemothorax
2. Into the pericardial sac
3. Directly out of the wound site

Not all penetrating injuries to the heart are fatal and many lives can be saved by prompt attention and transportation to hospital.

The management of such patients includes:
1. Treatment of haemorrhagic shock
2. Assessment of other injuries
3. Appropriate investigations
4. Treatment of cardiac tamponade
5. Exploratory surgery

The assessment and treatment of haemorrhagic shock should be carried out as described earlier in the chapter. If there is a wounding instrument, do not remove if for it may by its presence be minimizing blood loss. Removal should only take place under direct vision at surgery. On arrival at hospital the surgical team should be mobilized and made available even whilst the decision regarding surgery is being made in order that valuable time is not lost.

There are associated injuries which should always be looked for following this type of trauma. They are:
1. Sucking wound of the chest
2. Tension pneumothorax
3. Haemopneumothorax
   These can cause further severe cardiorespiratory embarrassment. Their management is discussed in Chapter 8.

The appropriate investigations should include:
1. Chest X-rays for evidence of pneumothorax, haemothorax
2. ECG for myocardial damage
3. Blood gas analysis
4. Grouping and cross-matching of blood

Cardiac tamponade is caused by fluid, in this case blood, entering the pericardial sac. This produces compression of the heart, thereby reducing its filling capacity during diastole. This means that there is less blood ejected with each beat and the cardiac output falls. Cardiac tamponade can be diagnosed by:

1. Tachycardia
2. Lowered blood pressure
3. A raised jugular venous pressure
4. Paradoxical pulse (weaker on inspiration)

One must have a high index of suspicion for this condition. Exploratory surgery through a left anterolateral thoracotomy is indicated for evacuation of the pericardial sac.

Other situations which warrant surgery are:
1. Continued bleeding through the wound
2. A large sucking chest wound
3. A large haemopneumothorax

Trauma to the great vessels

There are two categories of injury:
1. Penetrating aortic wounds
2. Traumatic aortic rupture

Penetrating aortic wounds follow stabbings, gunshot wounds, fractured ribs and any other projectile wound in that area of the body. There is a massive and rapid blood loss often resulting in early death. Those patients who survive long enough to reach hospital will have X-ray evidence of a left haemothorax and a widened mediastinum. Treatment consists of resuscitation and urgent surgery through a left thoracotomy to repair the damaged blood vessel.

Traumatic rupture of the aorta follows acute deceleration accidents such as motor vehicle accidents or a heavy fall. The tear usually occurs at a point just beyond the origin of the subclavian artery. The tear may be complete or partial. If complete, the blood loss is massive, and the outcome often fatal. However, if the outer layer of the aorta (adventitia) remains intact then an aneurysm (sac) may develop and the patient can survive for a long time. There are often other injuries associated with this lesion including limb and spinal fractures and other chest trauma.

Initially the clinical symptoms may be minimal, however, as the aneurysmal sac develops the patient may complain of:
1. Severe back pain
2. Shortness of breath
3. Difficulty in swallowing
4. Paralysis of legs (because the blood supply to the spinal cord is compromised)

The aneurysm may rupture at any time producing:
1. Increase of back pain
2. Shortness of breath
3. Haemorrhagic shock

Radiological evidence of a widened mediastinum and special X-rays to outline the aorta will confirm the diagnosis.

The treatment of this condition is to resect and replace the damaged aorta with a graft. This operation carries a high mortality.

Chapter 11

The Cardiovascular System. II. Non-trauma

G. K. Davies

ANEURYSMS

An aneurysm is a local dilatation in an artery. The aneurysmal sac begins at a point of weakness where degenerative changes have occurred in the medial layer of the vessel wall.

Aortic aneurysms

Aortic aneurysms are described as saccular, fusiform or dissecting and are illustrated in *Fig.* 11.1.

Thoracic aneurysms

The causes of thoracic aneurysms include hypertension, syphilis and rare congenital disorders.

Many saccular and fusiform aneurysms remain asymptomatic. However, they may rupture and haemorrhage with fatal consequences. Dissecting aneurysms may also rupture with fatal results. In the early stages the spread of the dissection may be limited by the use of hypotensive drugs. These decrease the intraluminal pressure which is causing the tear. Excision and re-anastomosis can be performed but carries a high mortality.

Abdominal aneurysms

Abdominal aneurysms are usually secondary to atherosclerosis. They commonly occur in males over 50. Like thoracic aneurysms they enlarge over time and may dissect and/or rupture at any time.

Classically the patient with a leaking abdominal aortic aneurysm presents with sudden onset of severe abdominal and back pain. On examination he may be shocked because of blood loss and resuscitation

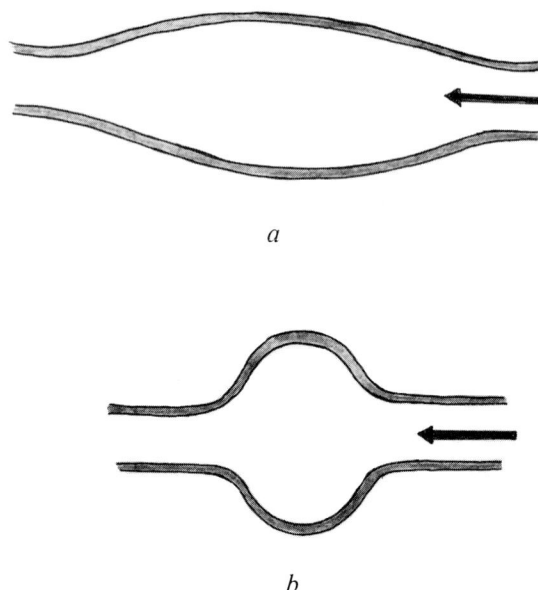

Fig. 11.1. Aneurysms. *a*, Fusiform type. *b*, Saccular type.

may be necessary before a diagnosis is established. Careful examination of the abdomen will demonstrate a pulsatile mass to the left of the midline. It is often tender. Pulses below the level of the aneurysm may or may not be present. Plain abdominal X-ray may show a rim of calcification around the aneurysm.

Full resuscitation procedures and preparation for emergency surgery should begin immediately once the diagnosis is made.

Surgery is required to control haemorrhage and replace the damaged aorta with a graft. This can be an extremely bloody operation with patients having their circulatory volume replaced once or even twice. Mortality varies from 30 to 60 per cent. The use of a 'G-suit' to reduce 'shock' may be feasible (*see* Chapter 19).

ARTERIAL HYPERTENSION

The generally accepted upper limit of normal blood pressure is 140/90 mmHg. There is an increase with age. Transient rises may occur during times of emotional stress, exercise and cold. The systolic pressure is a function of the work of the left ventricle. The diastolic pressure reflects the resistance of the arteriolar vessels.

When the blood pressure is above the expected normal this is called hypertension. Usually systolic and diastolic pressures are both raised.

Hypertension can be classified into *primary* or *secondary*.

Primary or essential hypertension is the commonest. The exact cause is not known but there is correlation with certain factors, including diet, smoking, emotional stress and heredity.

Secondary hypertension is a raised blood pressure secondary to another cause and includes:

Renal hypertension
Endocrine
    Cushing's disease
    Conn's syndrome
    Phaeochromocytoma
    Diabetes
Vascular
    Coarctation of aorta
Pregnancy
    Eclampsia and pre-eclampsia

The treatment of secondary hypertension is the treatment of the precipitating factor.

Primary hypertension may remain asymptomatic for many years. However, when symptoms do occur they are as a result of the disease process affecting major organs.

Atherosclerosis results in thickening and laying down of plaques on the vessel walls which may ulcerate or calcify, and then form the sites of arterial thrombosis. These thromboses may result in occlusion at those sites causing infarction of tissue. A piece may dislodge and travel to distant sites with the same result. Common sites are the coronary, cerebral, mesenteric to the intestines and peripheral arteries to the limbs.

With increasing strain put on the heart plus an increasingly less efficient blood supply to that organ the patient will exhibit signs and symptoms of cardiac failure.

Cerebral thrombosis or haemorrhage may manifest itself as a cerebrovascular accident.

Progressive cerebral deterioration may occur leading to general deterioration of the intellect. The eyes and kidneys likewise undergo progressive deterioration.

The treatment of primary hypertension includes:

Diet and smoking restrictions
Avoidance of stress factors

Table 11.1 **Common oral antihypertensive drugs**

Mode of action	Example
Diuretics	Frusemide
	Spironolactone
Arteriolar dilators	Hydralazine
Central sympathetic action	Methyldopa
	Clonidine
β-Blockers	Propanolol

Drug therapy (see Table 11.1).
Severe hypertension may occur because of developing malignant hypertension or because of acute withdrawal of antihypertensive therapy. Malignant hypertension usually presents with acute organ failure as a result of acceleration of the disease process. Common presenting signs and symptoms include:
Headache
Nausea and vomiting
Visual disturbances and mental confusion
Shortness of breath
Chest pain
Abdominal pain
On examination the blood pressure will often rise above 220 mmHg systolic and 120 mmHg diastolic.

Whatever the cause of the severe hypertension treatment includes immediate hypotensive drug therapy. Initially this should be given parenterally and then maintained by the oral route.

Commonly used intravenous vasodilators for control of hypertension are listed in Table 11.2.

MYOCARDIAL INFARCTION

Ischaemic heart disease is the commonest single cause of death in the U.K. Many causative factors have been implicated including hypertension, obesity, smoking, stress, diabetes and other endocrine disorders.

The disease causes narrowing of the coronary arteries, limiting the blood supply and hence the oxygen supply to the heart muscle. If the heart has to work harder, thus requiring more oxygen, the blood supply may be insufficient and the heart muscle becomes hypoxic. The results are angina, arrhythmias and acute heart failure.

Table 11.2 Vasodilators

Site and mechanism of action	Drugs
Autonomic ganglia with sympathetic blockade	Trimetaphan Pentolinium
By blocking alpha-adrenergic receptors at vascular smooth muscle	Phentolamine
By relaxing vascular smooth muscle	Sodium nitroprusside Hydralazine Nitrates
Combination of alpha-and beta-receptor blockade	Labetolol

The heart works harder when there is an increase in:
1. Heart rate (as in the response to exercise, anxiety, pain or some drugs.
2. Blood pressure (as in anxiety, pain, renal failure, hypertension).
3. Preload (blood returning to the heart, e.g. transfusion of fluids or blood).
4. Contractility (pumping action of the heart, e.g. anxiety, cardiac stimulant drugs such as digoxin, adrenaline etc.).

In severe ischaemic heart disease the natural progress is for one or more of the coronary arteries to become totally blocked leading to death of heart muscle. This is called myocardial infarction.

Clinical features of myocardial infarction
1. Persistent crushing pain in the chest often radiating to left arm and into neck and jaw
2. Nausea and vomiting
3. Fatigue
4. Palpitations

The diagnosis is confirmed by:
1. Electrocardiographic evidence of damaged heart muscle (*Fig.* 11.2)
2. Raised cardiac enzymes

The complications of myocardial infarction can be immediate or late.

Immediate
1. Death
2. Acute heart failure

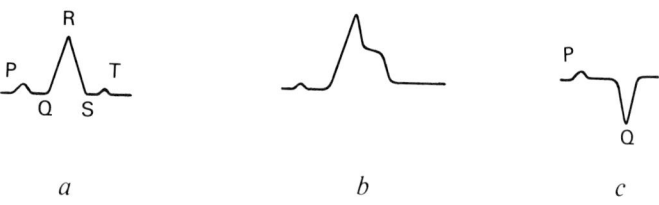

Fig. 11.2. a, Normal ECG. b, S–T elevation, i.e. cardiac injury. c, Persistent Q wave, i.e. infarction.

3. Dysrhythmias
4. Rupture of heart
5. Low output syndrome (cardiogenic shock)

Late
1. Re-infarction
2. Deep vein thrombosis
3. Cerebrovascular accidents
4. Aneurysms of heart
5. Ventricular septal defects
6. Post-infarction syndrome—a hypersensitivity reaction to the damaged myocardium.

The complications that demand immediate attention are:
1. Pain
2. Dysrhythmias
3. Heart failure
4. Cardiogenic shock

More than 50 per cent of all 'heart attack' victims die within the first 2 hours, many because of dysrhythmias. Therefore, prompt and efficient treatment is necessary.

In recognition of this fact there has been an increase in the number of Mobile Coronary Care Units (MCCU). For a MCCU to be effective there should be a two-way voice communication between the emergency attendants and medical personnel back at the hospital.

The purpose of the MCCU is to stabilize the patient's condition and provide continuity of care until arrival at the hospital. The usual format should be followed:
1. An airway should be established
2. 100 per cent oxygen administered
3. An intravenous line inserted
4. Relief of pain
5. ECG monitored
6. Treatment of dysrhythmias

THE CARDIOVASCULAR SYSTEM. II. NON-TRAUMA

Treatment of complications

Pain
The pain is secondary to the ischaemia of heart muscle. The analgesics of choice are morphine or diamorphine because:
1. They are powerful analgesics
2. They may be good anxiolytics
3. They produce venodilatation, thus reducing venous return to the heart and allaying the tendency to left ventricular failure and pulmonary oedema

Dysrhythmias
These not only occur after a myocardial infarction but can also associate with:
1. Acid–base imbalance
2. Disturbance of conducting tissue
3. Drug intoxication, e.g. digitalis

Normal sinus rhythm (Trace 1)

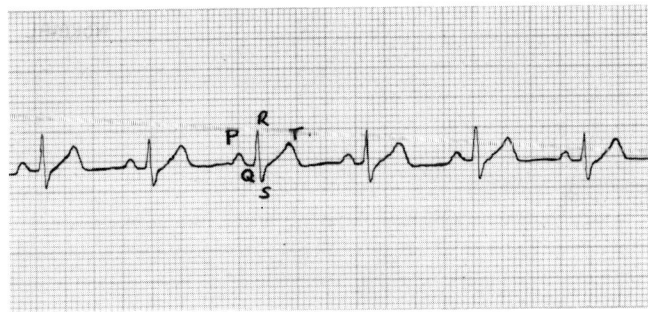

Trace 1

P = Atrial contraction
P–R interval = Time of conduction from sino-atrial node to ventricular muscle (normal 0·12–0·2 sec)
QRS = Ventricular contraction
T = Ventricular repolarization
When interpreting an ECG it is important to ascertain certain facts. Is there normal sinus rhythm? Can one see P waves? To calculate the rate approximately, the number of large squares on the paper (5 mm) between each R wave can be divided into three hundred. In *Trace* 1 the heart rate is approximately 75 beats/min.

Are the atria and ventricles contracting at the same rate? (if prolonged this is indicative of a heart block).
If the rhythm is irregular is there a discernible pattern? Dysrhythmias can be classified into:
1. Tachycardias (faster than normal rate)
2. Bradycardias (slower than normal rate)
3. Irregular

Sinus tachycardia (Trace 2)

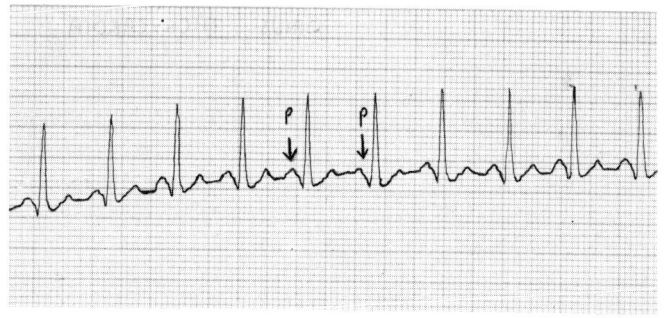

Trace 2

The heart rate is 110–140 beats/min, the PQRST configuration being normal.

This dysrhythmia may be associated with exercise. Some of the common pathological causes are stress, heavy alcohol or tobacco intake, heart failure or thyrotoxicosis.

Treatment
Remedy the underlying cause.

Paroxysmal supraventricular tachycardia (Trace 3)

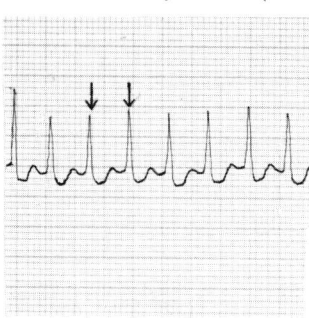

Trace 3

The heart rate is 140–200 beats/min and the QRS configuration is normal, but the P wave may or may not be seen, indicating that the pacemaker is not ventricular but arises above the ventricles either at the AV junction or in the atria.

This often comes on without any warning. It is not immediately fatal but can cause myocardial damage due to increased demand for oxygen.

Treatment

Carotid sinus massage (this produces vagal stimulation and a reduction in rate)

DC shock

β-Blockers

Verapamil

Sinus Bradycardia (Trace 4)

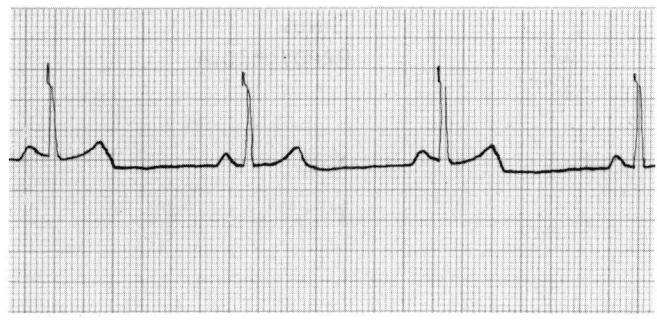

Trace 4

Note the regularity of evidence of p waves with a rate of 40–50/min.

The heart rate is 60 beats/min or below, the PQRST configuration is normal implying that the SA node is the pacemaker.

This dysrhythmia may be physiological, and seen in the resting state, e.g. an athlete, or it may be pathological due to ischaemia, increased vagal tone, drugs (e.g. β-blocker), and in certain disease states such as myxoedema.

Treatment

The underlying cause must be treated if possible. Atropine is the drug of choice in this condition.

Heart block

There are three types of heart block. All of them are pathological.
1. *First degree (1°) heart block.* The heart rate may be normal but the P–R interval is larger than normal (0·20 sec).
2. *Second degree (2°) heart block.* 2° heart block is divided into two types:

a. *Wenckebach Phenomenon* (Type I) (*see Trace* 5)
Characterized by an increasingly lengthening P–R interval which terminates in a non-conducted P wave in a repetitive pattern.
b. *Mobits* (Type II)
The P–R interval is constant and it may or may not be prolonged. However, there are two or more P waves to each QRS. The P–P interval is constant as is the R–R interval.
3. *Third degree* (*3°*) *heart block.* (*see Trace* 6). Also known as complete heart block. The AV node does not transmit impulses from the atria to the ventricles. The SA node is firing at its own rate of 70–90 beats/min and the His–Purkinje (conducting) system (because it has inherent automaticity) is firing at a rate of 15–40 beats/min. This results in a totally disconnected PQRST. The P–R interval is inconstant, and there may be any number of P waves seen between each QRS.

Causes of the heart blocks are myocardial infarction or ischaemia, electrolyte disturbances, certain drugs and cardiomyopathy.
The treatment for heart blocks is:
1. Atropine.
2. Isoprenaline
3. Cardiac pacing.

Wenckebach phenomenon (Trace 5)

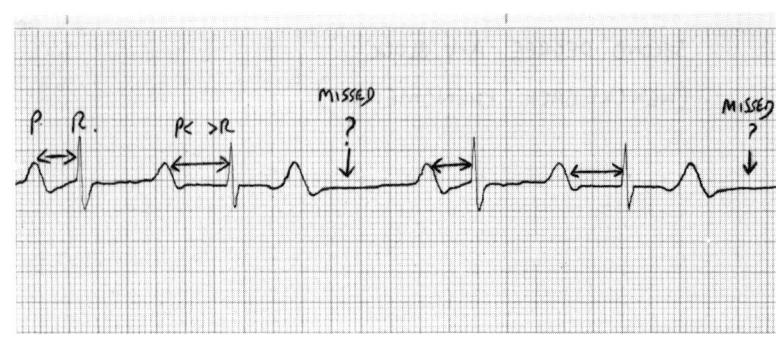

Trace 5

Note the P–R interval increases for two beats and then a 'dropped beat' occurs.

Complete heart block (Trace 6)

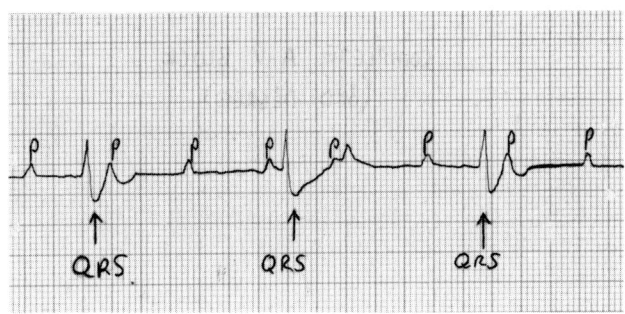

Trace 6

Note that the P waves are regular (approximately 100/min) and the QRS complexes are regular at approximately 70/min. This means that the atria and ventricles are beating completely independently of one another.

Treatment
  Atropine
  Isoprenaline
  Cardiac pacing

Premature atrial ectopic beats
These may be seen in normal hearts. There is a normal PQRST configuration which is premature and out of step with sinus rhythm.

Atrial fibrillation
This condition is always pathological. The atria are not beating rhythmically but are quivering at a rate of 400–600 times/min due to many *ectopic foci* in the atria superseding the SA node. As a result there are no P waves but a fine fibrillatory line is seen. The AV node is refractory to most of the impulses, but allows some to pass through and depolarize the ventricles, resulting in an *irregular ventricular response*. The pulse is characteristic and is described as 'irregularly irregular' (both in time and volume). The causes are many, but they include ischaemia, digitalis toxicity, mitral valve disease, cardiomyopathy, pulmonary embolism and thyrotoxicosis.

Atrial fibrillation with slow ventricular rate (Trace 7)

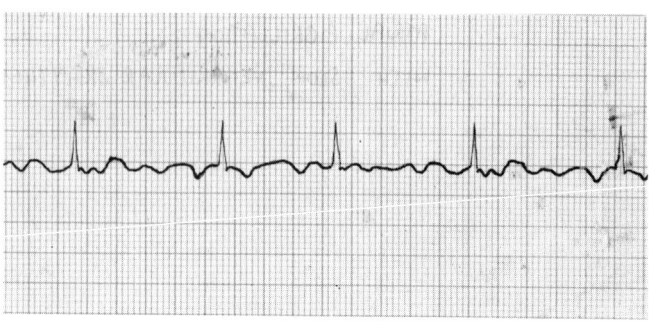

Trace 7

Treatment
1. Digitalis to decrease the ventricular rate if greater than 100 beats/min.
2. Synchronous DC shock in an emergency or in resistant cases where the circulation is compromised.

Atrial flutter (Trace 8)

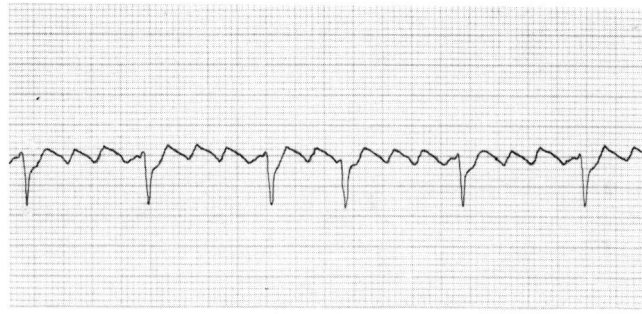

Trace 8

This dysrhythmia is always pathological. The atrial rate is 200–400 and a typical 'saw tooth' atrial pattern is seen. As the atrial rate is slower than in atrial fibrillation, the ventricular response is more orderly. The AV node may be refractory to every second, third or fourth stimulus, therefore giving atrial flutter with 2 : 1, 3 : 1, 4 : 1 etc. block. On the other hand, the response may be more haphazard giving atrial flutter with varying degrees of block. The causes of atrial flutter are the same as those of atrial fibrillation.

Treatment
1. Synchronous DC shock if the rate is fast.
2. Digitalis.

Ventricular ectopic beats

Ventricular ectopics are complexes occurring due to an irritable or ectopic focus in the ventricles of the heart which discharges prematurely, i.e. before the SA node.

The complex is always premature (*see Trace* 9) and is not preceded by a P wave. The QRS is of a bizarre configuration and its duration is longer than usual (over 0·10 sec) due to the abnormal route of ventricular depolarization. It is also followed by a full *compensatory pause*. (This is due to the SA node firing regularly and taking over again after the ventricular ectopic, and may be seen by measuring the R–R intervals of the complexes preceding and following the ectopic in comparison to three R waves of normal sinus rhythm.)

Some types of ventricular ectopics have more serious implication than others, in that they may predispose to more serious dysrhythmias. When ventricular ectopics are paired, the second ectopic may meet with refractory tissue and cause ventricular fibrillation.

In the *R on T phenomenon*, the ectopic falls upon the T wave (during the relative refractory period of repolarization) and may again cause ventricular fibrillation.

Multifocal ventricular ectopics (*see trace* 10) show that there is more than one ectopic focus in the ventricle and may be recognized by ectopics of a different shape and size.

The causes of ventricular ectopics are varied but include stress, hypoxia, myocardial infarction or ischaemia and metabolic disturbances.

Unifocal ventricular ectopic beats (Trace 9)

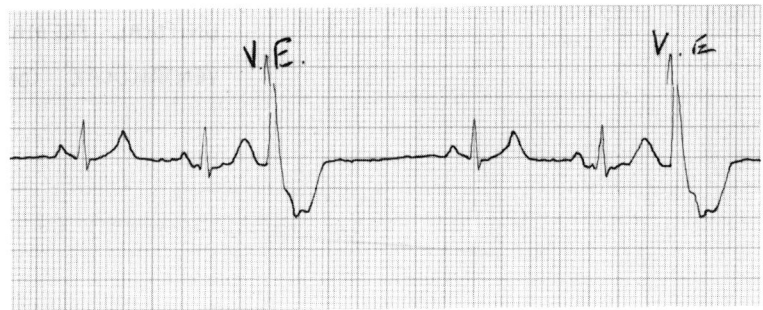

Trace 9

These denote an irritable focus. They require treatment if: there are more than 6/min, they are multifocal, or there is an R on T phenomenon present, i.e. the R wave is very close to the T wave of the last beat. Ventricular fibrillation may be precipitated.

Treatment
 Lignocaine
 If they persist check the serum potassium level

Multifocal ventricular ectopics (Trace 10)

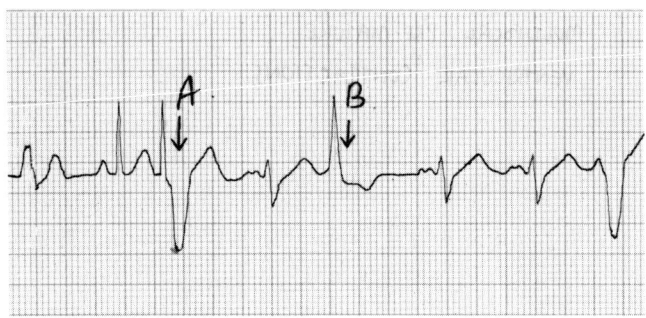

Trace 10

Ventricular tachycardia (Trace 11)

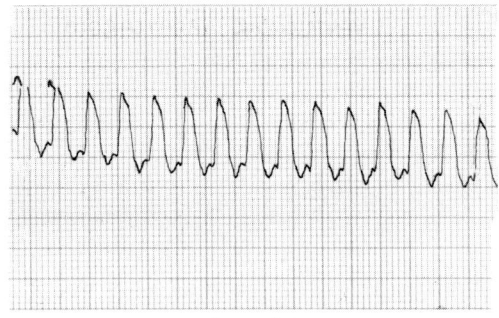

Trace 11

This usually occurs as a result of an ectopic focus taking over as the cardiac pacemaker. The heart rate is rapid, there are sometimes disconnected P waves scattered with the complexes and the complexes are broad and bizarre.

The causes, with the exception of stress, are the same as those of ventricular ectopic beats.

Like ventricular fibrillation, ventricular tachycardia can lead to death due to inefficient pumping of the heart.

Treatment
 DC shock
 Lignocaine

Ventricular fibrillation (Trace 12)

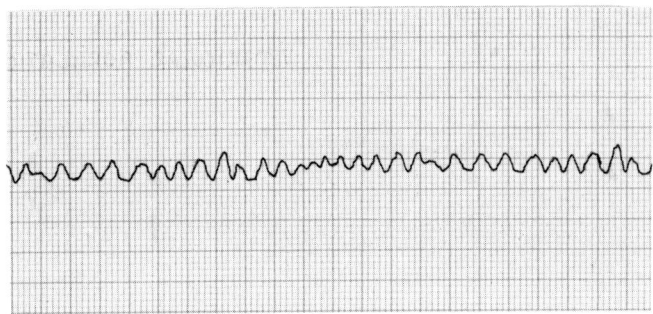

Trace 12

Ventricular fibrillation represents chaotic electrical activity. Myocardial cells are depolarizing but not in a unified fashion; the heart muscle is quivering. It is seen on the ECG as a fibrillatory line. It may be a coarse line indicating more activity than that which is seen as fine fibrillation. Coarse fibrillation is more amenable to treatment than fine. Ventricular fibrillation is fatal unless urgent treatment is instituted.

Treatment
  DC shock
  Effectiveness of shock can be increased by adrenaline or calcium.
  Sodium bicarbonate can be used to correct metabolic acidosis.

Ventricular standstill (Trace 13)

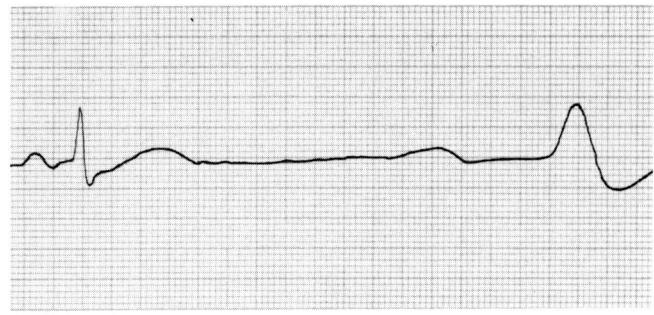

Trace 13

It is important to note the widening of the complexes and the slow rate.

Treatment
The rate may be improved by drugs such as atropine or isoprenaline.
The contractility may be improved with calcium.
However, the most effective treatment is cardiac pacing.

Ventricular standstill leading to asystole (Trace 14)

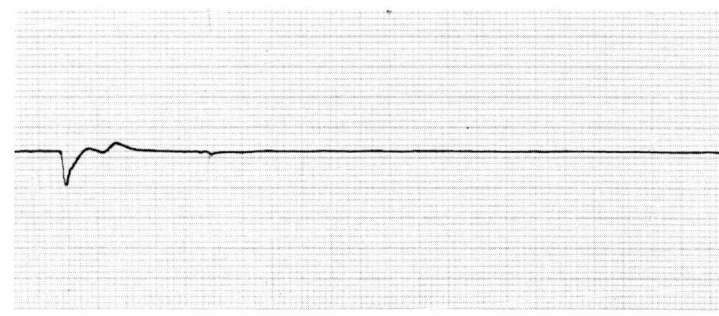

Trace 14

Treatment
Initially cardiopulmonary resuscitation (*see* Chapter 7) will be necessary and then cardiac pacing.

Ventricular bigeminy (Trace 15)

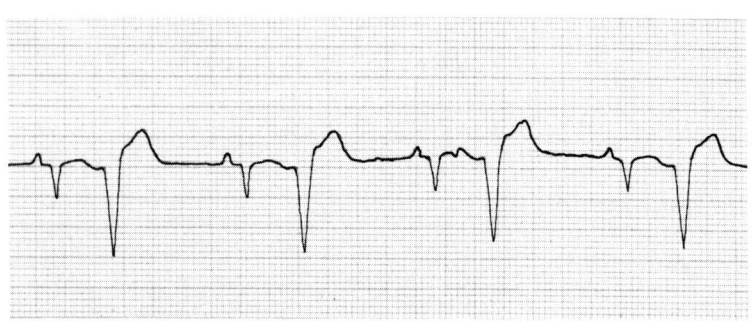

Trace 15

Causes include digitalis overdose, hypertension, hypercarbia (carbon dioxide retention).
Treatment
The underlying cause has to be identified and treated.

Rhythm strip of patient being paced (Trace 16)

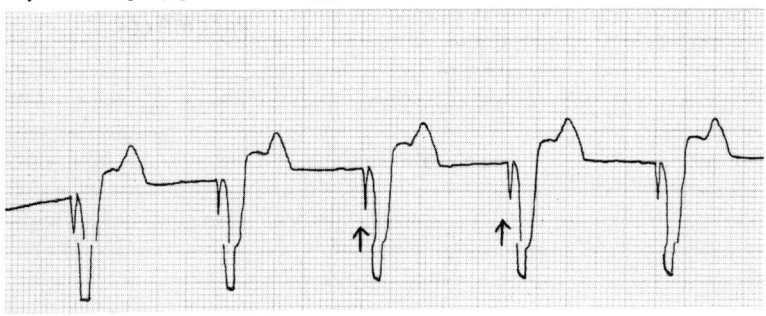

Trace 16

Note pacing 'blip'.

Muscle trembling (Trace 17)

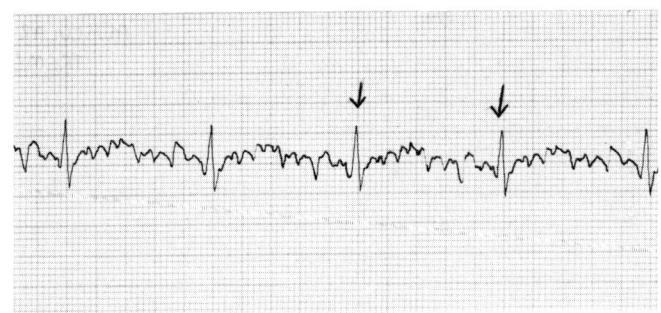

Trace 17

This shows gross irregularity, but note that the QRS complexes are regular. This is caused by a cold patient who is shivering.

Cardiac failure

This is the inability of the heart to pump sufficient blood around the body tissues. Right or left heart failure may occur in isolation or together. Right heart failure, often secondary to lung disease, is dealt with in Chapter 9. The causes of left heart failure include: myocardial ischaemia, hypertension and valvular disease.

The onset of heart failure may be insidious or acute. Starling's law states that the volume of blood ejected is proportional to the amount the muscle fibres are stretched at the end of diastole. In chronic conditions the heart can compensate by increasing its muscle bulk (hypertrophy). However, in acute conditions, e.g. fast dysrhythmias or myocardial infarction, it is unable to do so. That is, the heart muscle has gone over the top of Starling's curve and the ejection fraction and stroke volume decline as the cardiac muscle fibres are stretched.

Clinical signs and symptoms of left heart failure (LVF; left ventricular failure)

1. Dyspnoea (shortness of breath) — At first only on effort. Later at rest, made worse by lying down. Due to fluid accumulating in the lung.
2. Pulmonary oedema — Increasing fluid accumulation. Respiratory distress and wheeze. Frothy pink sputum production.
3. X-ray — Characteristic signs of cardiac enlargement and pulmonary oedema.

Treatment
1. Treatment of the underlying cause
2. Oxygen therapy
3. Rest
4. Morphine or diamorphine (alleviation of LVF by venodilatation)
5. Diuretics

Further reading

Evans R. (1981) *Emergency Medicine.* London, Butterworth.
The Merck Manual (1982) 14th ed. Merck, Sharpe & Dohme.

Chapter 12

The Abdomen

R. A. Warren

INTRODUCTION

The purpose of this chapter is twofold: first, to give a general account of those abdominal conditions arising spontaneously and as a result of injury; second, to try to help those paramedical personnel who, in special circumstances, may have to deal with an abdominal emergency. This second aspect will concentrate on deciding which acute abdominal problems require urgent medical assistance, and those which are less urgent. It is interesting to consider that of every 10 patients presenting to a hospital with abdominal pain, 9 will not require surgery.

GENERAL CONSIDERATIONS

Anatomy

The terminology can be somewhat confusing; the terms abdomen, peritoneal cavity, or abdomen and pelvis are not strictly interchangeable. By convention, the abdomen consists of all those organs contained within the peritoneal cavity (the alimentary system) and those organs lying behind the peritoneal cavity adjacent to the lumbar spine and muscles of the back (the kidneys, ureters, aorta and vena cava). The term pelvis in this context refers to the pelvic contents, e.g. bladder and rectum, and not to the bony pelvis, which is dealt with in Chapter 13. By convention again, the male genitalia are regarded as part of the abdomen and will be mentioned in this chapter. In the female the uterus, Fallopian tubes and ovaries are also contained within the pelvis and may be the source of abdominal pain.

No detailed anatomy will be described here. However, it is helpful to study *Fig.* 12.1 as it gives some idea of the position of the organs which will be referred to and, by implication, the site at which pain from an individual organ might be felt (*see below*—'Abdominal Examination').

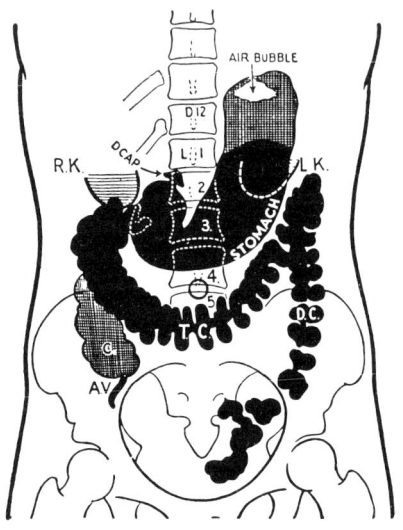

Fig. 12.1. Abdominal viscera. The position of the stomach, first part of the duodenum, large intestine and kidneys is outlined in relation to the bony landmarks. These positions are variable. RK, Right kidney; LK, Left kidney; DCAP, Duodenal cap; TC, Transverse colon; DC, Descending colon; AV, Appendix vermiformis.

Pain

The usual presenting symptom with an abdominal problem is pain. Two types of pain are usually described, colic and peritoneal. This division is useful, as the nature of the pain gives some idea as to the likely cause and urgency of treatment.

Colicky pain is caused by spasm in a muscular tube such as the intestine or ureter. This occurs most often if it is obstructed — as an attempt to try to clear the obstruction. A good example is biliary colic. This occurs because the muscle in the bile duct goes into spasm in an attempt to dislodge a gallstone which has become stuck in the duct. Colicky pain builds up slowly over several seconds or minutes, rises to a peak, then dies down a little. Even though the pain is very unpleasant, the

THE ABDOMEN

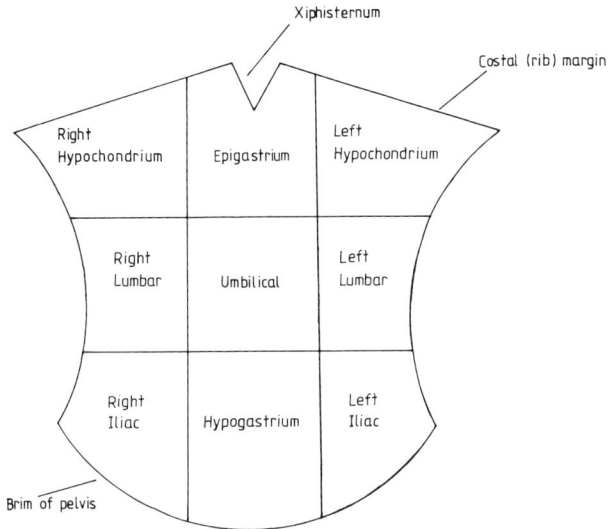

Fig. 12.2. The regions of the abdomen.

patient is unlikely to come to any great harm—in the short term at least.

The situation is very different with peritoneal pain. Such pain may be caused by blood, pus or bowel contents which escape and irritate the peritoneum lining the abdominal cavity. An infection can spread very rapidly through the peritoneal cavity, noxious substances such as bacteria and the poisons they produce can pass rapidly into the bloodstream with potentially fatal consequences. Peritoneal pain always requires much more urgent action than colicky pain. Usually, surgery is performed to find the cause of the peritonitis and remedy it.

The patient with peritoneal pain lies quite still, often with knees drawn up. Any movement worsens the peritoneal irritation thereby aggravating the pain. Even gentle pressure with a hand on the abdomen causes intense pain, the muscles of the abdominal wall being felt to go into spasm beneath the examining fingers; this is called 'guarding'.

Mention must be made of the phenomenon of referred pain. In fetal life some organs migrate from their original positions in the body and take their nerve supply with them. Because of this, when disease occurs in these organs, pain is felt not where the organ lies in the patient, but where the organ lay in fetal life. The best known example of referred pain occurs in appendicitis. The appendix lies in the right iliac fossa (*Fig.* 12.2), but in the early stages of inflammation of the appendix the pain is felt in the umbilical region where the appendix lay in fetal life.

Intestinal obstruction
This refers to obstruction of the alimentary tract anywhere along its length. As the tract is obstructed, four features occur:
1. Colicky pain due to spasm of the bowel muscle attempting to overcome the obstruction.
2. Abdominal distension due to a build up of gas and intestinal contents which cannot pass the obstruction.
3. Vomiting occurs when the build up of intestinal contents above the obstruction is so great that they have to be regurgitated.
4. Constipation is inevitable as nothing can pass through the obstructed bowel.

There are many causes of intestinal obstruction. Good examples are trapping of the bowel inside a hernia and blockage of the bowel by a tumour.

Obviously, the treatment of intestinal obstruction is to remove the cause, but there are general principles to be observed. Vomiting is a feature of almost all serious acute abdominal conditions. In obstruction of the small intestine it may be severe. The patient cannot take anything by mouth, and he is losing large quantities of fluid and electrolyte in the vomit. Replacement of these fluids and electrolytes via an intravenous infusion is the key to successful management. The patient can be made more comfortable by passing a fine plastic tube through the nose into the stomach (nasogastric tube). The stomach contents can be aspirated (and the volume measured) saving the patient the unpleasantness of vomiting.

In the severely shocked patient human plasma or an artificial substitute may be given. If much blood has been lost, it must be replaced (*see* Chapter 4).

Antibiotics have a critical role to play in peritonitis. If peritonitis is suspected suitable antibiotics should be given by the intravenous route.

Surgery often has an important role to play, and the various procedures will be mentioned briefly as the individual diseases are described.

Pain relief must be given a high priority. Morphine, pethidine, buprenorphine and similar drugs are effective if the pain is severe (*see* Chapter 5).

ASSESSMENT OF THE PATIENT WITH AN ACUTE ABDOMINAL CONDITION

Conventionally this is divided into history, examination and special tests.

THE ABDOMEN

History
If the patient has been injured, the site, nature and severity of the injury are of major importance. They should be established with as much accuracy as possible from the patient or witness. The site of injury will give a clue to those organs likely to have been damaged (*see Figs.* 12.1 and 12.2 and *Table* 12.1).

With abdominal pain in the absence of injury the type of pain (peritoneal or colicky) should also be established.

The presence of vomiting should be noted, together with its severity and the nature of the vomitus. Inquiry should also be made as to bowel habit, that is constipation or diarrhoea (*see* intestinal obstruction, gastroenteritis and Crohn's disease). Likewise, the patient should be asked about any problem with urination. Blood in the urine (haematuria), pain on passing urine (dysuria) and frequency of urination all imply disease in the urinary system. In women of childbearing age, inquiry should be made into the possibility of pregnancy and the presence of any vaginal discharge (*see* Chapter 18). Previous surgery or investigation for abdominal complaints should be noted.

Examination
General
The patient's general condition is important. Special attention should be paid to the heart rate, blood pressure and temperature. The presence of shock (*see* Chapter 19) should be treated appropriately and vigorously.

Abdominal examination
Inspection will show distension, hernia or scars which might help the diagnosis. Gentle palpation (feeling with pressure from the fingers and palm) will reveal areas of tenderness, masses inside the abdomen, and guarding of the abdominal wall muscles in peritonitis. (The abdomen is divided into nine areas for descriptive purposes (*see Fig.* 12.2), which is useful in describing the location of pain or tenderness to somebody else). Auscultation (listening with a stethoscope) is helpful in intestinal obstruction when, due to spasm of the bowel muscle, the normal 'gurgling' sounds of the bowel are increased. In cases of peritonitis the bowel is paralysed (paralytic ileus) and no bowel sounds can be heard, or perhaps just faint tinkling noises.

Special tests
Peritoneal lavage is very useful in cases of abdominal trauma. A plastic catheter is inserted through the anterior abdominal wall and into the peritoneal cavity; 0.9 per cent saline solution is run in through the catheter into the peritoneal cavity, and after a few minutes is retrieved. If

the saline is stained with blood or intestinal contents it is good evidence that damage has occurred and urgent surgery is required.

SPECIFIC CONDITIONS—ABDOMINAL TRAUMA

Two points need emphasizing; first, injuries to other parts of the body (especially the head and chest) should be searched for; secondly, that the patient's general condition is of great importance.

Organs most likely to be damaged in the upper abdomen are the liver and spleen, which are prone to tears as a result of blunt injury. They lie in the right and left hypochondrium, respectively. Both are vascular, and a tear can produce torrential bleeding. The patient may be shocked with peritoneal pain in the upper abdomen. Treatment consists of rapid administration of intravenous fluid, blood transfusion and urgent surgery. When the spleen is damaged it will be removed (splenectomy) as it is difficult to repair and not essential for life. This is not true of the liver and tears here should be repaired. It may be necessary to remove part of the liver (hepatectomy) but fortunately the liver's powers of regeneration are remarkable.

Damage to the kidney may occur if the blow is to the side or back. As the kidney lies behind the peritoneum bleeding does not occur into the peritoneal cavity though a large amount of blood may collect around the kidney (perinephric haematoma). The patient is tender in the lumbar region and hypochondrium and there is usually blood in the urine (haematuria). Minor degrees of damage will heal spontaneously but more serious injury requires surgery to repair the damage or remove the kidney (nephrectomy).

Injury to the lower abdomen can produce a fracture of the bony pelvis (Chapter 13). Such a fracture is likely to cause damage to the bladder or urethra necessitating surgical repair. If the patient cannot pass urine spontaneously he should not be catheterized as this may cause further damage. In such a case, access to the bladder can be achieved by passing a catheter through the abdominal wall.

Stab injuries may also injure the liver and the spleen and treatment is along the lines described above. In addition, as contamination has occurred, antibiotics should be given.

SPECIFIC CONDITIONS ARISING SPONTANEOUSLY

Appendicitis (inflammation of the appendix)

This occurs at all ages, most often in a child or young adult. The inflammation is bacterial. The appendix lies in the right iliac fossa, but initially pain is referred to the umbilical region. After 12–24 hours when the overlying peritoneum is irritated, the pain is felt in the right iliac fossa.

There is marked tenderness and guarding. Treatment is to remove the inflamed appendix (appendicectomy). If there is any delay antibiotics and analgesia should be given.

The danger from untreated appendicitis is of perforation of the inflamed organ leading to potentially fatal peritonitis.

Cholecystitis (inflammation of the gallbladder)

This is also due to bacteria and is nearly always associated with gallstones. Most commonly the disease occurs in young overweight women. The patient is feverish, nauseated and vomiting with pain in the right hypochondrium.

Treatment includes antibiotics and pain relief. If vomiting is severe a nasogastric tube should be passed and fluid and electrolyte given by intravenous infusion. The gallbladder should be removed surgically (cholecystectomy) some weeks after the acute inflammation has subsided to prevent further attacks.

Pancreatitis (inflammation of the pancreas)

This is commonest in patients with gallstones and in alcoholics. The pancreas is inflamed, the patient experiencing epigastric pain and vomiting. Treatment is to rest the organ by passing a nasogastric tube to empty the stomach and duodenum. Fluid and electrolyte replacement is given by the intravenous route, and strong analgesia must be given.

Pancreatitis may be a relatively mild disease recurring often, leaving the patient well between attacks, or it may be severe and rapidly fatal during its first attack.

Peptic ulcer

These most commonly occur in the duodenum and also in the stomach. They occur because of a breakdown in the normal defences of the alimentary tract resulting in damage by its own acid and digestive juices. The patient presents with epigastric pain and vomiting. He is not often 'shocked', and there may be a little epigastric tenderness. The pain is usually relieved by antacids and often there is a history of previous attacks.

Treatment is with antacids or H_2 antagonists (cimetidine, ranitidine, see Vol. 1, Chapter 38). These latter drugs have been so successful that they have drastically reduced surgery for peptic ulcer.

Two complications of peptic ulcer must be mentioned. First, a peptic ulcer may erode into a blood vessel causing vomiting of blood (haematemesis) and passage of altered blood in the faeces (melaena) which is jet black. This bleeding usually settles spontaneously, but surgery may be needed. Secondly, a peptic ulcer may perforate through the stomach or duodenum causing peritonitis. Surgery is indicated to clean out the peritoneal cavity and close the perforation.

Pyelonephritis (inflammation of the kidney and renal pelvis)
This is bacterial in nature. The patient may vomit and has pain in the hypochondrium and lumbar regions. When this condition occurs on the right side it can be difficult to distinguish from cholecystitis. Microscopic examination of the urine shows bacteria and pus cells. Treatment is with antibiotics.

Renal colic (ureteric colic)
This is caused by a stone lodging in the ureter. Sudden severe waves of colicky pain pass from the lumbar region to the groin. Vomiting can be profuse. There is usually blood in the urine (haematuria).

Treatment is with analgesics until the spasm passes off. The stone is often passed spontaneously, but if not, it can be removed surgically.

Lymphadenitis (inflammation of the lymph nodes)
This is common in children and may be indistinguishable from appendicitis. An infection of the throat can cause painful enlargement of the lymph nodes in the abdomen as well as those in the neck. Treatment is with analgesics. If there is doubt, it is safest to diagnose appendicitis and remove the appendix.

Gastroenteritis (inflammation of the stomach and bowel)
This is common in its mildest form as 'twenty-four hour gastric 'flu' '. There is vomiting, diarrhoea and colicky abdominal pain. There is little abdominal tenderness and the patient is not 'shocked'. In severe cases, intravenous fluid replacement and antibiotics may be needed, but this is unusual. Young babies must be referred for medical advice in all but the mildest cases, because fluid and electrolyte balance requires expert management in a baby.

Mesenteric infarction
This occurs mostly in the elderly and is usually due to obstruction of the blood supply to the bowel by atheroma. Pain and 'shock' are profound. Treatment includes surgical removal of the gangrenous bowel, but this may have to be so extensive as to be a hopeless procedure.

Hernia
A hernia is a protrusion of an organ or part of an organ through a narrow opening in which it may become trapped. There are many sorts of hernia but inguinal and femoral herniae are amongst the most common and present as a swelling in the groin. They may cause no trouble for years, but then bowel or other tissue may become trapped. The blood supply to

THE ABDOMEN

the trapped tissues may be cut off—strangulation—leading to gangrene. This is very painful and if the hernia contains bowel the patient may present with intestinal obstruction. Treatment consists of surgical repair.

Acute retention of urine

This occurs most commonly in old men due to enlargement of the prostate gland at the base of the bladder. This enlargement obstructs the passage of urine and very painful bladder distension occurs. Treatment includes passage of a catheter into the bladder to relieve the obstruction. Eventually, the prostate gland can be removed surgically (prostatectomy).

Torsion of the testis

This occurs in boys and young men when the testis twists on itself cutting off the blood supply. Pain is sudden and excruciating. The condition requires urgent surgery to untwist the testis and restore its blood supply. If not, gangrene rapidly supervenes necessitating removal of the testis (orchidectomy).

Epididymo-orchitis (inflammation of the testis and epididymis)

This may be difficult to distinguish from torsion. Pain is less severe and there may be evidence of a urinary infection. If there is any doubt the testis should be explored surgically to exclude torsion.

Medical conditions presenting as abdominal pain

Pain from myocardial infarction (Chapter 11) may be felt in the epigastrium. The most important medical condition leading to diagnostic problems is diabetes. It often presents with abdominal pain and vomiting, so the urine should always be checked for glycosuria (glucose in the urine).

Finally, mention must be made of 'Fraudulent Abdomen'. Occasionally, for psychiatric or manipulative reasons, patients who are dependent on narcotic drugs feign abdominal pain in the hope of being given a dose of morphine or pethidine. A patient with such a history should not be given narcotic drugs unless thought absolutely necessary by an experienced doctor. If no history is available, any patient with multiple small scars over the veins of the arms and legs should be viewed with suspicion, as these are highly suggestive of drug abuse.

Further reading

Elmslie R. G. and Ludbrook J. (1976) *An Introduction to Surgery: 100 Topics.* 2nd ed. Chapters 35, 37 and 38. London, Heinemann.

Wilson D. H. and Hall M. H. (1979) *The Casualty Officer's Handbook.* 4th ed. Chapters 8 and 21. London, Butterworth.

Rutherford W. H., Nelson F. G., Weston P. A. M. et al. (1980) *Accident and Emergency Medicine.* Chapter 19. London, Pitman.

Chapter 13

The Musculoskeletal System

D. I. Rowley

The musculoskeletal system consists of the bones and joints along with their associated muscles and ligaments.

TRAUMA

Most injuries to the musculoskeletal system are not life-threatening and most take second place to the trauma which may prejudice vital functions. There are a small number of exceptions to this rule and these may be called the 'dangerous injuries' and will be discussed below. All musculoskeletal injuries in the long term may have far-reaching effects on the social amd economic well-being of the patient and so must receive careful consideration early in treatment, once survival of the patient has been secured. The aims of immediate care of these injuries should be to reduce pain, prevent further damage and to keep open wounds from becoming contaminated.

PRIORITIES

Musculoskeletal injuries have been divided into three groups and only the first requires high priority in the early assessment and management of the patient. The conditions in this first 'dangerous' group must be looked for positively because if they are missed the injury may be worse or the life of the patient put in jeopardy. Any of these injuries can occur in isolation but usually are part of a multiple injury.

The subdivision described below is an aid to deciding the order of priority at the scene of accident. All these injuries are secondary to the correction of airway and circulation impairment.

Group 1. Dangerous injuries
1. Maxillofacial
2. Spinal
3. Pelvis
4. Ribs

Group 2. Urgent injuries
1. Open wounds with free bleeding
2. Limb injuries with evidence of circulatory impairment

Group 3. Non-urgent injuries
1. All 'closed' limb injuries
2. Most 'open' limb injuries

GROUP 1. DANGEROUS INJURIES

1. Maxillofacial injuries

Pathological anatomy
The face should be regarded as being a separate bony shelf slung under the front of the skull and closely related to its sloping front. Through the bony face pass the air and food passages.

Injuries
A significant blow to the face will cause bleeding and swelling from the resultant soft-tissue and bony injury. A severe blow may result in displacement of the bony face relative to the rest of the skull.

Significance
  a. Such injuries may be associated with unconsciousness and consequent loss of gag reflex. Bleeding into the air passages may result in airway obstruction because of the absence of protective reflexes.
  b. Severe displaced fractures may result in physical blockages to the air passages by distorted bones.
  c. Open injuries may be associated with dangerous bleeding from major vessels, such as the facial artery.

Immediate treatment
The unconscious patient should be kept head down and on his side to aid drainage of blood out of the nose and mouth. If available, suction should be used frequently but gently. If, in very severe injuries, despite all routine care of the airway, the patient still cannot breathe then the teeth or gums should be grasped and pulled gently up and out to free the airway. Bleeding from open wounds may be controlled by direct pressure through a clean pad.

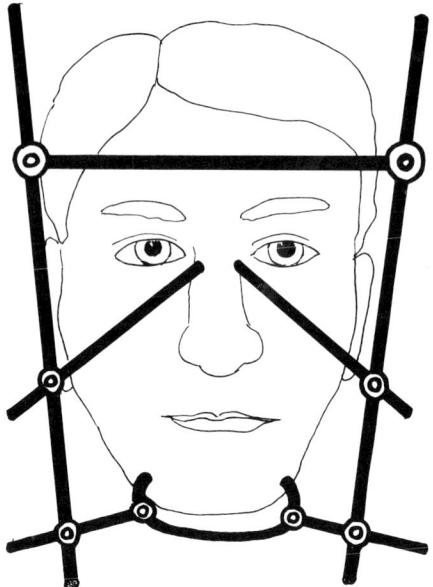

Fig. 13.1. Metal rods used to stabilize the maxilla and mandible.

Hospital care

The airway must be secured by endotracheal intubation or tracheostomy. The patient may need to be maintained on ventilation for a few days until swelling settles. Displaced and unstable fractures need to be stabilized either by fixation with wire or by an external fixator (*Fig.* 13.1).

2. Spinal injury

Pathological anatomy

The spinal cord is protected in front (anteriorly) by the vertebral bodies which also support the weight of the body. Behind (posteriorly) the spinal cord is surrounded by the neural arches and spinous processes. The interlocking of the arches by the facet joints and the surrounding ligaments make the whole structure stable (*Fig.* 13.2).

Injuries

Vertical forces resulting from a fall or an object falling on a patient from above will tend to damage the vertebral bodies, crushing them (*Fig.* 13.3). The fracture is stable because the posterior joints and ligaments are intact. These injuries may be produced by quite minor falls in the elderly because their bones are weak.

THE MUSCULOSKELETAL SYSTEM

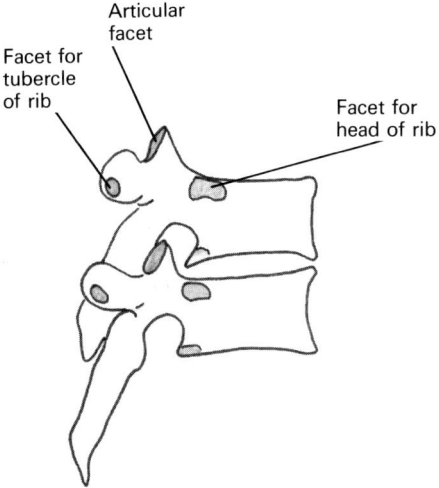

Fig. 13.2. Two thoracic vertebrae showing facets.

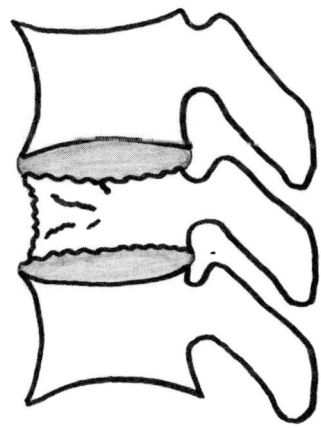

Fig. 13.3. Diagrammatic representation of a crush fracture of a vertebra.

Twisting and flexing forces damage the posterior facet joints and tear the surrounding ligaments. This makes the spine unstable, particularly if it is subsequently bent forwards. The unstable bones can move on each other (*Fig.* 13.4) and can damage the spinal cord at the time of injury.

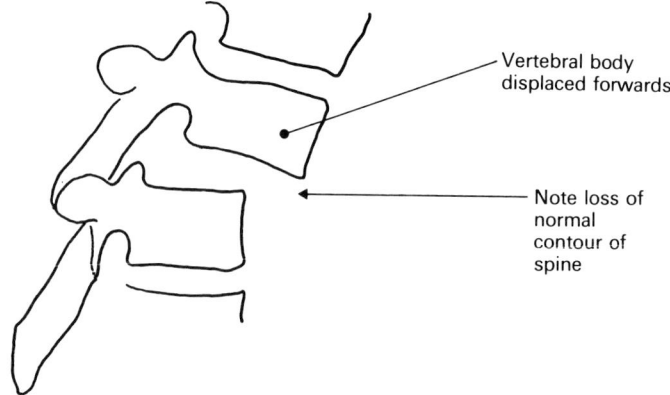

Fig. 13.4. Destabilizing injury due to flexion and rotation. One facet joint is often disrupted.

Because the bones are unstable this may allow cord damage at a later time when the patient is moved.

The more violent the accident then the more likely the spine is to be damaged. If the accident has made the patient unconscious then it is best to assume he has a spinal injury until he can be examined and X-rayed in hospital. This is doubly important because an unconscious patient will be unable to complain of pain, paralysis or loss of sensation, nor will he have protective muscle spasm to help support his injured back. The conscious patient will be able to complain of all these things and will be able to tell his rescuers if their actions are making these symptoms worse. Back or neck pain in the absence of paralysis or sensory change may *still be a sign of unstable spinal injury.*

Immediate treatment

a. The conscious patient

Gentle and slow handling, avoiding flexing and twisting movements, is required. Careful attention must be paid to any increase in pain or sensory disturbance of the patient. If these rules are obeyed the patient is unlikely to allow his rescuers to make him worse. If possible, the patient should be moved in the position in which he has been found after fitting a soft collar to his neck and a board to his back (spinal board). If space does not permit this he must be laid on his back, wearing a collar, with padding in the small of his back. Whilst moving him someone should be allocated to guard his neck, keeping it in a neutral position or slightly extended. If he needs to be turned then a number of people will be required to move him in 'one piece'.

THE MUSCULOSKELETAL SYSTEM

b. The unconscious patient

Extreme care is required in every case, but the unconscious patient requires yet more vigilance. The patient will be unable to tell his rescuers if they are causing him further pain. If possible, it is far safer to move the patient in the position in which he is found. Many helpers will be needed for this. However, care must be taken to keep the airway clear despite the difficulties in transport.

Hospital care

If the patient is already paralysed he will have no sensation below the injury and no control of bowel or bladder function. His breathing may be limited if his chest muscles are paralysed, although most patients are able to breathe adequately so long as the nerve supply to the diaphragm is intact (C3, 4, 5). Later, he is liable to develop chest or urine infections and his skin may break down. It may be advisable to operate on his back to fix the bones in position, although it is impossible to repair the nerve damage. Highly specialized nursing care will be required.

If the patient is not paralysed nursing care will be infinitely easier. He can be rested in bed in a moulded plaster until his bones heal, but it may be advisable to fix the bones with screws and rods, so making his nursing simpler.

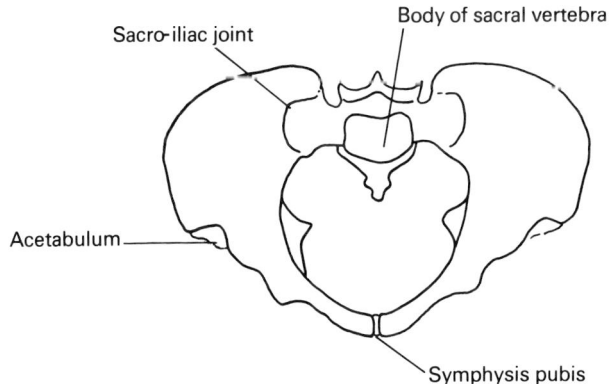

Fig. 13.5. The normal pelvis.

3. Pelvic injuries
Pathological anatomy

The pelvis is a bony ring transferring the weight from the back to the legs (*Fig.* 13.5). Pelvic bones have a very rich blood supply and on the inside wall is situated an extensive network of veins draining blood from the legs and viscera.

Injuries

The smaller bones at the front of the pelvis are commonly injured in the elderly when the bone is weak. A single break in the bony ring does not make it unstable and, though painful, these injuries are not dangerous.

In more violent accidents the bony ring may be broken in two or more places making the whole pelvis unstable (*Fig.* 13.6). A great deal of

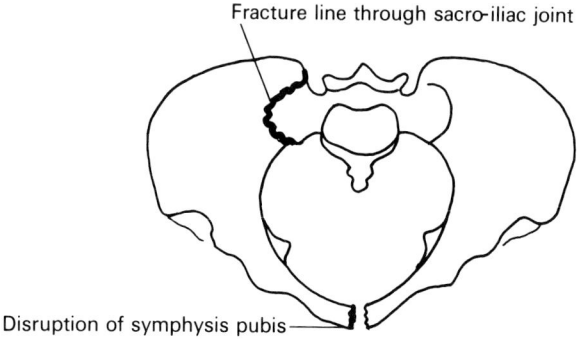

Fig. 13.6. Pelvic fracture through sacro-iliac joint and symphysis pubis. The pelvis is made unstable since the pelvic ring is disrupted in two places, one above the level of the hip.

trauma is required to do this and the venous networks are usually torn. The viscera are also liable to injury in this situation.

Significance

In the more severe injuries bleeding will be massive, but no external blood loss will be seen. The blood will be lost from the circulation into the soft tissues at the back of the pelvic and abdominal cavity, so no swelling is normally visible. The associated visceral injuries are potentially life-threatening.

Immediate treatment

Recognition of the injury may be difficult but if the patient complains of pain when the pelvis is examined or the legs are moved then an injury should be suspected. The patient should be moved with legs and pelvis in 'one piece'. He should be transferred to hospital as soon as possible with an intravenous infusion. Trapped casualties may require volume replacement and pain relief at the accident site.

THE MUSCULOSKELETAL SYSTEM

Hospital care
Replacement of blood loss is of first priority. There is no place for surgery to stop bleeding, but, initially, slings can be used to control it. Thereafter a decision can be made to continue to treat the patient in slings, or fix the fractures with an external scaffold or with plates.

GROUP 2. URGENT INJURIES

Once vital functions have been secured then attention can be focused on open injuries. Clearly severe bleeding from open wounds will be obvious and early action taken. Such bleeding is rare and most bleeding needs only elevation and direct pressure whilst the airway and circulation to vital organs are attended to.

1. Open wounds with free bleeding (*See* Chapter 10)

2. Limb injuries with evidence of circulatory impairment

Pathological anatomy
Vessels lie next to bones and can be injured by the broken bone, causing them to be blocked or torn.

Significance
The limb will look pale and the veins be collapsed. No pulsation will be felt and the limb will be cool. The patient may complain of pain, numbness and inability to use the limb.

Early recognition is important. After only a few hours the situation will be irreversible and the limb below the damage will die (gangrene).

Immediate treatment
This consists of controlling the bleeding and transport to hospital.

Hospital care
Careful X-ray examination followed by surgical exploration and repair is urgently required.

GROUP 3. NON-URGENT INJURY

In the field it is best to consider the limb as a whole unit rather than think of injuries to bone, nerves, muscles and tendons, etc., separately. In the acute situation it will not be possible to decide in great detail what has been injured and in an attempt to do so the significance of the injury as a whole may be lost. The most obvious fractures and wounds may not be the most serious and so it is important to develop a systematic approach.

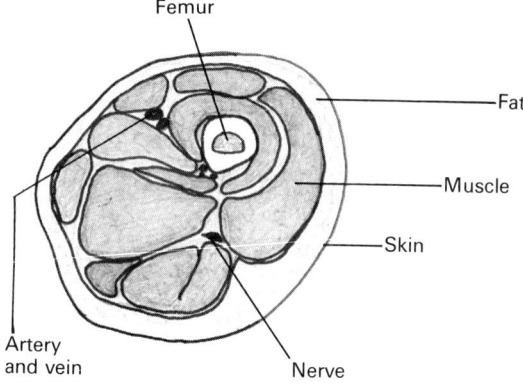

Fig. 13.7. The thigh in cross-section.

'Open' and 'closed' limb injuries
Pathological anatomy
The arm and leg are complex structures but their overall plan is quite simple and should be thought of like a joint of meat in cross-section (*Fig.* 13.7).

Starting from the outside the tissues can be damaged to varying degrees down to and including bone. Intervening skin fat, muscle, tendon, nerves and vessels may be caught in the violence. Equally a broken bone can damage the same structures up to and including the skin from inside. When examining any injury this simple plan should be remembered and the question 'what has happened to the structures underneath?' always asked.

Injury
In general, large direct forces are required to break bones transversely, obliquely or into a number of parts (*Fig.* 13.8) with, consequently, more damage to the soft tissues. Twisting forces causing spiral fractures do not need to be large and soft-tissue injury, although significant, will be less. Spiral fractures are the commonest type of bony injury.

Significance
All limb injuries may be classified as *open* or *closed*. An open injury in association with a broken bone used to be called a 'compound fracture'.

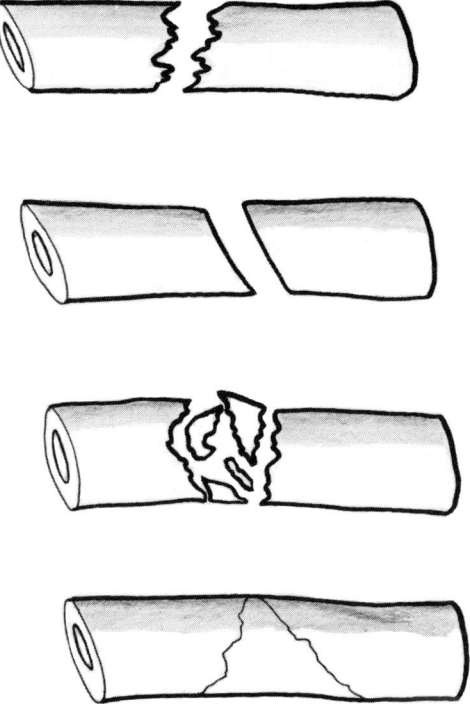

Fig. 13.8. Different forms of fracture.

Open injuries
'Untidy' open injuries imply a lot of potential damage deeper down, possibly including the bone. The open wounds will be contaminated by micro-organisms and dirt and are potentially a source of infection. The problems of swelling will be more severe than in closed injuries because the forces involved are greater. The significance of swelling is discussed below.

Closed injuries
Damage to skin and fat may not be very obvious early, but very bruised skin may slough many days later. Muscle injury will result in a lot of swelling that may impair an already damaged blood flow.
 Broken bones will bleed, e.g. a closed fracture of the femur will lead to 3 units of blood being lost from the circulation. This bleeding will add to swelling and excessive movements may allow the unstable bone ends to damage surrounding structures (compartment syndrome).

Assessment
Pain, swelling and discoloration of the skin signifies injury. Difficult, limited or painful movement suggests a fracture. There is no place for trying to elicit *crepitus* (a grating feeling on moving the bone) in assessing these injuries.

Immediate treatment
In open injuries clean dry dressings and direct pressure are all that are required in the early stages. Once this has been achieved they should be treated as closed injuries. All significant closed limb injuries should be splinted whether a fracture is suspected or not. This will reduce pain and swelling and reduce the risk of making the injury worse. Early elevation will reduce or even prevent swelling. Splintage should be as simple as possible, using wood, plastic or malleable wire; if not available, then an injured leg can be tied to the other or an injured arm to the chest wall, or a sling used.

Complex splints are often difficult to put on and pressurized splints applied over-zealously to a swollen limb can restrict blood supply and are no substitute for elevation.

A note on dislocations
All the above principles of limb care can be applied to dislocations. There is no place for blind, unskilled reduction of dislocations at the scene of accidents.

Fractures may be produced making subsequent treatment very difficult and surrounding soft tissue, particularly nerves and arteries, can be damaged.

Hospital care
Open injuries
All wounds require formal surgical exploration. All dead and contaminated tissue must be removed to reduce the risk of infection. Antibiotics and tetanus toxoid may be required but are less important than adequate surgery. Severe wounds may be better left open for a few days or allowed to close spontaneously without stitches. Definitive treatment must be delayed until only healthy soft tissue remains. As soon as possible tendons and nerves should be repaired.

Closed injuries
Excessive swelling may prevent early complete treatment, as the blood supply to the soft tissues may not be adequate to allow healing. Following closed or open (surgical) reduction of the fracture the bones can be held in alignment in three ways:
1. External splintage
2. Internal splintage
3. Traction

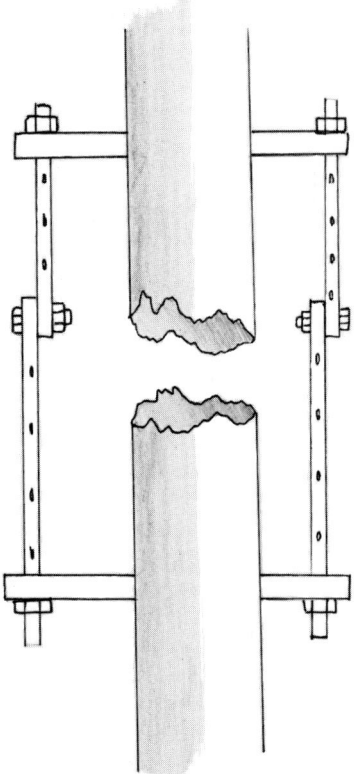

Fig. 13.9. External bracing of a fractured bone using a metal frame.

1. External splintage
   a. Plaster-of-Paris—this is the commonest method of treating low velocity injuries. The bones are restored to position and held in the plaster until they unite. It is dangerous to *completely* enclose a swollen limb in the early stages as further swelling may result in circulatory impairment. A simple slab is often used as a temporary measure. The joints have to be immobilized and the muscles, therefore, remain unused. To prevent stiffness and limb-wasting, physiotherapy is needed whilst the limb is in plaster. This is followed by more vigorous exercise and mobilization once the fracture has united.
   b. External fixation (*Fig.* 13.9) frames are useful where there has been a lot of soft-tissue damage including swelling or open wounds.

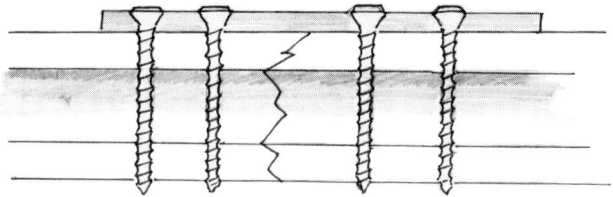

Fig. 13.10. Internal fixation using a plate and screws.

Simple enclosure in plaster in the presence of extensive soft-tissue damage is hazardous. Pins in the bone held on an external scaffold will hold the bones in reasonable position whilst allowing access to deal with the soft-tissue element of the injury.
2. Internal Splintage
Any bone may be fixed with screws (*Fig.* 13.10) and plates on the outside or nails and pins in the marrow cavity. It is particularly useful to do this where the precise realignment of a bone is important for normal limb function, such as around joints. It can be used in order to get a patient mobile quickly and is particularly useful in the elderly where prolonged immobilization renders them at risk from chest infection, deep vein thrombosis and bed sores. The operative techniques are difficult and there are many hazards. For example, if a fracture becomes infected following fixation it is very difficult to treat.
3. Traction (*Fig.* 13.11)
Limbs do not need to be fully immobilized for bones to heal. If the bones are put in a reasonable position the surrounding muscles will hold them there. Traction is a procedure where weights are attached to the limb, so making the muscles contract and hold the fracture. The complex pulley systems as in *Fig.* 13.12 are merely arrangements to allow the patient to exercise his joints whilst the pull is maintained in line with the limb whatever position the limb is in.

Complications of fractures
Pulmonary embolus
Prolonged immobilization in bed may lead to deep venous thrombosis and pulmonary embolus (*see* Chapter 9).

Fat embolus
Following fractures, particularly long bones, patients may develop respiratory distress and renal failure. This is often attributed to

THE MUSCULOSKELETAL SYSTEM

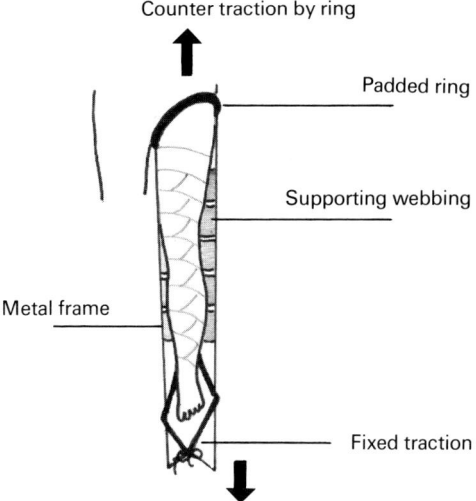

Fig. 13.11. Thomas' splint traction system.

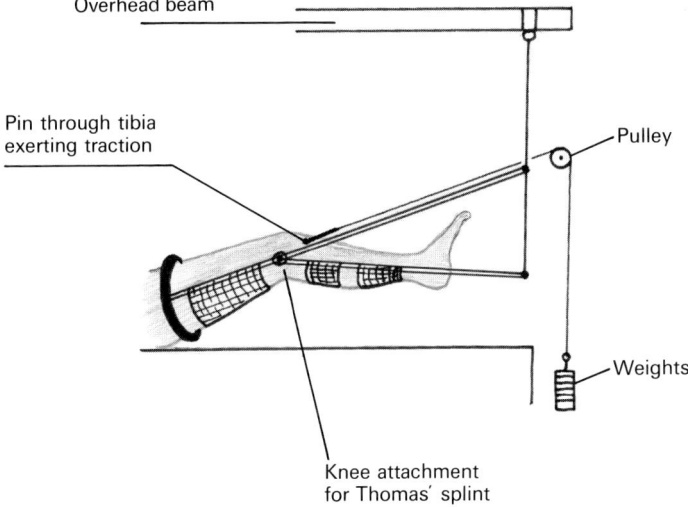

Fig. 13.12. A system of traction using weights.

embolization of fat from the bone marrow. Free fat may be found in the urine in such cases.

Treatment is supportive following admission to an Intensive Therapy Unit (ITU).

Further reading

Apley A. G. (1982) *A System of Orthopaedics and Fractures.* London, Butterworth.
Duckworth T. (1980) *Lecture Notes on Orthopaedics and Fractures.* Oxford, Blackwell Scientific Publication.
Rockwood C. A. and Green D. P. (ed.) (1975) *Fractures.* Philadelphia, Lippincott.

Chapter 14

The Nervous System. I. Trauma

A. C. Crosby and J. R. Paskins

Head injuries are the commonest reason for admission to hospital, and currently about 100 000 people a year are admitted with 1500 of those suffering significant physical and mental disability.

Three problems face the paramedical staff who find themselves dealing with a head-injured patient:
1. What is the level of consciousness and what is its significance?
2. How severe is the injury to the patient and what immediate complications may develop?
3. What other injuries are also present, and how do they influence the action that must be taken?

CONSCIOUS LEVEL

There is nearly always a change in consciousness following head injury. This may range from mild confusion through restlessness and unreasonable behaviour to profound coma.

By establishing the patient's conscious level at an early stage and reassessing it at frequent and regular intervals any deterioration can be rapidly appreciated and acted on.

There now exist specially prepared scales on which a patient's responses to external stimuli can be charted. One such example is the Glasgow Coma Scale (*see Table* 15.1).

One cause of rapid decrease in conscious level is the generalized fit or grand mal convulsion. This is an indication that the brain is being subjected to anoxia or pressure, or that the patient is prone to epilepsy. The fits may occur repeatedly and are a very serious sign.

The significance of level of consciousness lies in its rate and direction of change. Rapid deterioration requires a rapid response rather than inertia in the hope that the situation may somehow improve.

SEVERITY

A blow to the head imparts energy through the soft tissues and bone into the tissues of the brain itself. The brain is shaken and if the blow is severe enough the brain cells will cease to function and possibly die. Blood vessels may rupture and the fine control of the blood supply within the brain is disturbed, leading to swelling and bruising.

Following an injury it is important to know if a patient has been unconscious, because even a short period of being 'knocked out' indicates that the damage may be severe enough to cause complications. Fortunately, those who suffer only transient loss of consciousness are much less likely to develop serious problems, but all head injuries are potentially dangerous and even apparently minor episodes have been known to prove fatal in some circumstances.

One useful guide is the presence of *amnesia*. A patient who cannot remember the events which preceded his accident has probably received a blow that left him unconscious. The period of memory loss may be only a few minutes, though in more severe cases the amnesia affects memory function for events which span days both before and after the injury.

The danger from head injury comes from the patient's inability to care properly for himself. This may entail anything from inappropriate actions when confused, to choking on his own vomit when unconscious. To this is added the danger of bleeding within the skull. Haemorrhage may occur around the meningeal linings that surround the brain and when it does the collection of blood compresses the brain. The first effect of this is to diminish the patient's consciousness. As bleeding progresses the patient deteriorates further until he dies.

The brain is surrounded by three layers of membranes. Closest to the brain is the pia mater, a fine layer on the surface. Above this is the arachnoid mater which is closely associated with the fine blood vessels on the brain surface. The outermost layer is called the dura mater and is adherent to the inside of the skull vault. It is the toughest layer and affords the brain some protection.

Bleeding may occur:
1. Beneath the arachnoid: *Subarachnoid haemorrhage*
2. Beneath the dura: *Subdural haemorrhage*
3. Between the dura and the skull: *Extradural haemorrhage*

The commonest forms of haemorrhage after injury are the acute subdural and acute extradural haemorrhages. Direct impact and rotational forces may tear the delicate subdural veins, or an artery running along the inside of the skull may be torn when the bone fractures.

The extradural haematoma may have a particularly deceptive presentation. The patient suffers a blow which knocks him out. After a few minutes he recovers and seems all right. Subsequently he again lapses into unconsciousness. This phenomenon is known as the *lucid interval*. What has happened is that the injury was severe enough to tear a blood vessel on the surface of the dura and concuss the patient for a period. The recovery from the concussion is then followed by steady deterioration as the extradural haematoma collects.

It is not possible to predict which patients with apparently minor injuries will develop such a haematoma, but it is known that the presence of a skull fracture greatly increases the risk. Because of this it is a routine policy to admit to hospital all patients who have been concussed or have skull fractures. Other patients who have head injuries are warned of the possible effects of their injury and those relatives or friends with them told to return the patient to hospital if any of the signs of cerebral compression (vomiting, confusion or coma) develop.

Major head injury

If there is severe brain damage the patient will not recover consciousness quickly. The acceleration and deceleration forces cause tearing and bruising of the brain with destruction of brain cells and swelling of the brain tissue. This swelling is known as *cerebral oedema*.

The patient's coma may be profound enough to jeopardize the protective reflexes of the airway. Even if the patient does not asphyxiate the loss of airway control will rapidly worsen the effects of cerebral oedema because the rising carbon dioxide level in the blood provokes an increase in cerebral blood flow. The rising pressure within the skull has similar effects to that occurring following a haemorrhage, i.e. the brain is compressed and eventually ceases to function.

Thus the single most useful action of the emergency care team is to ensure a clear airway by suction and the insertion of an artificial airway. Oxygen given by mask will improve the situation but cannot by itself overcome the effects of an airway blocked by vomit, blood and saliva.

ASSOCIATED INJURY

Skull fractures

A direct blow may cause a depressed fracture, akin to the top of an egg that has been struck by a spoon. These are difficult to feel beneath bruised scalp and matted hair, but show up on a skull X-ray. Even if not severe enough to warrant surgery the patient is admitted for observation.

Fractures may also develop across the base of the skull, tearing into the cavities of the nose and ears. Though not all bleeding from the nose and ears means a fracture of this sort, the possibility should be borne in mind.

Scalp wounds

Profuse bleeding can be controlled by firm pressure. It is difficult to place sutures in the field, though this may be necessary if temporary control of a large flap is required.

Facial injuries

These may result in a threat to the airway, particularly when the jaw is involved. Bleeding is controlled by firm local pressure.

Neck injury

A force sufficient to concuss the patient may also damage the vertebrae in the neck. An unconscious patient will lack the ability to alert his rescuers to the pain in his neck, and will also lack any voluntary limitation of neck movement, and for this reason should always be treated as if a neck injury was present. The neck must be carefully stabilized before moving or lifting.

Chest and abdomen

The anoxia caused by a chest injury will worsen a head-injured patient's condition and it is easy to overlook such an injury when a patient is confused, uncooperative or bleeding. Similarly, an unconscious patient will not complain of pain in the event of an abdominal injury. Both of these conditions cause a considerable increase in the mortality amongst head-injury patients, and it must be remembered that whereas head injury is only occasionally swiftly fatal, intrathoracic or abdominal bleeding frequently causes death.

SPINAL CORD INJURY

The spinal cord runs from the base of the brain down the spinal canal. Discrete areas exist within it along which pass sensory messages from peripheral nerves and motor commands to the muscles.

Like the brain, the cells within the cord cannot regenerate. For all practical purposes damage is permanent.

Spinal fractures

These are the commonest cause of spinal cord damage, and the worst type is the transection in which there is complete division of the cord. This may happen instantly, at the time of the accident, or later because the fracture was unstable and the patient was moved without proper spinal support. In other circumstances the cord may only be bruised and a full recovery is possible. For this reason always treat a spinal injury as if the patient was fully recoverable. Similarly, a patient may be conscious, unparalysed and even be capable of neck or back movement,

THE NERVOUS SYSTEM. I. TRAUMA

yet have an unstable spinal fracture that leaves him paralysed as soon as he is moved at the scene of the accident.

The symptoms of cord damage are numbness and paralysis below the level of the injury. Cervical damage is particularly dangerous because not only may all the limbs be paralysed (*tetraplegia*) but above about the fifth cervical vertebra the muscles of respiration will fail—with fatal results.

Cord damage may also result in circulatory collapse, as the sympathetic nerve pathways are interrupted and the blood vessels in the paralysed part of the body relax. Pulse rate and blood pressure both fall and the patient may lose consciousness or die as a result of this. Fluid replacement must be given with care, for a patient in this condition will easily become overloaded and develop pulmonary oedema.

PERIPHERAL NERVE INJURY

These nerves carry both sensory and motor impulses, and may be bruised, partially cut or totally divided at any point on their course.

If a peripheral nerve is damaged near its origin at the spinal canal the whole area supplied by the nerve will be rendered anaesthetic and the muscles of the area will not function.

Some sites are more prone to injury than others. Where a nerve runs close to the skin or a bone it may be cut by broken glass or a nearby fracture; bony injury at the elbow and lacerations at the wrist are two examples.

Another mechanism of injury is traction on the nerves, such as that which occurs when a motorcyclist is thrown onto his shoulder. The nerves to the arm are torn away from their origins in the spinal cord and the arm is left paralysed. The degree of recovery can sometimes be improved by surgical repair of the damaged nerves, but in general the nearer the injury is to the spinal cord, the worse the outlook.

SUMMARY
USEFUL RULES IN NERVOUS SYSTEM DAMAGE

1. Guard the unconscious patient's airway.
2. Signs of deteriorating conscious level must not be ignored. Do not wait and hope that things will improve.
3. Remember to look for problems associated with head injury, particularly in the neck, chest and abdomen.
4. Avoid assuming that recovery cannot take place, or that injury cannot have occurred.

Further reading
Jamieson K. G. (1971) *A First Notebook of Head Injury*. London, Butterworth.

Chapter 15

The Nervous System. II. Non-trauma

S. J. Mather and D. L. Edbrooke

Some conditions of interest to critical care personnel will be described.

A. HEADACHE

The brain itself has no pain receptors, but the cerebral blood vessels and parts of the dura have. The muscles and fascia overlying the skull are pain sensitive and are often a source of headache.

Common causes of headache
a. Psychogenic (emotional) causes
b. Vascular causes—typically a 'throbbing headache'
  i. *Intracranial vessels*
      Dilatation of intracranial vessels
        influenza and the common cold
        post-epilepsy headache
        histamine release (allergy)
        alcohol
        hypertension (of sudden onset)
  ii. *Dilatation of extracranial vessels*
      Migraine
      Chronic hypertension

c. Traction (stretching) on intracranial structures
    Cerebral tumour

d. **Inflammation**
   Meningitis
   Intracranial bleeding
     muscle spasm (infection or inflammation of cranial nerves)
     arteritis (e.g. inflamed temporal artery)

e. **Referred pain** (e.g. dental and sinus pain)

f. **Muscle spasm** due to nerve root compression
   Cervical spine lesions (e.g. spondylosis, arthritis)

g. **General fatigue.** This may have an emotional component or may involve muscle spasms or 'tension'.

Treatment

Often the cause cannot be determined and simple treatment of the symptom with mild analgesics is acceptable. If the headache is characteristic or persistent, investigation of the cause is required. Specific treatment may be available (e.g. for migraine). One must never forget that most headaches do not signify serious disease but that very occasionally they may be due to a serious but remediable cause. Thus any persistent headache should be thoroughly investigated.

B. COMA

Coma is defined differently by different authors, and somewhat arbitrarily. It is usually thought of as 'deep unconsciousness', but it can be graded according to reflex responses obtained from various stimuli.

The Glasgow Coma Scale

Various scales for assessing coma have been devised. One of the best known is the Glasgow Scale (Teasdale and Jennett, 1974). An example is shown in *Table* 15.1. It enables an observer, with no specialist training in neurological assessment, to make reproducible observations. Furthermore, data from different observers is also reproducible and may be pooled. This greatly increases the value of observations made on one patient by many people over a period of time.

Causes of coma
   Head injury
   Cerebrovascular accident
   Cerebral tumour
   Infection (meningitis, encephalitis)

Table 15.1. The Glasgow coma scale

Eye opening		
Spontaneous	4	
To speech	3	E
To pain	2	
Nil	1	
Best motor response		
Obeys	6	
Localizes	5	
Withdraws (flexion)	4	M
Abnormal flexion	3	
Extensor response	2	
Nil	1	
Verbal response		
Orientated	5	
Confused conversation	4	
Inappropriate words	3	V
Incomprehensible sounds	2	
Nil	1	
Coma score (responsiveness sum = 3–15 (E + M + V))		

Drug overdose (central depressants, opioites)
Hypothermia
Respiratory failure (CO_2 narcosis)
Diabetic coma (ketoacidosis)
Hypoglycaemia
Uraemia (renal failure)
Hepatic coma (liver failure)

Management of the patient in coma

As coma deepens, the protective reflexes are lost and the patient is then unable to maintain his airway or cough and remove secretions from the respiratory tract. If coma persists additional problems, such as pressure sores, become evident. Thus good nursing care and physiotherapy are *essential* to the care of the patient in coma. He will not survive without them.

The patient must be nursed in such a way as to preserve vital reflexes. In the absence of artificial airway support, this will be on one or other side in the 'recovery position' (*see Fig.* 6.5).

In the serious neurological case initial management must once again be directed towards preservation of life, i.e. maintenance of the airway, oxygenation and ventilation.

If coma lasts for any length of time tracheal intubation or tracheostomy may be required to protect the airway.

Brainstem reflexes

If the brainstem is damaged, the patient may be unable to breathe for himself or maintain his blood pressure. If this occurs the possibility of brainstem death must be considered.

If the brainstem dies, the patient is effectively dead, even if the heart is still beating.

Assessment regimes have been worked out to enable the diagnosis of brainstem death to be made. If brainstem death is proven, life-support machines and pharmacological support can ethically be withdrawn and the patient allowed to die with dignity, the relatives being spared any false hopes.

C. INFECTIONS OF THE NERVOUS SYSTEM

1. Meningitis

The most frequently encountered is *meningitis*. In this condition, it is the pia and arachnoid rather than the dura which become inflamed. (It may be noted here also that meningitis may occur without infection, e.g. in subarachnoid haemorrhage.)

Viral meningitis

This is the most common form of meningitis. Echo and coxsackie viruses are most often the causative organisms, but meningitis may also occur as part of the clinical picture of measles, mumps, glandular fever (infectious mononucleosis) and viral hepatitis as may encephalitis (inflammation of the brain itself).

Clinically, viral meningitis appears similar whatever the causative organism unless other parts of the body are affected (e.g. orchitis in mumps, the rash of measles). Viral meningitis carries a good prognosis and treatment is supportive, with antibiotics if indicated for secondary bacterial infection.

Pyogenic meningitis

This is bacterial meningitis which is usually due to spread from a focus elsewhere in the body, e.g. heart or lungs, but rarely may be confined to the meninges. The usual organisms are staphylococci, streptococci or haemophilus.

Meningococcal meningitis

Like pyogenic meningitis this was once common but is now rare due to the availability of antibiotics. It was seen in epidemics among children and those living in crowded surroundings. If septicaemia occurs, a haemorrhagic rash may follow. This may be followed by adrenal haemorrhage and pyogenic arthritis (pus in joint spaces). This is a severe illness.

Tuberculous meningitis
Again, once a common disease but now rare due to the availability of effective treatment for TB. It was usually due to spread from distant sites (e.g. lung or bone) or a tuberculous abscess in the brain.

Syphilis
Syphilis may be associated with meningitis as part of a wider picture of neurological disease. Any patient with neurological disease should have screening tests for syphilis.

General signs of meningitis
These are essentially those of meningeal irritation:
 a. Headache, lassitude and photophobia (the patient seeks a dark, quiet room);
 b. Neck rigidity, which may be very marked in children;
 c. Kernig's sign. This is positive when the roots of the spinal nerves are inflamed. If the thigh is flexed to 90° (hip flexion) the bent knee cannot then be straightened due to spasm of the extensors (hamstrings). (The spasm is due to stretching of inflamed sciatic nerve roots.)

Diagnosis
The optic fundi may display papilloedema, i.e. the optic nerve becomes protuberant where it enters the eye, due to raised cerebrospinal fluid pressure. If this is very marked, lumbar puncture and drainage of any significant quantity of spinal fluid may lead to 'coning' (herniation of the medulla through the foramen magnum) with fatal consequences. However, lumbar puncture is usually safely performed and the CSF examined for protein, glucose, cells and organisms. Specific findings can greatly aid diagnosis, especially serological and immunological tests. Bacteria may be cultured from CSF samples within a few hours or days in pyogenic meningitis.

Treatment
It is beyond the scope of this book to discuss in detail the treatment of all forms of meningitis. We have noted above that viral meningitis is usually self-limiting, but antibiotics may be given to combat secondary infection. If the causative organism is known in bacterial (pyogenic) meningitis, treatment is dictated by culture and sensitivity tests. There are specific antibiotics used for tuberculous meningitis, and syphilis is responsive to penicillin.

Prophylaxis
Infection may enter the nervous system, including the meninges, following trauma such as a fractured base of skull, when there may be

CSF leaks from the ear or nose. Antibiotics are usually given to prevent such infection occurring (prophylactic antibiotics).

2. Cerebral abscess

This is a pus-filled cavity within the brain. The possible causes are listed below:
  a. Local spread from an infected focus, e.g. middle ear or sinuses.
  b. Blood-borne spread from infected foci elsewhere in the body.
  c. Open (compound) fracture of the skull.
  d. Penetrating or missile injury.

Organisms
Bacteria such as staphylococci and streptococci but also fungi (actinomyces).

Clinical picture
Clouding of consciousness, headache, vomiting and eventually coma. This may occur early or late after head injury or an infection elsewhere. The abscess may become chronic with symptoms and signs of a 'space-occupying lesion' within the skull.

There may be personality changes. Chronic abscess may be mistaken for cerebral tumour.

Diagnosis
Radiology, CAT (or CT) scanning (computerized X-ray scanning) and electroencephalography are all used. The abscess may be accessible to drainage via a needle. The pus may then be cultured and the sensitivity of the organism to antibiotics determined.

Treatment
Antibiotics and drainage if possible.

3. Encephalitis

This is usually viral. Sometimes the virus can be determined by immunological tests or culture but in many cases the causative organism is unknown.

Clinical picture
This depends upon the organism involved, but usually there is a rapidly developing fever with headache and clouding of consciousness. There may be no focal neurological signs, but epileptiform fits may occur. Fits and coma indicate a poor prognosis.

Diagnosis
Examination of the CSF and serological tests. Often the organism is not identified.

Treatment
There is no specific treatment for most of these infections but herpes virus may respond to idoxuridine. Acyclovir is also used.

4. Poliomyelitis
In poliomyelitis the virus attacks the motor neurone (anterior horn cells of the spinal cord and motor cranial nuclei).

Infection is via the gut (enteroviruses). Young adults and older children appear most susceptible but the disease has almost died out since the introduction of immunization (see Vol. I, p. 326). If the motor neurone is sufficiently damaged it degenerates, the muscle it supplies becoming wasted.

Bulbar paralysis
If the motor cranial nerves are affected the patient may be unable to swallow or cough with resulting aspiration pneumonia. If the respiratory muscles are also involved the prognosis is poor as recurrent chest infections and respiratory failure are certain to occur.

Complete respiratory paralysis is inevitably fatal unless the patient is aided by a respirator. It was, in fact, the polio epidemics of the late 1940s and early 1950s which led to the rapid developments in artificial ventilation of the lungs at that time.

Immunization with first the Salk and then the Sabin (oral) poliomyelitis vaccine has virtually eradicated the disease. It is important, however, that the 'herd' immunity is kept up by the immunization of all infants, since sporadic cases still do occur.

Treatment
 a. Bed rest
 b. Physiotherapy
 c. Immunoglobulin
 d. Artificial ventilation, if required.

5. Tetanus
Tetanus results from the effects of the exotoxin of *Clostridium tetani* (see Vol. 1, p. 314). The tetanus bacilli grow well in puncture or stab wounds, under anaerobic conditions. They occur in the gut of many mammals and in the soil. The bacilli do not migrate, but the exotoxin enters the blood and eventually finds its way to the motor nerves. The incubation period is two days to several weeks. The earliest sign is often trismus (masseter spasm). This gives the disease its traditional name of

'lockjaw'. The rigidity spreads over the face and trunk; the back becomes arched and the mouth is drawn into a sort of smile—the 'risus sardonicus'. Convulsive spasms may occur, embarrassing respiration. Death may occur from asphyxia and aspiration pneumonia. Occasionally serious arrhythmias and blood pressure changes may occur.

Treatment
a. Wide excision of the wound.
b. Penicillin and other antibiotics for secondary infection.
c. Sedation, and artificial ventilation.
d. Attention to fluid and electrolyte balance and calorie intake.
e. (Antitetanus serum. Raised in horses, this may prove dangerous since it is a foreign protein and may cause anaphylaxis).

Prophylaxis
This terrible disease can be so easily prevented by immunization with tetanus toxoid, prepared by treating the toxin chemically. Following a course, the individual produces antibodies which persist at adequate levels for at least five years (*see* Vol. I, p. 315). This is a very safe preparation and adverse reactions are usually very mild.

D. CEREBROVASCULAR ACCIDENT

1. Cerebral arterial thrombosis
Arterial thrombosis does occur in children occasionally due to acute fever, but mostly in old people due to arterial disease. Compared with embolism and haemorrhage the onset is slow, with symptoms developing over several hours or days.

The patient may not lose consciousness, but there may be fitting. The signs depend on the area of the brain in which the thrombus lies.

Treatment
Neurosurgery followed by anticoagulants.

2. Cerebral embolus
Embolism occurs from such causes as dislodged clot from atrial fibrillation, detachment of mural thrombus (over a myocardial infarct) or from bacterial endocarditis. Air embolism or fat embolism may occur in traumatic injury. Any of these emboli will result in cerebral infarction (death of tissue) in the area supplied by the vessel.

The symptoms and signs occur suddenly. The embolism may break up and pass on with rapid recovery, or lead to clot formation behind it. There may be haemorrhage into adjacent tissue following vascular damage.

Treatment

Anticoagulation to prevent further clot formation and embolization. Atrial fibrillation or damaged heart valves may be remediable.

3. (Intra) cerebral haemorrhage

Predisposing causes are arterial disease, high blood pressure and aneurysm of the cerebral vessels. Haemorrhage may occur anywhere but two common sites are branches of the middle cerebral artery and the apontine vessels (in the brainstem). Such haemorrhage is usually fatal.

Unconsciousness occurs rapidly, but sudden headache may precede this. If the brainstem is subjected to pressure from above or haemorrhage within it, respiration, vasomotor tone (pulse and blood pressure) and temperature may be affected. There may be hemiplegia (paralysis of the limbs and muscles of the face on the opposite side. The muscles are spastic (stiff) after a brief period of diminished muscle tone.

Treatment

The main problem for critical care personnel is that of management of a patient in coma, who may be a spastic hemiplegic.

If a high blood pressure is known to be present this should be treated after arrival in hospital. If the source of haemorrhage can be found on investigation (specialized X-ray examinations and electroencephalography) it may be amenable to neurosurgery.

Physiotherapy should start as soon as possible.

Cerebral haemorrhage is often devastating in its effects.

Patients rarely recover consciousness after more than 48 hours of coma.

4. Subarachnoid haemorrhage

This may be due to one of several causes:

a. Ruptured aneurysm—usually at the base of the brain ('berry' aneurysm).
b. Bleeding from a vascular (arteriovenous) malformation.
  (*a*) or (*b*) may be precipitated by hypertension (high blood pressure).
c. Head injury.

Symptoms and signs are severe headache of sudden onset and vomiting with rapid progression to unconsciousness. There may be specific neurological signs (spasticity, weakness) due to damage to nerve tissue caused by the bleeding.

There is usually *neck rigidity* (due to meningeal irritation by the blood in the cerebrospinal fluid) and signs of *raised intracranial pressure* (cardiovascular and respiratory effects—bradycardia and irregular respiration, papilloedema (swollen optic discs) and retinal haemorrhage). The cerebrospinal fluid is uniformly bloodstained.

Treatment

Special X-rays to elicit the cause may be performed. If this is remediable (e.g. an aneurysm) neurosurgery to tie or clip off the aneurysm may be indicated. Not every case will benefit from surgery, however, and there is a high mortality. Other treatment will include bed rest, control of hypertension and then gradual rehabilitation.

E. EPILEPSY

An epileptic fit may vary greatly in its severity from a momentary disturbance of consciousness (petit mal) to a generalized convulsion (grand mal). There is a further type of *focal fit* where consciousness may not be lost. For example, there may be progressive involvement of the muscles of a limb or limbs (Jacksonian 'March'). A generalized convulsion may or may not follow.

Temporal lobe epilepsy is of this focal type where an hallucination of smell or taste occurs and the patient may relive a past experience—the *déja vu* phenomenon.

The cause of many epileptic phenomena is unknown but may be due to biochemical imbalance within the brain. There may be a family history, but where the cause cannot be precisely defined, the term *idiopathic epilepsy* is used.

Epileptic manifestations may be due to almost any intracranial pathology, e.g. cerebral tumour, abscess, cerebrovascular accident, head injury, missile injuries and congenital malformations.

Description of fits

Generalized epilepsy

1. *Grand mal*

These fits are easily recognized. There are several well-defined stages.

a. The prodrome. The patient may be aware of an impending fit. This stage does not always occur.

b. Tonic stage. The patient loses consciousness and falls. The muscles are held contracted in spasm, making breathing impossible. Cyanosis usually occurs.

c. Clonic stage. The sustained muscle spasm abates and is replaced by repetitive convulsive movements. Those of the jaw and tongue cause frothing at the mouth. Both tonic and clonic stages last about 30 sec each, during which the patient may be incontinent.

d. Relaxation. Following the clonic stage the muscles relax. Consciousness gradually returns after a period of apparently normal sleep. There may be confusion and loss of memory and the patient may complain of headache.

When full recovery of consciousness does not occur between convulsions the patient is said to be in 'status epilepticus'.

2. *Petit mal*

There are several varieties; attacks always begin in childhood. They usually take the form of a transient loss of consciousness in which the patient may just interrupt what he is saying for a few seconds and then carry on as though nothing had happened.

Occasionally these brief episodes of unconsciousness may be accompanied by jerky movements of the limbs or abrupt falls, the patient quickly recovering consciousness.

Focal epilepsy

These may also progress to a grand mal seizure. The particular area of the brain involved will determine whether the fit is associated with movement or disturbances of memory or sensation. *Temporal lobe* epilepsy is the commonest type of focal epilepsy. The patient very commonly experiences an 'aura' of taste or more often smell. Characteristic of this type of fit is, however, the *deja vu* phenomenon where the patient seems to feel intense familiarity with his surroundings or current experience. There are often distinct changes of mood. Many patients do not fully lose consciousness but feel as though they are in a dream-like state. They may carry out movements or even behave violently during this state but have no recall of it when the fit has passed. Many temporal lobe fits do not follow this classic pattern however, and the diagnosis may only be suspected from an aura of smell or taste.

Jacksonian epilepsy is a variety in which the main feature is the spread of movements, initially localized, to involve nearby areas. For example, movements of the hand may spread to involve the arm and then possibly the whole of one half of the body. This occurs because the neurones involved, as they discharge, stimulate others in the adjacent motor cortex which then become involved. This produces the classic 'Jacksonian March'. Again the typical pattern described does not always occur. The patient may or may not lose consciousness and may lose the use of the affected limbs following the fit (Todd's palsy).

The electroencephalogram (EEG) is important in *confirming* the diagnosis of epilepsy but may be of no use between attacks. The diagnosis is therefore based on the history. Especially useful are reliable accounts from relatives who have witnessed the fits. Some patients, for example, only fit during their sleep or when subjected to a 'trigger' such as flashing lights.

It is most important to establish the *cause* of the fitting as this may be remediable (e.g. cerebral tumour). In most cases, however, surgical treatment will not completely cure the fits and anticonvulsant therapy with drugs is almost always required.

Further reading

Harvey A. McG., Johns R. J., McKusick V. A. et al (1984) *The Principles and Practice of Medicine*, 21st ed. New York, Appleton-Century-Crofts.

Salter R. H. (1984) *Essential Clinical Medicine*, Bristol, Wright PSG.

Chapter 16

Damage to Special Senses

J. R. Paskins

THE EYE (*Fig.* 16.1)

Traumatic conditions

Injuries to the eye are the commonest ophthalmic emergency. Most are comparatively minor, but all are potentially serious in that the sight may be affected. Eye injuries themselves are rarely life-threatening. This is important when a victim of multiple injuries is seen. In these cases the injured eye should be protected with a shield and attention focused on control of bleeding and protection of the airway. The history of an eye injury must be taken. Sometimes the diagnosis becomes obvious, e.g. a patient might mention that just before the injury he had been chipping at stone or rust, and then a careful search will have to be made for an embedded or penetrating foreign body.

Examination of the eye starts with an assessment of visual acuity; in this way any subsequent loss of vision may be accurately measured.

Special diagnostic tools are not essential. It is important to have a good light and some means of magnification. It has to be remembered that whilst most eye problems will be comparatively easy to deal with, there will be some that require urgent specialist advice and treatment. First aid management of eye problems should be constantly reassessed so that any deterioration is quickly noticed and the patient referred to a specialist unit.

Lacerations around the eye

Skin on the face heals quickly. There are rarely any problems with infection and even small areas of skin loss will usually heal without serious scarring.

DAMAGE TO SPECIAL SENSES

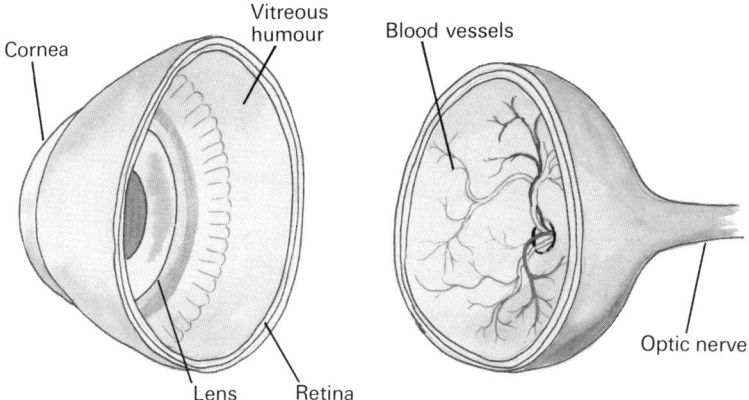

Fig. 16.1. The eye.

Foreign bodies

Bits of grit, metal and dust can be blown or rubbed into the eye. They can accumulate under the eyelids or embed themselves in the cornea or conjunctiva. If projected into the eye at high velocity they may actually penetrate the globe and cause disruption of the internal structure of the eye. This possibility must always be borne in mind, as loss of vision may result.

To examine an eye in order to find a foreign body the patient should be seated and the eye looked at with a bright light and magnification. Magnifying spectacles or a loupe are the most convenient tools but a simple magnifying glass will suffice.

The foreign body may simply be lying on the anterior surface of the eye, and can be wiped away with the corner of a clean handkerchief. If the object is not immediately apparent then the eye should be anaesthetized with 1 per cent amethocaine drops and the whole conjunctival and corneal surface examined. This will mean turning the upper lid inside out, as the inside surface of this lid is the most frequent site of hidden foreign bodies. To do this, stand behind the patient, pull the lid forward with the eyelashes and press a glass, plastic or wooden rod down on the outer surface of the lid. The eyelid is stiffened with a cartilaginous plate, rather like the peak of a school cap, and can be 'flicked' over.

If, after a full examination, the foreign body cannot be found it may be that it has already been wiped away, or washed away by tears. The patient's discomfort then will be due to a scratch or abrasion of the cornea or conjunctiva. Conjunctival abrasions, and even small lacerations, will usually heal quickly with no treatment.

Corneal abrasions are potentially serious. In order for it to be clearly seen, a corneal abrasion should be stained with fluorescein. Sterile fluorescein-impregnated strips (Fluorets) are available and easy to use. The orange end of the strip is placed under the upper lid of the anaesthetized eye and after a few moments it will be seen that the whole eyeball has turned bright orange. Any scratch on the corneal surface will now show up bright green, and can be easily seen with a torch and magnifier.

Corneal abrasions usually heal within 24-48 hours, and it is sufficient to rinse the eye with 0·5 per cent chloramphenicol drops and apply a pad for this time. The pad is important because the eye is anaesthetized by the amethocaine for some hours. If unprotected it could easily be damaged again without the patient feeling discomfort. A foreign body embedded in the cornea must be removed. If it cannot be dislodged with a moistened cotton wool bud, the patient should be taken to hospital straight away.

Perforating eye injuries

A foreign body which perforates the eye damages the internal structure and may cause the iris and its surrounding muscles to distort as fluid flows out of the eye chambers. This will cause disturbance or even loss of vision.

If there is a clear history of a high-velocity foreign body impact, even if the entry wound cannot be seen, it is essential to treat the eye as if it has been perforated.

The eyelids should be closed and a metal or plastic shield should be taped in place. Broad-spectrum antibiotics, such as a combination of ampicillin and flucloxacillin (Magnapen) should be started, and the patient should be transported to a specialist unit.

Contusions

The well-known 'black eye' results from bruising of the tissues around the margin of the orbit. The orbit is designed not only to hold the eye, but also to protect it. It is usually only the skin and soft tissues surrounding the eye which are damaged, unless the blow is with an object small enough to enter the bony orbit itself.

The swelling will sometimes make it difficult to examine the eye, but the eyelids should be opened and the eyeball checked to see whether the cornea is damaged, or whether there has been bleeding into the eyeball itself.

Damage confined to the skin and soft tissues can be safely left to settle on its own.

Blunt injury to the globe of the eye is shown by bleeding into the conjunctiva. There is sometimes bleeding into the anterior chamber, the space behind the cornea and in front of the iris. Conjunctival bleeding

DAMAGE TO SPECIAL SENSES

alone is not serious. However, it is important to be sure just how much of the conjunctiva is involved. A simple poke in the eye with a finger will cause a well-defined area of bleeding. If the patient moves his eye from side to side it is usually possible to see normal white, or sclera, behind or to one side of the haemorrhage. If, however, there has also been a fracture of the skull, there may be haemorrhage covering the entire white of the eye, and no rear limit to the bleeding will be seen.

'Blow-out' fractures

The eyeball contains fluid. If one surface is compressed, the other surfaces expand. A blow with a fist, or round object like a squash ball on the front of the eye will cause the rest of the eye to expand and push against the walls of the orbit. The floor is the weakest part, and may break under the strain and allow the muscles and fat under the eye to fall through the floor into the air-containing cavity below. This 'blow-out' fracture tends to trap the muscle which pulls the eye to look down. The patient becomes unable to look *up* properly, and so will complain of seeing two of everything (diplopia) when trying to look upwards. This double vision may take several days to develop, and when such an injury might have occurred the face should be X-rayed. Fractures of the bony orbit may be seen, or soft tissues may be present in the maxillary antrum, the normally empty air compartment under the eye.

Burns

In a fire where the face has been burned, the eyelids are often sufficient protection for the eyes which escape unscathed. However, in the event of a sudden flash, as in an explosion, the eyes will not have closed quickly enough, and the patient may sustain a heat or radiation burn. In any burn involving the face, the eyes must be examined so that any tissue loss from the front of the eyes can be seen.

Flash burns

These usually result from an over-exposure to ultraviolet radiation. Welders, and those using sun-lamps are often affected. So called 'snow-blindness' caused by sunlight at high altitude or reflected off snow and ice is the same disorder. The symptoms are pain, redness of the eyes, excessive watering and pain or discomfort made worse by bright light (photophobia). On examination the cornea will be dull, and if stained with fluorescein pinpoints of green stain will be seen, showing that there is widespread damage of the corneal epithelium. No treatment other than rest and reassurance is necessary. In most cases the patient can be told that normal vision will return in a day or two. Pain is best controlled by aspirin or paracetamol tablets, as local anaesthetic drops may delay healing. If there has been severe tissue loss, or the eye has been contaminated, then specialist advice should be obtained.

Chemical burns

Caustic (alkaline) substances cause more damage than acids. Caustic solutions continue to damage tissue for as long as they are in contact, whereas acids tend to be neutralized and inactivated when they have destroyed surface tissue. Treatment for any chemical burn must be immediate and prolonged. The eye is simply washed out with lots of water. The washing must be thorough; the head may, for example, be plunged into a bucket of water and the eyelids forced open. A more refined washout can be given with 0·9 per cent saline and a standard intravenous giving set. Washing should continue for several minutes until it is certain that all contaminant has been removed. There will sometimes be foreign bodies present as well, and all these have to be removed.

Further treatment will depend on the degree of damage. If the cornea is only slightly damaged then rest and pain-killers may suffice. However, the coatings of the eye may have been so badly eroded that the eye may later burst. All but the most minor chemical burns will need referral to an eye specialist.

Heat burns

The treatment is the same as for chemical burns. The eye should be irrigated, and foreign bodies removed. It is most important to prevent the eye from drying out, so after irrigation it may be necessary to tape plastic sheeting, like a blindfold across the eyes. Alternatively, antibiotic ointment can be put in the eyes, which are then closed with adhesive tape.

The eye—non-traumatic conditions

Most eye problems not related to injury will cause the patient to complain of a red, painful eye. This may be caused by a mild disorder such as conjunctivitis, or the results of a serious intra-ocular disease such as glaucoma. It is important to be able to recognize which conditions need to be treated by the specialist, as delay in management can lead to loss of sight.

As with injuries, accurate diagnosis depends on careful examination and close questioning of the patient.

Infections around the eye

The stye is the commonest of these. It is simply an infection, usually caused by staphylococci, of the follicle, or root, of an eye lash. Treatment is to remove the lash, and bathe the affected part in salt water. This will promote the discharge of pus from the follicle, and allow spontaneous healing. Antibiotics are not required. Meibomian cysts may sometimes look like styes. These are small pea-like swellings occurring in the eye lid. The cyst is a collection of an oily secretion from glands in the eye lids. Unlike styes they are rarely painful. They need to be removed surgically but do not present an urgent problem.

More serious deep-seated infection may occur around the eye. The patient will present with swelling, like a 'black eye', but the swelling is hot, red and very painful. This infection in the skin and soft tissues of the orbit may be life-threatening. If not treated the infection may spread posteriorly into the membranes, or meninges, of the brain. Immediate bed rest and antibiotics are required, and it may be necessary to operate to drain pus.

The viral infection shingles, herpes zoster ophthalmicus, can occur around the eye. It presents with painful blisters around the orbit and sometimes over the eye itself. It is particularly important to be aware of this condition because it may present simply as a rather larger than usual corneal abrasion of irregular outline. There may be a temptation to treat such ulcers with steroid drops. If the ulcer is caused by herpes virus there will be a catastrophic deterioration following steroids, and the eye may be lost.

The red eye

The commonest cause is inflammation of the outer covering of the eye, the conjunctiva. Conjunctivitis can be due to infection with bacteria or viruses. In the first case there is a thick creamy discharge of pus mixed with the tears; with viral infections the discharge is thin and watery. In simple conjunctivitis from whatever cause, the cornea, and the sclera immediately surrounding it are spared from the inflammation. Sight is not affected. The complaint will be of painful eyes and lids and excessive watering.

There is no danger to vision, and the condition will usually settle on its own. Regular bathing of the eyes with saline will help, and if the infection is clearly caused by bacteria then chloramphenicol eye drops or ointment will speed recovery.

Sometimes close examination will show that there is very little reddening of the eye except for that part just around the cornea. The conjunctiva of the eyelids is not involved and may look normal. This circumcorneal inflammation is a sign of trouble inside the eye. It may even be possible to see a collection of pus behind the cornea.

The patient will complain of severe pain and watering. Light, especially, may hurt the eyes, and the lids will either be blinking constantly or the patient will be unable to open his eyes properly at all.

There is no satisfactory first aid treatment for these conditions. They require specialist attention if the sight is to be saved.

Glaucoma, a condition in which the fluid fails to drain properly from the anterior chamber of the eye can also present as an emergency red eye. The patient will complain of severe pain, poor vision and a very red and hard eye. The hardness of the eye can be crudely measured by pressing over the closed top lid. Pressing one's own eye will give an idea of what it should feel like, and the glaucomatous eye will be found to be quite a bit harder, and very much more tender.

Immediate referral is essential.

Detached retina

This condition is not common. It is, however, particularly likely to occur in those with very short sight. These people have very long eyeballs, more like lemons than oranges, and the retina is not as well attached as usual. Normally the retina is stuck like wallpaper across the back of the inside of the globe. It may come unstuck at one corner, or be torn, as the result of quite mild trauma.

The patient experiences a dimming of vision, sometimes with flashes of coloured light, and seeks advice when repeated rubbing of the eye or cleaning of the spectacles fails to restore normal vision.

If the eye is examined with an ophthalmoscope the retina may be seen as a filmy floating grey curtain.

Treatment is surgical. The torn part is 'welded' back together and tacked to the back of the eye using a laser. If treated promptly normal sight will return.

EAR AND NOSE EMERGENCIES

The ear (*Fig.* 16.2)

The ear has three distinct parts: the outer ear which includes the auditory canal down to the ear drum; the middle ear, a tiny cavern within the skull which contains the three small bones of the auditory chain (the incus, malleus and stapes); and the inner ear which contains the sense organs which detect sound and control balance. These three parts will be considered separately.

The outer ear

Blows to the pinna, the visible shell-like structure which collects and reflects sound, can cause bleeding under the skin and the membrane which covers the cartilaginous skeleton of the ear, the perichondrium. This haematoma, if allowed to remain, causes scarring which will eventually lead to the well-known 'cauliflower ear'. The collection of blood has to be drained surgically under full aseptic conditions or inflammation of the cartilage, perichondritis, may result. Perichondritis may also follow lacerations to the pinna, and all of these need to be thoroughly cleaned and all dead or damaged tissue excised. In addition to this surgical treatment any severe wound of the outer ear should also be treated with antibiotics.

DAMAGE TO SPECIAL SENSES

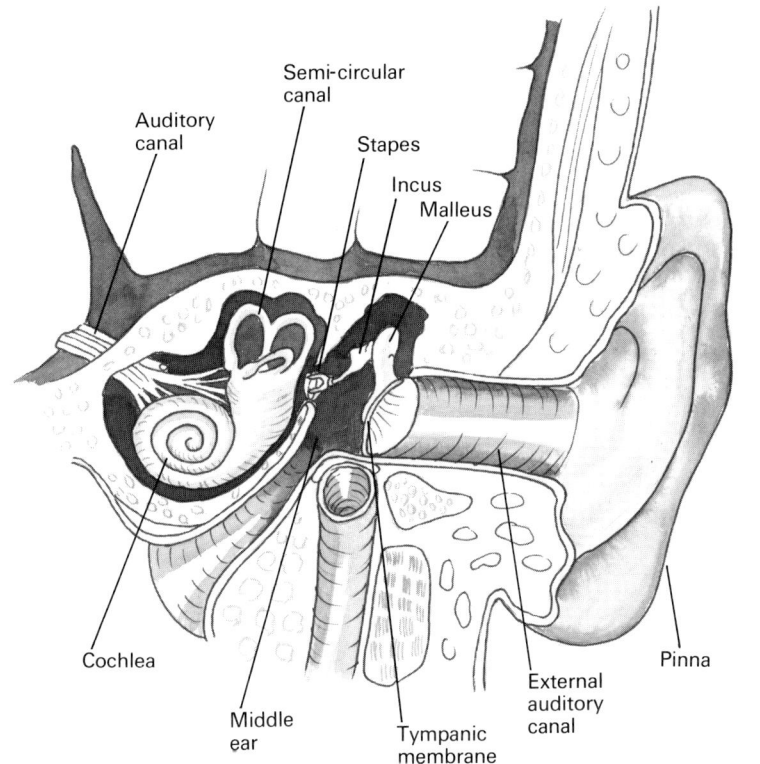

Fig. 16.2. The ear.

Foreign bodies sometimes find their way into the auditory canal and may lead to sudden deafness. They are often difficult to remove, but as they rarely need to be removed as an emergency, skilled help can usually be obtained.

Wax collects in the normal ear and is not usually a problem. However, a collection of hard wax, especially if mixed with dirt or dust can cause deafness, and should be softened with olive oil or proprietary drops (Cerumol) before removal by syringing.

The middle ear

The cavity of the middle ear is normally at atmospheric pressure. The Eustachian tube, which connects the middle ear to the back of the throat is normally patent, and allows the pressures inside the ear and outside to equalize. Changes of atmospheric pressure, such as occur when going up in an aeroplane or fast lift, cause a sensation in the middle ear. This sensation disappears when the ears 'pop'. This 'popping' is the Eustachian tube opening to allow the excess pressure to bleed from the middle ear. Most people can blow up the middle ear by closing their nose and mouth and blowing out their cheeks. The resulting high pressure in the ear is then relieved by swallowing, which opens the throat end of the Eustachian tube.

Because the middle ear is so sensitive to changes in environmental pressure, sudden changes in pressure, such as occur during the blast wave of an explosion, may actually rupture the most fragile part of the system, the tympanic membrane or ear drum. It is even possible for the ear drum to be ruptured by a blow to the outer ear, especially with a cupped hand, and self-inflicted ear drum rupture is not unknown.

Obviously the ear drum is also vulnerable to direct trauma. The careless use of a hairclip to clean out foreign bodies or wax is a common cause of damage.

If the perforation is small and there is no obvious infection of the canal then the hole will usually heal on its own. The canal should be sealed with cotton wool and petroleum jelly and the patient sent to an ear, nose and throat (ENT) specialist.

Continued exposure to abnormal pressure differences results in pain and deafness. This is called otitic barotrauma and may be a problem for divers, fliers and those in decompression chambers. This condition is usually managed in hospital, but immediate relief of pain can be obtained by puncture of the eardrum with a sterile hypodermic needle.

The inner ear

This is usually only damaged by trauma to the skull or by exposure to excessive noise. Gunfire, explosions or other very loud noises may cause deafness and ringing in the ears (tinnitus). There is usually a quick return of normal hearing, but the tinnitus may last longer. Severe deafness, or a slow recovery may need to be treated in hospital, and is certainly worthy of referral to an ENT surgeon.

Fractures of the skull near its base often extend into the bony and cartilaginous parts of the ear. This will cause deafness, dizziness and bleeding from the ear. There will also be a leak of cerebrospinal fluid from the ear, but as this will probably be mixed with blood it may be overlooked unless thought about. If fluid drips continuously from the ear then it is very likely to contain cerebrospinal fluid (CSF) as it does not then clot as well as pure blood.

Any patient with a head injury and bleeding from the ear, or for that matter the nose, should be assumed to have a basal skull fracture. These may be difficult to see on an X-ray, and if in doubt the patient should be carefully watched and started on antibiotics.

DAMAGE TO SPECIAL SENSES

Non-traumatic conditions of the ear

Most non-traumatic ear emergencies present as pain in the ear. It has to be remembered though that about half of all earaches have nothing to do with the ear at all and are the result of problems in the neck, face and upper chest.

The outer ear

The auditory canal may become infected (otitis externa). At first this will cause itching, and the patient tries to relieve this by scratching. This usually makes matters worse, and a discharge of clear fluid and sometimes pus will develop. Isolated boils may also occur in the canal. These conditions are very painful as the skin is sensitive and tightly attached to the cartilage underneath so that swelling very quickly pulls on nerve endings.

Infections in the outer ear need to be treated with analgesics first of all. Boils can be incised. Otitis externa should be treated by frequent cleaning of the ear with antiseptic and cotton wool buds. The patient has to be discouraged from scratching the ear. If the lymph glands around the ear are swollen, or the patient is generally ill, then a broad-spectrum antibiotic will be needed.

The middle ear

Infections of the middle ear, otitis media, may follow otitic barotrauma, but are more usually associated with throat and chest infections and are common in children. The patient feels ill, with a high temperature and an increasing throbbing pain deep in the ear. If the eardrum can be seen with an auriscope it may be found to be reddened or even bulging outwards. The pain is caused by the increased pressure in the middle ear as fluid and trapped air collect. To relieve the pressure the drum can be incised, or more simply the Eustachian tube can be unblocked. The lower end of the tube, which opens into the back of the throat, is often closed by the swelling which accompanies the respiratory tract infection. Anti-histamines, decongestants, and nasal decongestant drops usually reduce the swelling and allow the tube to open and the middle ear to drain. The patient will usually respond rapidly to a broad-spectrum antibiotic, and this may be enough on its own.

If untreated, otitis media may spread through the bone of the middle ear cavity causing pain and redness behind the ear as infection enters the mastoid air cells at the base of the skull. This is a surgical emergency and needs prompt skilled attention.

The inner ear

Emergencies affecting the inner ear are not common. The most frequently seen condition is a combination of dizziness, nausea and vomiting which is known as vertigo.

Vertigo is usually short lasting. The patient often recovers in a few hours. Bed rest, anti-emetic drugs which will stop the sickness, and antihistamines are often sufficient. If an attack does not settle in a few hours it is possible that a much more serious condition is affecting the labyrinth, the collection of organs which control balance, and specialist help will be required.

Trauma to the nose

The nose, by virtue of its position, is particularly vulnerable to injury. It comprises a small bony and a larger cartilaginous framework surrounding air passages with a very sensitive membrane. The lining of the nose is richly supplied with blood. Most traumatic and some non-traumatic conditions present as nose bleeds (epistaxis).

Broken nose

The bones of the nose are easily broken by direct violence. The cartilage which makes up the rest of the nasal skeleton can also be damaged. Often there will be so much swelling that the shape cannot clearly be seen, but sometimes the nose can be seen to deviate to one side or the other. This sort of fracture, with misalignment of the nose, will need reduction or straightening. This may be done at any time up to about 10–14 days after the injury. It may even be done straight away after the injury if the patient's sensitivities are dimmed enough to allow reduction without an anaesthetic.

Diagnosis is not difficult. X-rays are not really needed, but will often confirm the presence of a fracture.

It is more important to look inside the nose than to worry about its outside shape. The nose is divided into two halves by a central cartilaginous plate, the septum. Like the cartilage of the ear this plate is covered with perichondrium, bleeding into which gives rise to a large potentially dangerous swelling. This septal haematoma, if left, can cause infection and collapse of the bridge of the nose. A swollen septum is a sign that drainage of the haematoma is required, and surgical advice should be obtained.

Nose bleeds

Nose bleeds may be so trivial that they are of only passing interest to the patient, or so severe that life is threatened. As mentioned above, the lining of the nose, particularly over the septum, is richly supplied with blood vessels. Four major vessels come together near the front of the septum. This area, known as Little's area, is a common site of bleeding. In older people bleeding from the nose tends to occur deep in the recesses of the nasal cavity and can be difficult to treat.

Bleeding from Little's area can nearly always be stopped by pinching the front of the nose, just above the nostrils, between thumb and forefinger. The patient should sit, leaning forward, gripping his own nose tightly for several minutes. Even if the bleeding is not completely stopped, it may be possible to see the bleeding point when the force of the haemorrhage has subsided. Continued bleeding should be controlled by cautery of the area with silver nitrate or a hot wire.

If this is not possible, or fails, then the nose should be packed. Ribbon gauze impregnated with BIPP (bismuth iodoform paraffin paste) should be used. The paste has an antiseptic effect and prevents the pack from becoming too offensive.

The layers of the nasal packing have to fill the entire cavity, which is larger at the back than at the front. The nasal cavity should be anaesthetized with a local anaesthetic spray before packing. Once in place, nasal packs have to be watched carefully. It is quite possible for them to slip backwards and obstruct the airway. A patient with a nasal pack should not be allowed to leave hospital.

Epistaxis usually occurs as the result of trauma, but it is also a feature of some disorders of blood clotting and high blood pressure.

Fractures of the base of the skull often cause leakage of CSF. If the fracture has been at the front of the skull then CSF will leak from the nose. As in the case of leakage from the ear, bloodstained CSF leaking from the nose can be distinguished from pure blood by its poor clotting.

Patients with frontal basal fractures may also lose their sense of smell. At the base of the skull, behind the bridge of the nose, is a small, eggshell thin plate of bone. The plate is perforated like a tea-bag and through these small holes emerge the olfactory nerve roots which supply the sense of smell. Basal skull fractures in this region often include this plate (cribriform plate) and thus disrupt or divide some or all of the nerve roots. This leads to instant and irreversible loss of the sense of smell.

Foreign bodies

Children and, to a lesser extent, adults, will sometimes put small objects into the nostrils. These can be difficult to remove. If they are solid objects, e.g. beads, then they may cause nothing more than mild irritation and a blocked nose. Porous objects, however, like bits of paper or sponge, cause a continuing offensive nasal discharge.

Foreign bodies should be removed as soon as possible as they may suddenly dislodge and be inhaled with disastrous results.

Unless the object is easily reached with blunt forceps or other suitable instrument, the patient should be referred to an ENT specialist.

Further reading

Bankes J. L. K. (1982) *Clinical Ophthalmology: A Text and Colour Atlas*. Edinburgh, Churchill Livingstone.

Duguid I. M. and Berry Anne A. (1971) *Ophthalmology*. London, Hodder & Stoughton.
Pracy R., Siegler J. and Stell P. M. (1974) *A Short Textbook: Ear, Nose and Throat*. London, Hodder & Stoughton.
Smyth G. D. L. (1978) *Diagnostic Ear, Nose and Throat*. Oxford, Oxford Medical Publications.
Trevor-Roper, Patrick D. (1975) *Lecture Notes on Ophthalmology*. Blackwell Scientific Publications.

Chapter 17

Disorders of the Endocrine System

J. V. Mundy

TRAUMA

Damage to the pituitary gland following head injury can be suspected from certain clinical signs. The patient is usually comatose immediately following the accident, and commonly has sustained injury to the frontal region together with widespread fractures. In some cases there is damage to the optic nerves or oculomotor nerves. The specific signs suggesting pituitary or hypothalamic damage include:

1. *Hypothermia.* Temperatures as low as 32°C have been recorded.
2. *Slow pulse and low blood pressure.*
3. *Slow respiratory rate and reduced muscular tone.*

Treatment

Treatment should be aimed at maintaining a normal temperature. Hydrocortisone (100 mg once or twice daily) may be required and often has a dramatic effect in restoring blood pressure. Long-acting corticotrophins (ACTH) may be required after the acute period. In the later stages thyroxine may be indicated.

Pituitary and hypothalamic injury is likely to be accompanied by other severe brain damage, but it is quite clear that recognition of injury to these structures, followed by appropriate supportive treatment will help some patients to survive the most critical period after injury.

DIABETES INSIPIDUS

This syndrome may develop after head injury. It involves the passage of large quantities of dilute urine. In the conscious patient with an intact 'thirst mechanism', drinking large quantities of fluid corrects the deficit and keeps the patient healthy. In the unconscious patient it is necessary to provide an increased fluid intake, perhaps up to 5 litres daily. In severe cases it may be necessary to administer synthetic antidiuretic hormone.

DIABETES MELLITUS

In Great Britain 1–2 per cent of people suffer from diabetes (the term 'diabetes' is taken to mean diabetes mellitus). The main feature of the disease is a disorder of carbohydrate metabolism associated with a lack of insulin, leading to high blood sugar levels.

During the course of the disease damage may occur in many organ systems, including arterial, cardiac, renal and neurological systems, and in the eyes and skin.

Diabetes mellitus is classified into two main types:

TYPE 1	TYPE 2
Acute onset	Gradual onset
Mostly young people	Mostly older people
Usually thin	Usually fat
Always require insulin	Rarely require insulin to maintain life

A diabetic state may also develop during pregnancy and when patients are receiving steroid medication.

Biochemical consequences of diabetes mellitus

The effect of insulin is to facilitate the transfer of glucose across the cell membrane. It also acts in the cell to:
 1. Promote the build up of glycogen (the storage form of glucose).
 2. Promote protein synthesis.
 3. Inhibit breakdown of fats.

Insulin deficiency therefore results in glycogen, protein and fat breakdown (*Fig.* 17.1).

Protein degradation releases amino acids which may be 'glucogenic' (produce glucose through further metabolism) or 'ketogenic' (produce ketones, e.g. acetone). Breakdown of glycogen, together with gluconeogenesis (production of glucose from glucogenic amino acids) raises the plasma glucose. Lipolysis (breakdown of fat) releases triglycerides, which are broken down to glycerol. This substance is also glucogenic.

Free fatty acids, also products of triglyceride breakdown, are converted to acetyl coenzyme A, which eventually may be metabolized to β-hydroxybutyrate or acetone (ketone bodies) (*see Fig.* 17.1).

The main features of insulin deficiency, therefore, are a raised plasma glucose concentration (hyperglycaemia) and ketoacidosis (acidosis due to increased levels of ketone bodies in the blood).

DISORDERS OF THE ENDOCRINE SYSTEM

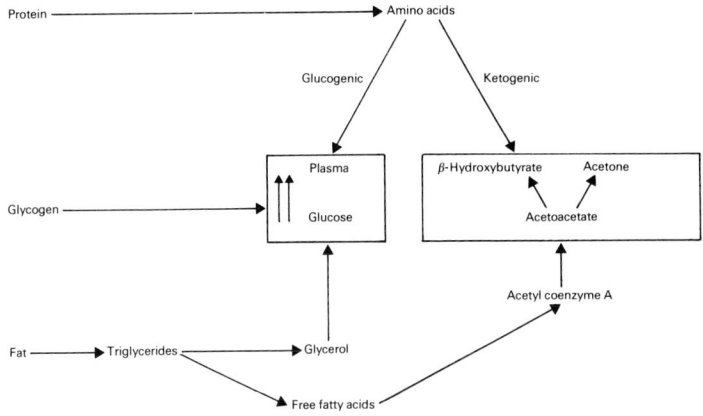

Fig. 17.1. Substrate utilization.

Pathological consequences of diabetes mellitus

Prolonged hyperglycaemia, which occurs in poorly controlled diabetes, may cause biochemical changes in many tissues. The glycoproteins of cell basement membranes become excessively and abnormally glycosylated (combined with the sugar), resulting in their becoming thickened; this can be readily observed in the glomeruli of the kidney.

Sorbitol, which is the sugar alcohol of glucose, may accumulate in the lens of the eye, giving rise to cataracts and is possibly also involved in the development of some forms of diabetes-induced nerve damage (diabetic neuropathy).

Alterations in metabolism also play a part in the process of large blood vessel damage of diabetes, especially the hyperlipidaemia (high level of blood fats) which follows altered fat metabolism.

Diagnosis and monitoring of diabetes mellitus

Screening for diabetes is conveniently carried out by testing the urine for glucose with a 'Clinistix' or similar reagent strip. Glucose is not normally found in the urine of healthy individuals. The point at which glucose 'spills over' from the blood into the urine is called the renal threshold for glucose and is about 10 mmol/L (180 mg/100 ml) the normal range of random blood sugars lies between 2·8 and 7·3 mmol/L (50 and 131 mg/100 ml)).

Measurement of blood sugar is preferable to urine testing and this can be done easily using glucose oxidase reagent strips, e.g. 'Dextrostix'. A single large drop of blood obtained from a finger prick is sufficient.

Formal diagnosis of diabetes can be made using the glucose tolerance test: 50 g of glucose are taken orally and blood and urine samples estimated for glucose at half-hourly intervals for 2 hours. A blood sugar value of greater than 10 mmol/L (180 mg/100 ml) then indicates diabetes mellitus.

Clinical features
Type 1
Increasing hyperglycaemia raises the plasma osmolality leading to excessive production of urine and consequently frequent drinking because of extreme thirst. The presence of excess glucose in the body fluids encourages bacterial and fungal growth. The absence of insulin prevents the build up of protein from amino acids so that muscular wasting and weight loss occur. Eventually large amounts of acetyl coenzyme A lead to the production of ketone bodies in excess, resulting in ketoacidosis, followed by coma.

Type 2
Any of the features of type 1 diabetes may occur but ketoacidosis is an uncommon and late feature. Weight gain is common. Infections, particularly in the skin folds, occur. Because the onset is slow and insidious many patients present with late features such as neuropathy, foot ulceration and cataract.

Late features of diabetes mellitus include:

1. Arterial disease
Atheroma produced by altered lipid metabolism produces:
   a. Coronary artery disease (angina, myocardial infarction).
   b. Cerebrovascular disease (strokes).
   c. Peripheral vessel disease (poor healing, ulceration, retinal damage).

2. Heart disease
Due to:
   a. Coronary artery disease as in (a) above.
   b. Damage to the autonomic nerves producing abnormal cardiac rhythm.
   c. Cardiomyopathy (a weakness of cardiac muscle) due to metabolically abnormal myocardial cells.

3. Skin disease
Small vessel disease causes ischaemic skin and mucous membranes, increasing the tendency to infection.

4. Sensory neuropathy

Damage to sensory nerves occurs particularly in poorly controlled diabetics. It is probably due to abnormal metabolism in the nerve. Commonly the long nerves are affected first, causing numbness or pain in the feet. In the elderly this may lead to the development of extensive ulcers, infected toenails and other lesions. Because of the lack of pain sensation injuries pass unnoticed.

5. Autonomic neuropathy

Involvement of the sympathetic and parasympathetic nervous systems occurs increasingly as the disease progresses. The following are consequences of diabetic autonomic neuropathy:
   Postural hypotension (fainting on rising from bed for example)
   Irregular heart rate
   Impotence
   Retention of urine
   Loss of ability to sweat
   Pupillary abnormalities
   Diarrhoea or constipation
   It is important to be aware of the existence of autonomic neuropathy in diabetics about to undergo surgery as there is a risk of cardiac arrest or autonomic instability.

6. Kidney disease

Infective conditions are common, especially cystitis. Other conditions include:
   Acute pyelonephritis
   Abscess formation around the kidney
   Direct damage to the glomeruli or renal tubules
   Blood vessel damage within the kidney

7. The eye

Diabetes is the most common cause of blindness among young adults in the UK. Diabetic damage to the eye includes:
   Extra-ocular muscle weakness
   Glaucoma
   Cataract
   Retinopathy

Treatment of diabetes mellitus

There are three main aspects to the treatment of diabetes—diet, oral hypoglycaemic agents and insulin.

1. Diet

Intelligent management of the diet is the mainstay of the treatment of all diabetic patients. The diet may be restricted in terms of grams of carbohydrate or total calories. As well as achieving a suitable balance with protein and fat it is important to achieve an adequate supply of vitamins and minerals. All diabetics, especially those newly diagnosed, should be seen and advised by a dietitian.

The exact diet will depend upon the age, build and occupation of the patient and the type of diabetes.

2. Drugs

a. Oral hypoglycaemic agents

These drugs are used virtually exclusively in type 2 diabetes. Type 2 diabetics suffer from a relative lack of insulin, i.e., insulin is not released in sufficient quantities from the pancreas or it is not utilized correctly at cellular level.

Oral hypoglycaemic agents help either to stimulate release of insulin from the pancreas (e.g. tolbutamide, chlorpropamide—two drugs from the sulphonylurea group) or promote the peripheral utilization of insulin (e.g. metformin—a biguanide, *see also* Vol. 1, Chapter 35). The biguanide drugs also have the useful property of suppressing appetite. These drugs are therefore valuable in the obese, middle-aged diabetic who has failed to respond to restriction of carbohydrate alone.

b. Insulin

In the past in the UK insulin was available in concentrations of 20, 40 and 80 international units per ml. At the time of writing patients are being converted to the new standard 'U100' insulin (100 units per ml). This will make calculation of the dose simpler and safer for the patient.

Not only does the strength of insulin preparations vary but also their duration of action. Insulins can be classified into 'short', 'medium' and 'long' acting (from 4 to 36 hours). This allows for 24-hour insulin cover with flexibility for meals and exercise.

The end product of conventional insulin manufacture (pork and beef insulin) contains many impurities. A purified monocomponent insulin is mostly used now.

When introducing insulin, full explanation and instruction are essential. The patient must be supervized closely until he can manage his own injections. It is most important that the injection is made at the correct depth, avoiding veins.

Injection sites should be 'rotated' so that the same piece of skin is not in constant use. Failure to do this may lead to erratic absorption of the drug and tissue damage (fat necrosis).

The management of diabetic patients

The aim is to achieve as near normal blood sugar levels as possible. Many patients with type 2 diabetes may be controlled with a suitable diet alone and then reviewed every 6 months. Patients with blood sugars consistently above 10 mmol/L (180 mg/100 ml) should be started on a small dose of an oral hypoglycaemic agent, the dose being gradually increased to achieve control.

Patients with type 1 diabetes require insulin. Young patients usually require twice-daily injections of insulin to maintain the best possible control. When commencing insulin therapy the patient should be admitted to hospital to enable requirements to be assessed and injection technique taught. After adjustments have been made and the control established, the patient is allowed home and reviewed monthly in the clinic. Regular checks are made on the optic fundi, the cardiovascular system, the skin (particularly of the feet) and peripheral nerves.

Coma in diabetes

a. *Hypoglycaemia*

This results from:
Overdosage with insulin
Overdosage with oral hypoglycaemic agents
Insufficient carbohydrate intake

Symptoms appear when, typically, the blood sugar falls below about 2·5 mmol/L (45 mg/100 ml). If the patient has damage to the autonomic nervous system symptoms may be minimal. The symptoms are caused by lack of glucose in the brain and activation of the sympathetic nervous system. The symptoms are:
Sweating
Tachycardia
Tremor
Dilated pupils
Peripheral vasoconstriction
Hunger-disturbed behaviour, often aggression
Dizziness, progressing to:
Loss of consciousness

The onset of hypoglycaemia is rapid and the diagnosis can be quickly confirmed by measuring the blood glucose using glucose oxidase strips (e.g. Dextrostix). Patients who are unconscious or uncooperative require intravenous glucose solution (25 g or 50 ml of 50 per cent solution). In a conscious patient, 50 g of dextrose may be given orally. If the patient is unconscious and a vein cannot be found glucagon 1 mg injected intramuscularly will restore consciousness for long enough to allow glucose to be given orally.

In patients who are likely to have frequent attacks of hypoglycaemia a supply of glucagon may be given to a friend or relative to give to the patient if necessary.

Hyperglycaemic coma

This appears to be occurring less frequently, perhaps due to better education of patients. It may be a presenting feature or develop during treatment. Hyperglycaemic coma is often precipitated by infections, especially renal, respiratory or gastrointestinal. It may also occur during myocardial infarction and cerebrovascular accidents.

The onset is gradual (hours to days), the patient may be confused, drowsy, severely dehydrated and have a strong smell of acetone on the breath. He may be overbreathing (due to the acidosis) and the blood pressure may be low. Often the patient has not been eating properly and has stopped taking insulin.

The treatment of ketoacidosis aims:
1. To correct dehydration
2. To lower the blood glucose
3. To maintain a normal plasma potassium

The acidosis is usually corrected by these measures alone and rarely requires specific treatment with, e.g., bicarbonate.

Correction of dehydration is life saving and a reliable intravenous infusion should be set up immediately. Hartmann's solution is poorly tolerated and 0·9 per cent saline is the fluid of choice. The volume infused should be carefully monitored and the provision of a central venous line is recommended.

Initial investigations should include:
1. Blood glucose (laboratory sample)
2. Plasma electrolytes, especially sodium and potassium
3. Arterial blood gas analysis
4. Packed cell volume (haematocrit)
5. Full blood count
6. Chest radiograph
7. Cultures of blood, urine, sputum and from any areas of sepsis

Further management depends upon the clinical state of the patient and their response to initial rehydration.

A constant infusion of insulin is usually administered to control the blood sugar.

Regular blood sugar and plasma potassium estimations should be made and potassium supplements given as necessary.

Infection may precipitate poor control of the diabetic state and if suspected should be treated with a suitable antibiotic, given intravenously.

ADDISON'S DISEASE

This is the name given to the rare syndrome of primary failure of the adrenal cortex. There are a number of causes of Addison's disease, but in about 50 per cent of cases no cause can be found.

Causes of primary hypoadrenalism
1. Autoimmune destruction of adrenal cortex
2. Tuberculosis
3. Infiltrations
4. Metastatic cancer (secondary spread, usually from breast or bronchus)

Clinical features
There is a deficiency of both glucocorticoids and mineralocorticoids. Symptoms are vague at first, this phase lasting for several months. Lack of glucocorticoids causes fatigue, weakness and weight loss.

Later in the course of the illness the patient may develop loss of appetite, abdominal pain, nausea, vomiting and diarrhoea.

Lack of mineralocorticoid leads to excess urinary sodium loss. Salt-craving may be a feature in many cases, but if salt is not supplied there is hypotension, often manifest as postural falls in blood pressure when a patient stands up, with resulting dizziness and tachycardia

The plasma level of adrenocorticotrophic hormone (ACTH) is high because the negative feedback provided by cortisol is absent or reduced.

ACTH also stimulates the pigment-producing cells (melanocytes) and pigmentation of the skin and mucous membranes develops. The pigmentation is a typical brown-grey colour and is best seen in exposed areas, skin creases, friction areas and in the mouth.

Treatment
Glucocortoid therapy should as near as possible follow the normal diurnal requirement of steroids; an example of maintenance therapy is cortisone 25 mg in the morning and 12·5 mg at night.

Mineralocorticoid replacement is also necessary and fludrocortisone 50-100 mg is given in a once daily dose.

CUSHING'S DISEASE

This uncommon condition was described by the famous American neurosurgeon, whose name it bears. There are three similar disorders with differing pathologies:

1. *Cushing's Disease.* This term is used when the primary abnormality is a disorder of the pituitary or hypothalamus, usually a tumour causing excess production of ACTH.

2. *Cushing's Syndrome.* Used when there is an adrenal tumour.
3. *'Cushingoid'.* This term describes the features of patients who have developed the features of Cushing's syndrome while being treated with steroids.

Apart from development of Cushingoid features following treatment with steroids, this disorder is very rare and is the result of excess corticosteroids.

Clinical presentation
1. Alteration in appearance caused by redistribution of body fat, 'mooning' of the face, obesity of the trunk, with a buffalo hump. The term 'lemon on matchsticks' has been used to describe Cushingoid patients.
2. Muscle weakness caused by protein breakdown, wide purple striae (streaks in the skin) on the abdomen, thighs and buttocks, and easy bruising.
3. Osteoporosis ('thinning' of the bones) with backache and vertebral collapse.
4. Disturbance of carbohydrate metabolism which may become frank diabetes.
5. Electrolyte disturbance with sodium retention and potassium loss.
6. Hypertension related to sodium retention.
7. Masculinization of females with amenorrhoea (absence of menstruation), development of facial hair, deep voice and acne.
8. Mental disturbance—depression or mania and occasional exaggeration of previous psychiatric abnormalities.

Investigation of Cushing's disease
The investigation is complex but first of all requires confirmation of raised plasma cortisol levels with lack of normal diurnal variation.

Treatment
Adrenal tumours should be removed, following which replacement steroids will be required for a short time because the normal gland will have been suppressed by the lack of ACTH. Bilateral adrenalectomy should be performed for adrenal hyperplasia. Full doses of replacement steroids will be required for the rest of the patient's life. The treatment of hypothalamic and pituitary disease is more difficult. Surgery to the pituitary gland usually produces a cure but requires postoperative hormone replacement not only for adrenal and thyroid glands, but also for the sex hormones. The latter can be a major problem in young people.

DISORDERS OF THE ENDOCRINE SYSTEM

THYROID DISEASE

Thyroid disease is relatively common. Enlargement of the thyroid of varying degrees is frequent especially in women. Both hypothyroidism and hyperthyroidism are relatively common. Thyroid cancer is rare.

Hypothyroidism (myxoedema)

This results from a low level of circulating thyroid hormone, either free thyroxine (T4) or tri-iodothyronine (T3). The term 'myxoedema' means that there is a deposit of mucopolysaccharide beneath the skin, producing swelling of subcutaneous tissues.

Causes of hypothyroidism

1. Thyroiditis.
2. Destructive therapy for hyperthyroidism or carcinoma by operation or radioactive iodine.
3. Failure of development of thyroid gland. This may cause cretinism in infancy.
4. Large or prolonged doses of antithyroid agents e.g. iodine.

The onset of hypothyroidism is slow and may be difficult to distinguish from depression. The condition may be far advanced before diagnosis is made. The most important symptoms are:

- Intolerance of cold
- Reduced energy
- Physical tiredness
- Slow thinking
- Increase in weight
- Hoarseness of the voice
- Reduced sweating
- Dry, rough skin
- Thinning hair
- Deafness
- Constipation
- Muscular pains
- 'Pins and needles'

The patient has a typical facial appearance with pallor and puffiness around the eyes. Ths skin is cold, movements are slow, there is a slow pulse and slowing of the recovery phase of the ankle jerk reflexes. Ischaemic heart disease is common. Central nervous system involvement may produce intellectual impairment and dementia (myxoedema madness) and coma (with hypothermia).

Investigations

These may show:
Low free thyroxine index
Raised serum cholesterol
Anaemia
Raised erythrocyte sedimentation rate
ECG shows low voltage with flattened or inverted T waves

Treatment
Thyroxine is given in doses of 0·05–0·3 mg a day. Patients should be warned that treatment is for life.

Hyperthyroidism

The clinical picture results from an excess of thyroid hormones, triiodothyronine (T3) and thyroxine (T4). There is a general acceleration of metabolism.
Symptoms include:
Preference for cold weather
Sweating
Excessive movement and irritability
Weight loss, despite increased appetite
Tremor and palpitations
Diarrhoea, abdominal pain and vomiting

In the elderly, cardiac features are more common and atrial fibrillation, cardiac enlargement and outright heart failure are prominent.

Physical examination reveals warm sweaty hands. The pulse is rapid even during sleep, an important difference from patients with an anxiety state, in whom the pulse slows during sleep.

Atrial fibrillation is often found in the older patient and hyperthyroidism must always be considered when atrial fibrillation has developed for no apparent reason.

A fine tremor of the outstretched hands is common and tendon reflexes are brisk. Wasting of the limb girdle muscles (shoulders and pelvis) may cause extreme weakness. Often the thyroid gland is generally enlarged and soft, but may also be irregularly enlarged and hard.

Eye lid retraction, protrusion of the eyeballs and lid-lag are commonly found, but are more severe in the form of hyperthyroidism called Graves' disease.

Investigation of thyrotoxicosis

This can be very complicated, but at least one test should be done before starting treatment to confirm and assess the diagnosis.
The tests available include:

T4	Basal TSH measurements
T3 (resin) uptake	T3 suppression test
Protein bound iodine (PBI)	TSH stimulation test
Free thyroxine index (FTI)	TRH test
^{132}I Uptake	

Less specific investigations include:
ECG
Chest X-ray
Basal metabolic rate

Treatment of hyperthyroidism
Three methods are available:
1. Antithyroid drugs (Carbimazole)
2. Radioactive iodine
3. Surgery

Further reading
Daggett P. R. (1981) *Clinical Endocrinology.* London, Arnold.
Oakley W. G., Pyke D. A. and Taylor K. W. (1980) *Diabetes and its Management.* Oxford, Blackwell Scientific Publications.
O'Riordan J. L. H., Malan P. G. and Gould R. P. (ed.) (1982) *Essentials of Endocrinology.* Oxford, Blackwell Scientific Publications.

Chapter 18

Pregnancy and Related Problems

M. J. Wolfe

THE PHYSIOLOGY OF PREGNANCY

In females who have passed puberty, ovulation occurs more or less regularly about once a month. During the menstrual cycle ova are developed into more mature forms known as *Graafian follicles*. The Graafian follicle moves gradually toward the surface of the ovary under the influence of the hormone FSH (follicle-stimulating hormone) from the pituitary gland. At about midcycle (for an average cycle of 28 days) the ovum is released into the peritoneal cavity. It is picked up by the fimbriae of the Fallopian tube, which it enters. If the ovum is fertilized by a sperm, this normally occurs in the Fallopian tube. If the ovum is not fertilized it passes down the tube into the uterine cavity where it is shed with the uterine lining (the endometrium) at menstruation.

If the ovum is fertilized, however, luteinizing hormone (LH) brings about conversion of the empty Graafian follicle into the corpus luteum. This corpus luteum then secretes *progesterone* which prevents the maturation of any further ova.

The fertilized ovum divides repeatedly until a small ball of cells rather like a blackberry is formed. This is called the *morula*. A cavity forms between the peripheral and central cells of the morula which now becomes known as the *blastocyst*. The outer layer of cells is destined to form the placenta. The embryo is formed within this layer of cells and eventually comes to lie in a fluid-filled cavity, the *amniotic cavity*, attached to the placenta by the *umbilical cord*. This process does not take place in the cavity of the uterus, however, since the fertilized embryo becomes *implanted* in the lining of the uterus when only a few cell divisions have taken place.

DIAGNOSIS OF PREGNANCY

Pregnancy cannot be certainly proven until a fetus has been detected, but it can be presumed to have occurred when the maternal changes of pregnancy such as amenorrhoea (cessation of periods), breast changes and uterine enlargement have occurred. These days hormonal pregnancy tests are used as reliable indicators of the presence of a pregnancy. They do not, however, guarantee that the pregnancy is developing normally. Most, but by no means all, women suffer nausea and vomiting in early pregnancy ('morning sickness') which is presumed to be due to high levels of the hormone HCG (human chorionic gonadotrophin). The hormonal pregnancy tests in common use rely upon the detection of HCG in the maternal urine, although certain tumours can produce HCG so the pregnancy test cannot prove the existence within the uterus of a normal fetus.

The fetal heart beat can be detected by ultrasonic techniques as early as the eighth week after the last period. Actual palpation of fetal parts is not usually possible before 20 weeks which is also the time at which fetal movement begins to be felt by the mother. The expected date of delivery of the fetus can be predicted at 40 weeks after the first day of the last menstrual period (LMP). Normal pregnancy is, however, accepted as 38–42 weeks.

The period of time over which the pregnancy continues is known as *gestation*. The average 40 weeks are conventionally divided into three more or less equal trimesters. The third trimester begins at 28 weeks and fetuses born after this time have a reasonable chance of survival. Most fetal weight gain occurs in the third trimester.

The mother of course gains a considerable amount of weight during her pregnancy (12–14 kg). Much of this is accumulated as fluid and fat, although there is an increase in the weight of the uterus. At term the fetus and placenta together weigh about 4 kg.

ANTENATAL CARE

Antenatal medical and nursing care is judged to be of great importance to the well-being of both mother and baby. Mothers should be encouraged to seek advice as soon as they think they are pregnant and to attend for regular visits throughout pregnancy.

Good antenatal care should detect the presence of any systemic disease such as cardiovascular, renal or endocrine problems, particularly diabetes. A careful watch is kept for obstetric complications which may be prevented or ameliorated by the clinician having advanced warning of their existence. Hypertension and pre-eclampsia (*see below*) are particularly important in this respect.

Below is given a list of common complaints associated with pregnancy.
1. Nausea and vomiting
2. Constipation
3. Reflux oesophagitis (heartburn)

4. Urinary frequency (sometimes accompanied by stress incontinence, i.e the voiding of urine when coughing or straining)
5. Vaginal discharge
6. Backache
7. Varicose veins
8. Mood changes

NORMAL LABOUR

'Labour' is the term given to the process whereby the fetus is expelled from the uterus into the outside world.

Anatomy

The uterine cervix acts as a sphincter or valve, keeping the fetus within the uterus until labour begins. The cervix is further closed with a plug of mucus, which is expelled at the onset of labour (the 'show').

After about twenty-four weeks of pregnancy the cervix begins to undergo certain changes. The cervical canal becomes shorter (*effacement*), and the cervical opening (internal and external os) become dilated. The extent to which these changes occur in individual women is very variable.

Uterine contractility

At about twenty weeks, the uterine muscle undergoes an increase in contractility and becomes progressively more sensitive to the effects of the hormone oxytocin. These contractions continue to increase as the pregnancy advances.

Labour

The onset of labour is characterized by the onset of regular contractions, which usually become frequent and painful, occurring every few minutes in established labour. Oxytocin is produced in increased amounts during labour.

The first stage of labour lasts from the onset of regular contractions to full dilatation (opening) of the cervix.

The second stage of labour is the period following full dilatation until birth of the baby.

The third stage of labour is the interval between the birth of the baby and delivery of the placenta.

First stage

The onset of regular contractions marks the beginning of the first stage. At the same time the uterus undergoes progressive sustained contraction, the uterus feeling hard when felt through the abdominal wall. As the contractions increase in severity they also increase in frequency. The pain is felt in the lower back, abdomen and thighs. Sometimes the back pain can be very uncomfortable indeed.

These contractions bring about dilatation of the cervix, which is accompanied by a 'show' of bloodstained mucus (the cervical mucus plug). The first stage of labour may last up to 24 hours (but in modern obstetric practice the obstetrician will rarely allow his patient to labour as long as this without intervention.

Toward the end of the first stage there is usually rupture of the membranes surrounding the fetus with a gush of amniotic fluid ('the waters'). The first stage of labour ends with full dilatation of the cervix.

Second stage

The character of the pain usually changes to one of expulsive character and the mother will want to push. Holding her breath increases the intra-abdominal pressure and, together with the action of the abdominal muscles and uterine contractions, brings about delivery of the child.

A full bladder or rectum will impede the passage of the fetal head through the pelvis and so an enema is usually given in early labour and the mother encouraged to empty her bladder.

As the head descends through the pelvis it rotates. Once the head has been delivered it will be seen to rotate through 90°, indicating that the baby's shoulders are descending (and rotating) through the pelvis. Once the shoulders are born, the trunk and limbs follow immediately. This point marks the end of the second stage.

Third stage

At the end of the third stage the uterus should have contracted down to a hard mass in the lower third of the abdomen. Contractions usually cease for a short time, after which small gushes of blood and renewed contractions indicate separation of the placenta. Sometimes, however, there is no bleeding.

The third stage usually lasts only a few minutes (about 20 in an average patient) but may exceed 1 hour in a patient having her first baby (primigravida).

It is now common practice to give drugs that will contract the uterus during the third stage of labour, to keep this stage as short as possible.

PRACTICAL CONSIDERATIONS FOR PARAMEDICAL PERSONNEL

1. Medical and surgical problems

Numerous conditions may be aggravated by the coexistence of pregnancy. In particular, the medical disorders of diabetes mellitus, idiopathic epilepsy, hypertension and cardiac valvular disease may all become less stable as a pregnancy advances. Surgical conditions, especially the abdominal ones of acute appendicitis, cholecystitis, torsion of an ovarian cyst and intestinal obstruction, may not necessarily have a higher incidence in pregnancy but their signs and symptoms may be masked, making diagnosis and eventual surgical management more difficult.

It must never be forgotten that the management of all conditions coexisting at the time of pregnancy, as well as those relating directly to the pregnancy itself, require consideration of the effects of treatment on two individuals—the mother and her fetus. Treatment given to one may well have an effect on the other. This is especially important around the time of delivery when careful consideration must be given to the choice of any anaesthetic technique and drugs which may be used.

2. Haemorrhage

A useful classification is as follows:

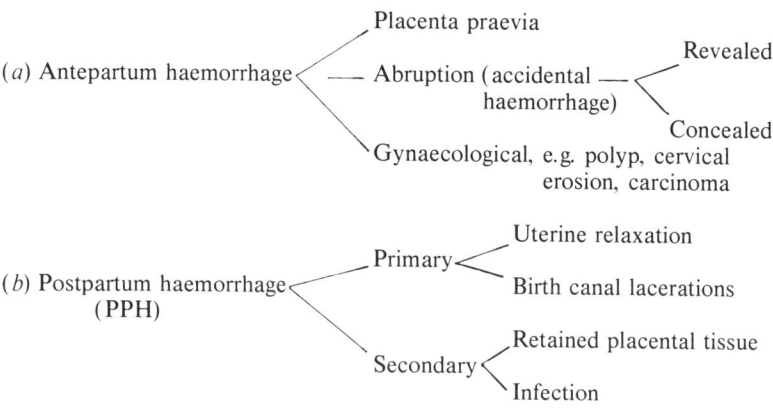

a. Antepartum haemorrhage (APH)

Placenta praevia is a condition in which the placenta has implanted around the outlet, or internal os, of the uterus. Premature separation of even a small amount of placental tissue can result in bleeding, which may be excessive, at any time throughout pregnancy. Indeed fresh blood loss through the cervix in pregnancy must always be considered as due to placenta praevia until proved otherwise.

With the more major types of placenta praevia where the os is fully covered by placental tissue the fetus cannot safely be delivered vaginally, and Caesarean section becomes essential. It may be extremely dangerous to perform a vaginal examination in this condition, and if such an examination is necessary it must be performed in the operating theatre with all obstetric, anaesthetic and nursing personnel at the ready to perform immediate Caesarean section if the placenta is damaged and haemorrhage results.

Abruption of the placenta or 'accidental' haemorrhage is a condition where bleeding occurs from a normally situated placenta, i.e. there is no placenta praevia. Partial separation of placental tissue from the uterine wall may occur at any time during pregnancy. If the resultant haemorrhage tracks down between the uterine wall and the membranes to escape through the cervix it is known as a *revealed* accidental haemorrhage. Bleeding which remains localized may result in separation of placental tissue from the uterine wall without visible blood loss. This is known as *concealed* accidental haemorrhage.

The patient with an APH of any amount needs immediate hospital admission for assessment, observation and to exclude placenta praevia. In many cases the bleeding will cease quickly and the patient may be allowed home again within a few days. Extensive bleeding can result in a complete loss of blood supply to the fetus resulting in its rapid death. The mother may be pale, with a tachycardia and hypotension, indicating a severe degree of shock. Blood loss is often far greater than the severity of clinical signs suggest. The uterus is invariably hard and tender to palpation. Urgent blood transfusion is essential in such cases.

Concealed bleeding is also serious in another respect. If extensive it may use up large quantities of coagulation factors resulting in a coagulation defect (often known as 'defibrination syndrome'). This may present dangers if surgical intervention is used to deliver the fetus since uncontrollable haemorrhage may ensue. Large quantities of fresh blood and clotting factors may be required.

Gynaecological causes of APH must not be overlooked. In particular, haemorrhage from cervical erosions, polyps or carcinomas must be considered.

b. Postpartum haemorrhage (PPH)

Uterine relaxation may arise from failure to deliver the placenta or from the retention of some placental fragments within the uterine cavity. Treatment requires removal of the placenta or retained fragments, using spinal or general anaesthesia if necessary. Uterine relaxation may also follow the previously uneventful delivery of the placenta and is often due to the use of oxytocic drugs to induce or accelerate labour. Manual compression of the relaxed uterus through the abdominal wall should bring about contraction of the uterine muscle. The further administration of oxytocic drugs such as ergometrine or oxytocin by injection may be useful.

Birth canal lacerations usually result from a difficult vaginal delivery necessitating the use of obstetric forceps, or the birth of an unduly large baby. Perineal tears, episiotomy, lacerations of the cervix or vaginal vault may all produce large haemorrhages.

Secondary PPH is usually due to the retention of fragments of placental tissue, membrane or blood clots within the uterine cavity. Light bleeding may respond to parenteral oxytocic drugs, but curettage (scraping) of the uterine cavity is usually required. A less common cause of secondary PPH is uterine infection and separation of slough from the placental site or following Caesarean section. It usually occurs 7–14 days after delivery.

3. Pre-eclampsia and eclampsia

These conditions may be referred to in some texts as 'toxaemia of pregnancy'. Mild forms of pre-eclampsia are quite common and are manifest by hypertension (in a previously normotensive individual), excessive weight gain, fluid retention and oedema (particularly noticeable as ankle and facial puffiness). Regular antenatal care may pick up these signs early and if the obstetrician is concerned he will admit the woman for bed rest and drug treatment of the hypertension if necessary. Should the early signs of pre-eclampsia be missed the severity of the condition may increase rapidly and fulminating pre-eclampsia or eclampsia (fits) may develop. There is increasing hypertension and proteinuria appears. Further deterioration results in drowsiness, headache, blurred vision, abdominal pain and vomiting. This is a critical state and even immediate treatment at this stage may not prevent the onset of eclamptic fits. Although manifest initially as generalized muscular twitchings they rapidly progress to severe grand-mal type seizures followed by a refractory state of variable duration. The patient may appear deceptively well between fits.

Eclampsia is a life-threatening situation for both mother and baby. Primary treatment must be rapid to control the fits and prevent asphyxia. Anticonvulsant drugs such as diazepam may be required in large doses. Nursing must be performed with the patient in the 'three-quarter prone' position and the airway protected with a mouth prop, oral airway or even endotracheal tube, depending on the level of consciousness. Further management may require control of the hypertension with drugs such as hydralazine or diazoxide; epidural analgesia may also be used. Finally, once the blood pressure and convulsions have been controlled the baby must be delivered expeditiously.

4. Prolapsed cord

If the membranes rupture spontaneously (or if they are ruptured artificially) and the baby's presenting part does not completely fill the lower uterine segment there is a danger of prolapse of a section of the umbilical cord through the cervix. The risk is greatest with malpresentation (e.g. breech, transverse lie or unengaged high head at term). The prolapsed cord may become compressed by the presenting part and the blood supply to the baby either partially or completely obstructed. Treatment must be urgent if the baby is to survive. A midwife or other appropriate assistant should nurse the patient in the 'knee-chest' position with a hand on the presenting part in an attempt to reduce the pressure on the cord. First-aid measures are designed to protect the fetus until Caesarean section can be performed, unless the cervix is fully dilated in which case a forceps or breech delivery may be possible.

5. Fetal distress

The normal fetal heart rate at term is 120–160 beats/min. Since the fetus's metabolism depends on an adequate supply of oxygen being allowed to diffuse across the placenta, reduction of the oxygen supply will produce fetal hypoxaemia and this is manifest by changes in the fetal heart rate, known as fetal distress. With the advent of modern technology and continuous fetal heart rate monitoring during labour it is possible to detect fetal distress very quickly. Mild fetal heart rate abnormalities are fairly common during labour and require only close supervision. If severe bradycardia develops or if there is passage of meconium it may be necessary to deliver the baby quickly before it risks permanent damage from prolonged asphyxia. If the mother's cervix is fully dilated a forceps or ventouse suction delivery may be performed; if not a Caesarean section is necessary.

Further reading

Donald I. (1979) *Practical Obstetric Problems.* 5th ed. London, Lloyd-Luke.
Llewellyn-Jones D. (1982) *Fundamentals of Obstetrics and Gynaecology,* Vol 1; *Obstetrics.* 3rd ed. London, Faber & Faber.
Myles Margaret F. (1981) *Textbook for Midwives.* 9th ed. Edinburgh, Churchill Livingstone.

Chapter 19

Shock and Thermal Injury

S. J. Mather and D. L. Edbrooke

SHOCK

'Shock' is a term which has been used for many decades to describe conditions ranging from simple faints to an illness leading to death. In more recent times the condition has been more precisely defined.

It is now defined in simple terms as 'a severe syndrome associated with abnormal cellular function'. This is usually the result of poor tissue perfusion due to an inadequate blood supply. It may, however, be due to the release of toxins in the body from bacteria.

Shock is classically subdivided into the following categories:
1. Hypovolaemic shock
2. Cardiogenic shock
3. Septic shock
4. Other causes

Hypovolaemic shock

This, by definition, is caused by a reduction in the blood volume. The reduction required to cause shock is usually in the order of *at least* 20 per cent.

It is also important to realize that the fluid loss does not only affect the vascular compartment but also the extracellular fluid compartment, and this, in turn, will affect the intracellular compartment (*see* Chapter 4).

The most obvious condition which can lead to hypovolaemic shock is acute blood loss from trauma. Massive blood loss can also occur from a variety of pathological conditions such as gastric ulceration.

SHOCK AND THERMAL INJURY

Cardiogenic shock
This form of shock is due to the inability of the myocardium to continue its pumping function due to damage usually caused by a large myocardial infarction. It is often termed 'pump failure'. In addition it is often associated with various dysrhythmias. It is characterized by a low systolic blood pressure and inadequate organ perfusion which produces mental impairment, a poor urine output and poor peripheral perfusion.

Septic shock
This is also known as bacteraemic, septicaemic and endotoxic shock. The shock state is produced by the presence of bacteria or their toxins in the bloodstream. It is due to overwhelming infection from any one of a variety of different organisms. It is seen commonly following abdominal surgery or severe respiratory infections. It must be stressed, however, that infection from any site can produce septicaemic shock.

If the body's defences are compromised by a disease process then any moderate infection can produce a severe state of septicaemic shock.

Shock from other causes
It is possible for a shock state to develop from other causes. Neurogenic shock has been described. This is due to the interruption of the normal sympathetic pathways which leads to intense vasodilatation. It is not commonly seen but can occur after spinal trauma. The shock states associated with head injuries are usually due to blood loss from other injuries and not a result of the head injury itself.

It is also possible to diagnose shock following acute metabolic disorders, for example acute hypoglycaemia.

Features of the shock state
a. Blood pressure
In early shock states the blood pressure can be normal. This is due to the compensation that the vascular bed can produce by vasoconstriction. This can be misleading because the blood pressure can drop precipitately when compensation is no longer possible. *A narrowing pulse pressure* is the best guide to falling stroke volume.

It is possible that the pulses may not be palpable in the arm due to intense vasoconstriction (*see* Chapter 2). In these patients the only possible way of monitoring the blood pressure may be to palpate a large artery. The best site is usually the femoral artery and it is necessary to record both the rate of the heart and also the volume of the pulse.

b. Heart rate
The use of the heart rate as a guide in the diagnosis of a shock state is open to considerable error as the heart rate can vary for a variety of

different reasons. To base any judgement on this parameter alone would be unwise.

c. Peripheral perfusion
As has been already described, the peripheral perfusion in hypovolaemic shock is impaired. The peripheral perfusion can be assessed at a variety of different sites. The commonest sites are in the ear lobe and nail bed. If gentle pressure is exerted and quickly released the 'colour' will quickly return. This is termed the capillary refill time. In the normal person this will take less than 2 sec. In a patient with hypovolaemic shock this time will be lengthened.

This test may be unreliable for a variety of different reasons. These include pre-existing arterial disease or simply the fact that the patient may have been in a cold environment for some time.

d. Urine output
As the blood volume is reduced in hypovolaemic shock the amount of blood available for distribution throughout the circulation will be reduced. Consequently the blood supply to the kidney will be reduced and this in turn will produce a reduction in the urine output. In the event of a severe shock state the urine output may completely stop and acute renal failure will ensue.

e. Acid–base changes
In the normal body cell, cellular metabolites (cellular waste products) are being continuously removed by the circulation. Most of these metabolites are acidic and if the circulation is impaired they will build up producing an acidosis. This acidosis is in itself harmful to the normal functioning of body cells.

f. Changes in the rate and depth of respiration
Shock states are in their own right powerful stimuli to respiration and can double the rate and depth of breathing.

In addition to this the metabolic acidosis produced can lead to a compensatory respiratory alkalosis, due to depletion of carbon dioxide in the blood by overbreathing.

g. Other changes
If hypotension develops this may lead to large changes in the fluid balance in the body. It has been established in studies on American soldiers during the Vietnam War that in 1 hour up to 1 litre of fluid can shift from the interstitial compartment to the vascular compartment if the shock state is untreated.

Another characteristic of the shock state is platelet aggregation. These clumps of platelets can severely impair flow in the capillaries.

SHOCK AND THERMAL INJURY

Once a diagnosis of shock has been made, it is next necessary to establish the cause of the shock state and then treat it. It is often difficult to distinguish the type of shock from the clinical features but a good idea of the probable cause can be obtained from the history immediately preceding the onset of shock.

Treatment of shock states

Once the diagnosis of hypovolaemic shock has been made it is of extreme importance to institute treatment immediately. The mortality of shock is related to the delay in treatment and the old maxim of 'too little too late' continues to be a problem.

a. Treatment of the cause

If an obvious cause for the onset of shock is apparent then it is mandatory to treat this. So, for example, if the patient has hypovolaemic shock due to blood loss it is first of all necessary to avert this. If the shock is due to septicaemia then it will not be possible to treat the primary cause in the field.

b. Oxygenation

In all cases of shock it is essential to administer oxygen. It is usually appropriate to give the oxygen by face mask but it may be necessary to consider intermittent positive-pressure ventilation (see Chapter 6).

c. Cardiac massage

This may be necessary in patients who are unable to produce a cardiac output large enough to produce pulses in the major arteries. Consequently it is vital to monitor a major arterial pulse (e.g. the femoral) at regular intervals.

d. Fluid replacement

In patients who are likely to develop the shock syndrome it is valuable to start fluid replacement early. It is, therefore, logical to replace immediately some fluid loss. If the fluid loss is visible the assessment of replacement volume is fairly simple. When the fluid loss is not visible the assessment of replacement volume is not quite so easy and will require both experience and measurement of cardiovascular parameters (see Chapter 4).

As a general rule it is usually possible in an adult to administer 500 ml of fluid over 30 min without any danger of overloading the circulation. This may avert or at least delay the onset of hypovolaemic shock and so 'buy time'. In cases of true hypovolaemic shock this volume of fluid will not be anywhere near enough but it is unwise to administer very large volumes of intravenous fluids without the ability to measure the effect on the vascular compartment. In general, however, enough should be given to restore the blood pressure to near normal levels. Fluid therapy is discussed in detail in Chapter 4.

This fluid regime can also be applied to patients with septicaemic shock but this is not the case in patients with cardiogenic shock. As has been described these patients have a 'pump failure' and the shock state is due to the myocardium itself and not to the amount of fluid in the circulation. It is therefore mandatory to administer fluids in these patients with great caution and as a rule of thumb it should not usually be necessary to exceed a maximum of 500 ml of crystalloid fluid.

e. Corticosteroids

The administration of corticosteroids to patients with a shock state is a subject of spirited debate in the medical profession. It is the opinion of the authors that they have a place in the treatment of shock states. It is, however, beyond doubt that their usefulness is very dependent on the time that they are given. It is necessary to administer them as soon as possible after the shock state has been recognized.

It is, therefore, possible that a case for the administration of corticosteroids by paramedical personnel could be supported.

Some other measures used in the hospital environment are included here for completeness.

f. Inotropic agents

These are drugs which can increase the force of contraction of the heart. They are very effective and are commonly used. Good examples include dopamine, dobutamine, adrenaline and digoxin.

g. Vasodilating drugs

These drugs cause peripheral vasodilatation and as such overcome the peripheral vasoconstriction. Good examples include sodium nitroprusside and isosorbide dinitrate.

h. Diuretics

As has been described, with the reduction in cardiac output the urine output falls and renal failure can result. This can be averted in some cases by the administration of diuretics such as frusemide. A bladder catheter should be inserted before this treatment is undertaken.

In conclusion it must be stressed that shock states carry a very high mortality and too often the maxim of 'too little too late' still applies. It is possible that by the early recognition and initial treatment of the shock state in the field the high mortality of this condition can be reduced.

Intravenous fluid therapy is the single most effective measure in these conditions.

SHOCK AND THERMAL INJURY

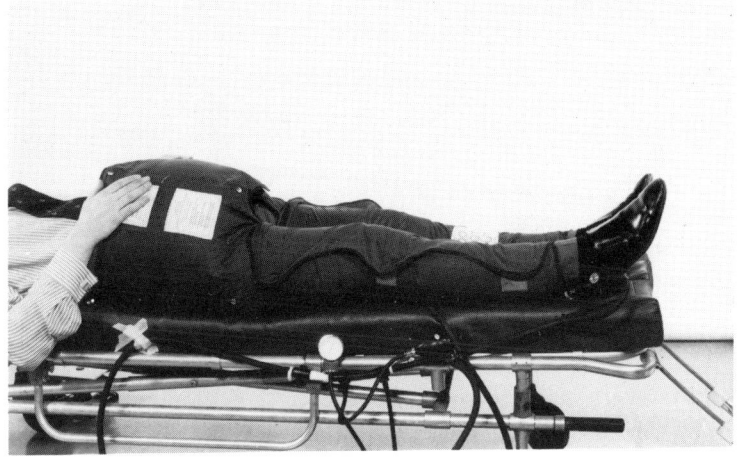

Fig. 19.1. Antigravity suit.

'*Antigravity suits*' (*Fig.* 19.1)

These suits are also called 'G' suits and 'Mast' suits.* They are designed to exert a positive pressure to the lower half of the body. The principle is that by inflating a suit with air or oxygen to a given pressure (usually about 20 mmHg) some venous blood in the lower part of the body will be returned to the circulation and thus increase the venous return to the heart. Consequently, the systemic blood pressure will rise. In addition, they have been found to reduce venous bleeding.

The origin of this type of equipment was in its application for pilots. They were developed to combat the 'G' forces exerted on the pilot during violent manoeuvres. By application of pressure to the lower half of the body it was found that loss of consciousness could be avoided in most cases.

Much research work has been undertaken in the USA and the result of this research has indicated that they are indeed of great value in the treatment of shock states, particularly hypovolaemic shock. They appear to have few disadvantages. For example they have little effect on respiratory function.

They have yet to gain wide acceptance in the UK but it is the authors' contention that they should be a standard part of the armamentarium of paramedical personnel.

---

*Mast = military anti-shock trousers.

IMMEDIATE CARE OF THERMAL AND CORROSIVE INJURIES

The physiological derangement associated with a major burn is complex and as yet incompletely understood. This is true whether the 'burn' is a true thermal injury (heat or cold) or a corrosive (acid or caustic) one.

Pre-1960 many patients with a burn area of greater than 50 per cent stood little chance of survival. Improvements in recent years are due to a greater understanding of the pathophysiology of burn injuries and the development of intensive monitoring facilities and 'burns centres'. In the burns centres, specialist expertise is immediately available in both the medical and nursing fields. Once the initial life-threatening episode has passed, there may follow a long period of rehabilitation. Extensive plastic surgery may be required to correct deformities which may necessitate many months of hospitalization. One must not forget the psychological trauma suffered by these patients. This, too, requires careful and thorough rehabilitation. Some patients may never work again; the domestic and financial problems may then become intolerable for the patient and his family.

Pathophysiology of burn injury
The burn results from the denaturation of cell protein and coagulation (like a boiled egg) which occurs at temperatures above 50°C.

Immediate care of burn injuries
Thermal and corrosive injuries should be immediately flushed with large quantities of cold water to reduce tissue temperature, or dilute the corrosive.

Specific neutralizing agents have a strictly secondary role.

Corrosive	*Dilution*	*Neutralization*
Acids		
Hydrochloric	water	sodium bicarbonate solution
Sulphuric	water	sodium bicarbonate solution
Trichloracetic	water	sodium bicarbonate solution
Hydrofluoric	water	calcium gluconate injection s.c.
Formic	water	calcium gluconate injection s.c.
Picric	water	calcium gluconate injection s.c.
Phenol (carbolic)	water	glycerol
Caustics		
Sodium hydroxide	water	weak acid e.g. dilute acetic acid
Potassium hydroxide	water	weak acid e.g. dilute acetic acid
Quicklime	water	weak acid e.g. dilute acetic acid
Ammonium hydroxide	water	weak acid e.g. dilute acetic acid

SHOCK AND THERMAL INJURY

Excluding corrosive injuries, the burn wound itself is not then the most important object of attention, apart from covering the site to reduce fluid losses and prevent infection. Initial management must be directed toward the maintenance of the airway, a normal circulating volume, cardiac output and renal perfusion.

The airway

Respiratory problems may result due to inhalation of smoke, fumes, steam or carbon monoxide. Thermal injury to the airway may cause rapid onset of laryngeal and pulmonary oedema. Soft-tissue oedema is maximal at 24–48 hours after the injury.

Immediate care of smoke or steam inhalation will include oxygen therapy and airway protection (*see* Chapter 6).

The burn wound

This is best initially treated with sterile occlusive dressings to prevent infection and minimize fluid loss. Sterile plastic bags may be the most effective for this purpose in burns of the extremities.

Volume replacement

Careful fluid replacement therapy is vital to the successful management of thermal injury.

Following a major burn there is movement of water and electrolytes from the extracellular fluid (including the plasma water) into injured cells. This produces a hypovolaemic state and, if unchecked, a fall in cardiac output and renal perfusion. If adequate volume replacement is achieved 'normalization' of body water compartments begins within 48 hours.

Initial extracellular fluid depletion is proportional to two variables. These are the depth, and more importantly, the area of the burn. The importance of accurate assessment of the burned area cannot be overstressed since fluid replacement predictions depend upon that knowledge.

Fluid replacement therapy

Most formulae require the surface area of the burn to be estimated. An equation incorporating this value is then used to calculate the fluid requirement. Some authorities advocate the use of crystalloids only but others favour administration of both crystalloid and colloid. It must be stressed, however, that the use of any one formula is secondary to the principle that constant modification will be required in the light of changing haemodynamic and biochemical values. Two examples of fluid replacement formulae are given below.

1. Parkland formula (Baxter & Shires)
First 24 hours:
Ringer-lactate 4 ml/kg × % burn, given at a rate of:
 half total volume in first 8 hours
 quarter in second 8 hours
 quarter in third 8 hours
Second 24 hours:
Areas 40% plus: human albumin solution as required to maintain urine output at least 0·5 ml/kg/hour.

2. Monafo formula
First 24 hours:
Hypertonic solution containing 250 mmol/l sodium
                              150 mmol/l chloride
                              150 mmol/l lactate
given at a rate of 3 ml/kg/hour. The rate is then adjusted to maintain a urine output of 0·5 ml/kg/hour.
Second 24 hours:
5% dextrose solution.

Other formulae, e.g. Brooke, Evans, Cope and Moore, have been worked out but the two most recent are presented here. The individual response of each patient tends to outweigh the small differences between the formulae. They are only *guides* to therapy and should be altered according to individual patient's requirements as judged by clinical assessment, estimates of circulating volume and urine output.

Assessment of burned areas

In adults the burned area can be roughly assessed by the 'Rule of Nines' (*see opposite*). This visualizes the body surface divided into areas, each comprising 9 per cent or multiples of 9 per cent, plus the perineum (1 per cent).

This 'rule' is not accurate in children since (especially in young infants) the head and neck represents much more than 18 per cent and each lower limb rather less. Tables are available which relate body surface area to age with relative percentage distribution of parts of the body (Lund and Browder tables). These should always be consulted in the case of children.

Acute gastric dilatation

This may become a real emergency as the dilated stomach splints the diaphragm and embarrasses respiration. (It is not unique to burns and occurs frequently after any major trauma.) In such patients early placement of a Ryle's or Levin tube will decompress the stomach and also allow antacids to be given (acid aspiration pneumonitis is a very real risk). *Stress ulcers* may also occur. Antacids and an H_2-receptor (histamine) antagonist such as cimetidine or ranitidine may be employed.

The Rule of Nines

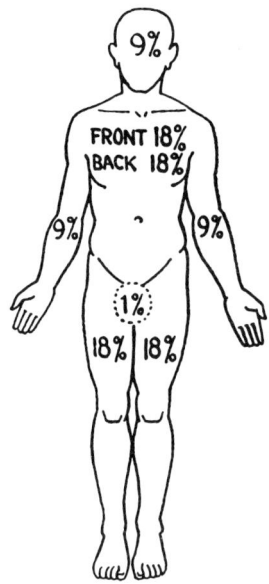

Head and neck	9%
Two upper limbs (2 × 9%)	18%
Each lower limb	18%
	+ 18%
Front of trunk	18%
Back of trunk	18%
Perineum	1%

Note: Does not apply to children

Bladder catheterization
The measurement of urine output is an accurate means of monitoring fluid therapy. Early catheterization is therefore essential.

Weighing
As soon as possible after admission to hospital the patient should be weighed. Adequate resuscitation should increase the body weight by

10–20 per cent in a major burn. This value gives a baseline from which to monitor progress.

Analgesia

Partial thickness burns are extremely painful; full thickness burns less so. Adequate analgesia must be given as soon as is practicable. Nitrous oxide in oxygen (as Entonox) is the safest agent in the presence of hypovolaemia (low circulating volume) but its administration may be difficult or impossible if facial burns have occurred.

Intravenous opioids such as morphine are widely used but care must be exercised since vasodilatation will follow and may cause a rapid fall in blood pressure. As with all patients in 'shock', all medication should be given intravenously.

The analgesic agent should be given intravenously, in small increments until adequate pain relief is achieved. The dose required varies enormously between individuals and is dependent upon the nature of the burn, other injuries and the age and fitness of the patient.

One must always bear in mind the possibility that respiratory depression may occur following the administration of powerful analgesics of the opioid type. Respiratory rate and depth must be monitored frequently and oxygen or assisted ventilation given as necessary.

Transport of the burned patient

Once the patient has been brought out of the hazardous environment (flame, smoke, fumes) his general state must be assessed by systems. As soon as possible an intravenous line should be started, even in those with relatively small burns (anything over 10 per cent) as veins present at this stage may rapidly disappear as fluid moves out of the circulation.

Any corrosive substance must be thoroughly diluted, the burn wound covered with sterile occlusive dressings (burns dressings if available), and the patient transported to the nearest Accident and Emergency Department. The patient should be stabilized before moving him since, at this stage, the burn wound takes second place to cardiorespiratory resuscitation.

ECG monitoring, if available, together with frequent assessment of the blood pressure and respiration is advisable during the journey.

Advance warning should be sent to the receiving hospital and the resuscitation team notified if the patient is 'shocked' or unstable.

It is beyond the scope of this book to discuss the late problems of thermal and corrosive injuries but a brief list of complications is given opposite.

Early
  Fluid loss
    water
    protein
  Blood loss
  Infection
    localized
    generalized (septicaemia)
  Development of a shock state
  Airway problems
  Adult respiratory distress syndrome
Late
  Eschar and scar formation
  Disfigurement
  Psychological trauma

Further reading
Hummel R. P. (ed.) (1982) *Clinical Burn Therapy. A Management and Prevention Guide.* Bristol, Wright-PSG.

Chapter 20

Paediatric Emergencies

N. R. Bennett

INTRODUCTION

Death during childhood is fortunately uncommon. Infant Mortality refers to deaths occurring during the first year of life. Although the Infant Mortality Rate has declined steadily over recent years, 50 per cent of all deaths before the age of 20 years occur during the first year of life, the main causes being birth injuries, congenital malformations, infection, asphyxia, accidents and injuries. After the first year of life the main causes of death are childhood cancers and trauma.

Accidents are the largest single cause of death in children between the ages of 1 and 15 years, and most of these occur either at home or on the road. Most children who are killed or injured in road accidents are pedestrians; serious injuries to children in cars are becoming less common as a result of the increasing use of safety restraints. The commonest causes of acccidents in the home are falls and poisoning; other important causes include burns, scalds and suffocation.

It is, therefore, clear that the rapid provision of skilled and appropriate immediate care by members of the emergency services can dramatically improve the outcome in many children who find themselves in some of the life-threatening situations which are described below.

CARDIOPULMONARY RESUSCITATION

Cardiopulmonary resuscitation is considered at the beginning of this chapter because many of the conditions to be discussed require the rapid restoration of respiratory and cardiac function. In addition, there are significant differences in resuscitation techniques when applied to

children. The signs of cessation of effective respiration and circulation in children are:
1. Gasping or absent respiration
2. Pallor or cyanosis
3. Absent peripheral pulses
4. Absent heart sounds
5. Dilatation of the pupils

Cardiopulmonary resuscitation should achieve the following objectives:
1. Airway opened
2. Breathing restored
3. Circulation restored

These steps should be initiated as soon as possible and followed in the order listed above; a child can be kept alive for a long time by efficient artificial respiration and cardiac massage thus allowing for transfer to hospital and definitive treatment.

The airway

The most important priority when confronted with an unconscious child is the airway. The commonest cause of cardiac arrest during childhood is hypoxia; this is due to factors such as the high oxygen consumption of small children, immaturity of lung function, and the ease with which the airways may become obstructed. Immediate clearance and opening of the airway may, therefore, allow respiration to restart and prevent a catastrophic chain of events ending in cardiac arrest.

Airway obstruction should be suspected if vigorous respiratory efforts result in a characteristic see-saw motion of the chest and abdomen or the production of gurgling or rattling noises from the throat. This may be caused by foreign material in the mouth or throat which should be rapidly cleared with the fingers or by other available means.

Ventilation

If the patient does not resume spontaneous breathing after the airway has been cleared and opened up, artificial ventilation should be started immediately using mouth-to-mouth respiration. In infants and small children the rescuer covers the patient's mouth and nose with his own mouth and blows gently to inflate the lungs at a rate of 20–30 breaths per minute. During this procedure the infant's head should be tilted gently back but extreme extension should be avoided. In older children the rescuer puts his mouth around the patient's mouth, occludes the nostrils and blows in exhaled air to inflate the lungs at a rate of about 12–20 breaths per minute. A further improvement is to use positive pressure-ventilation using one of the commercially available self-inflating bags which are made in adult and paediatric versions.

The most efficient way of maintaining the airway and ventilating a child is to perform endotracheal intubation and to connect the tracheal tube either to an anaesthetic breathing circuit or a self-inflating bag. This technique requires skill and it must be stressed that unless there is a person available who is expert in intubation of children, time should not be wasted in performing this manoeuvre; adequate oxygenation should be possible using the measures described above.

Cardiac massage

The diagnosis of cardiac arrest is made if there are no heart sounds to be heard, and the pupils are dilated or dilating.

Having made the diagnosis of cardiac arrest the patient should be placed on a firm surface. In neonates the fingers of one hand should be placed behind the chest and the sternum should be compressed with the thumb at a rate of about 120 per minute: in infants both hands should be placed behind the chest and the midsternum should be compressed using two thumbs at a rate of about 100 per minute; in children between 1 and 10 years the heel of one hand is placed over the midsternum which is compressed at a rate of about 60 per minute; over the age of 10 years two hands, one placed on top of the first, should be positioned over the lower third of the sternum. When properly performed external cardiac compression can produce systolic peaks greater than 100 mmHg and it should be possible to produce a palpable carotid or femoral pulse.

The technique must always be accompanied by artificial ventilation: a single operator should ventilate the lungs with two breaths and then compress the heart 15 times; if there are two operators 5 compressions of the heart should alternate with each breath.

Once the airway has been opened, artificial ventilation initiated and effective cardiac compression commenced, a plastic cannula is inserted into a vein and an ECG connected to the patient. Appropriate drugs such as calcium, adrenaline and sodium bicarbonate may be administered intravenously, and if necessary defibrillation of the heart performed.

POST-RESUSCITATION CARE

Following successful resuscitation there remain two problems which require careful management: the underlying cause of the cardiorespiratory arrest, and the sequelae of cardiorespiratory arrest. The immediate sequelae which require treatment may include metabolic acidosis, cardiovascular instability, renal failure and cerebral oedema. It is, therefore, imperative that these cases are admitted to the Intensive Care Unit for further management.

RESUSCITATION OF THE NEWBORN

Ambulance personnel may on occasions be involved in resuscitating a newborn infant of a mother who has gone into sudden labour and has delivered before reaching hospital.

The main priority in a newborn child is to clear the airways immediately after birth by gently sucking out the nose and mouth using a small suction catheter attached to a vacuum source or a mucus extractor.

If the child is pink, crying and has regular respiration within a minute of birth no further management should be required except to wipe the baby down and wrap him in a warm blanket; another way of maintaining body heat is to wrap the child in a silver foil blanket.

If the child is blue or grey but is otherwise making vigorous respiratory efforts he should be sucked out and given oxygen to breathe. If respiration is slow to commence it is customary to stimulate the child by gently flicking the heels.

If a child has not responded within one minute of birth and is blue or grey and has gasping or absent respiration or is limp, a small airway should be inserted and the lungs gently inflated with oxygen using a self-inflating bag and mask fitted with a valve which blows off at 30 cm H_2O; the chest should be auscultated and in the absence of heart sounds external cardiac massage commenced.

Respiratory difficulties may develop in babies some time after birth; the baby may appear to be 'working' rather hard, with indrawing of the ribs and grunting; there may be an increasing respiratory rate, or there may be episodes of apnoea.

Common causes of respiratory problems at this stage include surfactant deficiency (respiratory distress syndrome), pneumonia following aspiration of secretions at birth, septicaemia and cardiac problems.

These cases should be given oxygen, kept warm and transferred to a Special Care Baby Unit. No attempt should be made to feed a baby with severe respiratory problems.

SUDDEN INFANT DEATH SYNDROME (SIDS)

Sudden infant death syndrome (cot death) occurs during the first few months of life usually for no apparent reason: it accounts for about half of all deaths between the ages of 1 week and 2 years. The cause remains unknown. Brothers and sisters of victims of SIDS are themselves more likely to develop the syndrome. It should be remembered that a number of cases of apparent SIDS may in fact be victims of childhood abuse and have been deliberately asphyxiated by a parent, relative or child-minder.

Infants who for no apparent reason suffer an acute episode of apnoea, cyanosis or hypotonia and survive are referred to as 'near-miss' SIDS. If the child has recovered from the episode by the time medical or paramedical help has arrived he should nevertheless be transferred to hospital for observation and investigation.

If the child has not recovered by the time expert help arrives, the management is the same as for any child with severe respiratory difficulty.

HEAD INJURY

Any child with a head injury should be admitted to hospital if there has been loss of consciousness for even the shortest period of time. Small children show a wide variation in their response to head injury; they may initially appear to have suffered little harm but suddenly deteriorate. The principles of immediate management of children with head injury are the same as in adults; in the unconscious child immediate attention should be paid to the adequacy of the airway and ventilation. Where possible serious bleeding from associated injuries should be stopped. There may not necessarily be very much external evidence of injury, but any child who is draining clear watery fluid from the nose or ear or who is convulsing for no known reason should be suspected of having a head injury.

The essence of immediate management of head injuries lies in their rapid transfer to hospital before any further deterioration has occurred; great care should be exercised when moving the patient particularly if a neck injury is suspected; the usual measures to maintain the vital functions of airway, ventilation and circulation should where appropriate be employed.

MULTIPLE INJURIES

The initial assessment of children with multiple injuries is important in order to recognize any problems which may rapidly become life-threatening. The history, of course, is very important as it gives clues to injuries which might otherwise be missed. The severity of the child's condition may not be proportional to the apparent degree of trauma. It is, therefore, essential to make a rapid assessment in order to establish the correct sequence of actions to ensure survival. As usual, the state of the airway, breathing and circulation take overall priority.

If the child has sustained a chest injury and his respiration is grunting in character, he is cyanosed, and one side of the chest moves more than the other during respiration, a pneumothorax or haemopneumothorax should be suspected. Auscultation of the chest with a stethoscope should reveal any obvious inequality in ventilation between the two sides. Remember that small children can sustain violent chest injuries with severe lung contusion, pneumothorax and haemopneumothorax without necessarily fracturing ribs. In any patient who shows signs of inadequate respiration one should administer 100 per cent oxygen from a close fitting face mask and be prepared to take over ventilation at any time using a self-inflating bag.

Severe blood loss will lead to hypovolaemic shock. The signs of hypovolaemia are a cold, pale, sweaty skin, a fast thready pulse, hyperventilation, poor capillary refill and peripheral cyanosis. In addition, the child may be drowsy or restless. Management of the hypovolaemic child should include:
1. Prevention of further bleeding by appropriate means
2. Oxygen administration
3. Elevation of the legs
4. Maintenance of body temperature
5. Intravenous fluid replacement
6. External cardiac massage where appropriate

UPPER AIRWAYS OBSTRUCTION

Children are particularly at risk of developing upper airways obstruction on account of the relatively small size of their breathing passages. Obstruction may be partial and of gradual onset or complete and of sudden onset. Partial obstruction is usually associated with stridor which is a high pitched crowing noise occurring either during inspiration, expiration or both. The commonest acquired causes of stridor in children are acute laryngotracheobronchitis, acute epiglottitis and foreign body inhalation.

ACUTE LARYNGOTRACHEOBRONCHITIS

This is the commonest cause of stridor in small children occurring usually between the ages of 3 months and 3 years, and is due to a viral infection. Symptoms are relatively gradual in onset and are caused by swelling of the mucous membranes of the larynx. These cases usually have inspiratory stridor together with a characteristic brassy or barking cough and there may be a history of previous attacks. Any child with progressively worsening symptoms should be admitted to hospital. Invasive measures such as endotracheal intubation are rarely required and most cases respond to humidity, oxygen and other conservative measures.

ACUTE EPIGLOTTITIS

Unlike acute laryngotracheobronchitis, this condition is usually caused by bacterial infection with *Haemophilus influenzae*. It occurs typically in children aged between 18 months and 7 years and can lead to complete upper airway obstruction within hours of the onset of symptoms. Fortunately this is an uncommon condition, symptoms being caused by severe and rapid swelling of the epiglottis and surrounding tissues. The diagnosis can often be made from the history. The illness starts as a sore throat, cough or mild upper respiratory infection which progresses over a few hours to the full picture of acute epiglottitis in which there is severe pain on swallowing, muffling of the voice, drooling, fever, and the child sits forward in order to breathe.

These cases need immediate hospitalization and admission to an Intensive Care Unit where they will be intubated and commenced on high doses of intravenous antibiotics. During transfer to hospital the child should be kept as calm as possible and allowed to remain sitting up. Examination and frequent suction of the upper airway must be avoided since this may precipitate respiratory arrest.

FOREIGN BODY

The possibility of foreign body aspiration should be considered in any child who suddenly develops stridor, particularly if there has been an acute episode or history of choking. Although peanuts are most commonly involved, other objects inhaled include pen tops, screws, pins, needles and bones. As an immediate measure the child should be held upside down and the back slapped; if this fails and the child's breathing is totally obstructed the fingers may be swept around the inside of the child's mouth in order to dislodge any object which may have impacted above the larynx. All cases of suspected foreign body inhalation should be transferred for immediate hospital management.

POISONING

Poisoning accounts for about one-third of all childhood accidents occurring most commonly in those under the age of 4 years. This group is particularly attracted to brightly coloured tablets which may have been left within reach of the child by parents or elderly relatives. It is not uncommon for highly toxic liquids such as the weedkiller Paraquat to be contained in old lemonade bottles and hence be mistaken for a favourite soft drink.

The main groups of substances which are ingested by children are:
1. Tablets
2. Houshold and garden chemicals
3. Plants and berries

In the absence of any obvious evidence such as an empty bottle or medicine container or discoloration of the lips and tongue, the diagnosis of poisoning may not be considered. However, there should be a high index of suspicion in any child with symptoms such as coma, hyper- or hypoventilation, drowsiness or unusual muscle movements which cannot otherwise be explained.

Each year a small but significant number of children die from the effects of poisoning, although the chances of survival can be greatly improved by the application of the following basic principles of management which should be instituted as soon as possible and continued following admission to hospital.
1. Support the child's vital functions, paying particular attention to airway patency and adequacy of breathing: sedatives and tranquillizers may obtund laryngeal reflexes and depress ventilation; salicylates may cause hyperventilation.
2. Attempt to identify the poison: look for scattered pills and tablets, empty bottles or medicine containers, and hand them to medical or nursing staff on arrival at hospital; look inside the mouth for any unswallowed tablets or evidence of burns which would indicate ingestion of corrosives.
3. Prevent absorption: induce vomiting by stimulating the back of the throat except in:
   a. The child who is unconscious or convulsing
   b. The child who has ingested petroleum derivatives or corrosives
4. Transfer the child to hospital.

Following admission to hospital these principles of management are continued.

Supportive measures

Oxygen administration, endotracheal intubation and positive-pressure ventilation may be required if the child is so deeply comatose that his airway reflexes and respiration are seriously impaired.

Circulatory support in the form of plasma or inotropic agents may be required if there is severe hypotension: in other cases there may be cardiac failure which requires treatment. Dysrhythmias are particularly likely in cases of tricyclic antidepressant overdose.

Vomiting may be induced by the administration of Syrup of Ipecacuanha. If ingestion of the poison has occurred within the past 6 hours, gastric lavage should be performed through a large-bore nasogastric tube except in those cases where corrosives or petroleum products have been involved. Following gastric lavage activated charcoal may be administered via the nasogastric tube; this binds many substances such as salicylates, barbiturates, paracetamol and tricyclics and, therefore helps to prevent absorption of the remaining poison. If the ingested substance has been identified, it may be possible to administer a specific antidote, such as desferrioxamine in the case of iron poisoning, or to hasten the elimination of the poison from the body using such means as forced diuresis. These supportive measures should only be carried out under direct medical supervision.

DROWNING

Drowning may occur at any age, but toddlers are particularly at risk since they may stray and fall into swimming pools, fish ponds, lakes and rivers. The incidence of childhood drowning is higher in those countries such as North America where there are more domestic swimming pools. It is important to remember that small children can drown whilst paddling in quite shallow water since they may stumble and fall face down.

The immediate effects of total immersion are aspiration of water into the airways and lungs leading to asphyxia and eventual cardiac arrest; hypothermia follows rapidly in cold water. If the child is immersed for only a short period before rescue, water may have been prevented from entering the lungs because of laryngeal spasm.

There have been a number of incidents reported where full recovery has taken place following periods of drowning of 30–40 minutes. These have usually occurred after immersion in cold lakes in Canada and Northern Europe where the rapid development of hypothermia has helped to protect the brain. The chances of survival depend on the duration of the immersion, the temperature of the water, and the provision of prehospital care. The priorities when managing a victim of drowning are:

1. Remove the child from the water
2. Clear and drain the airways
3. Commence exhaled air artificial respiration or administer oxygen by positive-pressure ventilation if respiration is absent or inadequate
4. Apply cardiac massage if no heart beat is present

Remember that a child who is hypothermic as a result of falling into ice-cold water may be comatose, be without reflexes, have no heart beat and have dilated pupils. However, these cases may respond well to resuscitation and treatment. Immediate cardiorespiratory support should be commenced and continued during transfer to hospital.

Although rapid warming should be avoided during transfer, further drop in body temperature should be prevented because below 30 °C serious abnormalities in cardiac rhythm and myocardial depression occur.

THE DROWSY OR UNCONSCIOUS CHILD

The main causes of drowsiness or coma during childhood are listed here:

Trauma — Recent head injury
Intoxication — Drugs
　　　　　　　Alcohol

Neurological — Recent fit
　　　　　　　Meningitis
　　　　　　　Encephalitis
Infection　　 — Septicaemia
Metabolic　 — Severe dehydration
　　　　　　　Diabetic ketoacidosis
　　　　　　　Hypoglycaemia
　　　　　　　Reye's syndrome

The parents should be asked about the possibility of recent fits, head injury, drug ingestion, infection, vomiting and diarrhoea. Although the chief priority when dealing with a drowsy or unconscious child is to maintain the vital functions of airway patency, breathing and circulation during transfer to hospital, a quick examination may give clues as to the underlying cause. An assessment can be made of the level of consciousness, state of the pupils, adequacy and pattern of respiration, and presence of abnormal muscle movements.

THE CHILD HAVING A FIT

Fits in children often last only a few minutes and simple care may be all that is necessary. Medical intervention will be required if the fit is prolonged. Fits lasting more than 30 min can lead to permanent brain damage. The main causes of convulsions in children are shown in *Table* 20.1.

Table 20.1. **Principal causes of convulsions in children**

Neonates
　Perinatal asphyxia
　Birth trauma
　Cerebral haemorrhage
　Hypocalcaemia
　Hypoglycaemia
　Infection

Infants and older children
　Febrile convulsions
　Meningitis and encephalitis
　Epilepsy
　Dehydration
　Water overload
　Head injury
　Hypoglycaemia

The most urgent priority is to prevent hypoxia: the mouth must be cleared and constrictions around the neck and chest relieved. An airway or spatula should be positioned between the teeth, the child placed on the side and oxygen administered if available. Parents of a child who has frequent fits may have received instructions on provision of suitable immediate care and may even administer an appropriate anticonvulsant. Although prolonged convulsions will require anticonvulsants to be given by the intravenous route, early treatment may be commenced by the rectal administration of diazepam 0·5 mg/kg, after which the child will require continued supervision.

The child should then be transferred to hospital for futher treatment and investigations.

Febrile convulsions are the commonest cause of fits in children between the ages of 6 months and 5 years. Characteristically they present as a generalized fit of 5–10 min duration in a child who has recently developed an acute rise in body temperature. In addition to the measures already described, the child should be cooled by removing the clothes and sponging the surface of the body with tepid water. Although most children with febrile convulsions respond to these simple measures, some continue to fit and require anticonvulsant therapy.

BURNS

Burns are an important cause of accidental death in childhood. The majority of burn injuries occur at home to children under 5 years of age.

Scalds are an especially distressing form of injury which can occur when a child pulls a saucepan of water from a cooker or turns a hot tap on in the bath only to find that he cannot turn it off again. In a child who has just suffered a severe scald, symptomatic relief may be provided by the liberal application of cold water to the affected area.

House fires are particularly lethal since, in addition to external injury, there may also be airway burns and lung damage caused by inhalation of hot gases, carbon monoxide and toxic combustion products which are released from the foam filling of modern furniture. Extensive burns may therefore produce pain, airway problems and shock. In these cases clothing may still be smouldering or even alight. Water should be used to extinguish any flames, and lower the temperature of the clothing material, thus providing some symptomatic relief and reducing further burn damage. Water, however, is unsuitable where burning oil is involved such as in chip pan fires. Any child who has been in a smoke filled room should be immediately removed into the open air and given oxygen. Remember that he may have inhaled carbon monoxide and, therefore, look characteristically pink, and oxygen administration is even more important. One must remember that breathing may become rapidly obstructed by oedema of the upper airways if the child has sustained respiratory burn injuries. It is important to be suspicious of any child who has burns around his mouth, singed nasal hairs, a black tongue and is coughing up a sooty secretion.

A severely burnt child should be transferred to hospital as rapidly as possible. Pain relief may be provided by the administration of Entonox which, in addition to providing analgesia, will also allow the administration of supplemental oxygen. Further management of these cases centres around management of 'shock', by means of intravenous fluids to maintain circulatory blood volume, pain relief and airway care. Cases with severe airway burns may require tracheostomy at an early stage.

CHILD ABUSE

Child abuse is unfortunately quite common, affecting at least one child in one thousand. The highest incidence is in children under the age of 2 and, where injuries are inflicted, the term Non-accidental Injury (NAI) is used.

Paramedical personnel, such as ambulance crews, may be involved in providing immediate care for victims of NAI and features which should arouse suspicion are as follows:
Multiple bruises including black eyes
Fractures
Bite marks
Scalds and cigarette burns
Poisoning
Evidence of neglect
Delay in seeking medical attention
Unexplained injury
Implausible explanation of injury

If non-accidental injury is suspected, the child must be admitted to hospital, but considerable tact must be used when dealing with the parents. On no account should the parents be accused or made aware of one's suspicions. It is important to remember that the victim remains at risk from further injury until removed from that environment.

Further reading
Black J. A. (1979) *Paediatric Emergencies.* London, Butterworths.
Illingworth C. M. (1978) *The Diagnosis and Primary Care of Accidents and Emergencies in Children.* Oxford, Blackwell Scientific Publications.

Chapter 21

Toxicology and Common Poisoning

H. G. Schroeder

Poisoning by drugs or other toxic substances is very common, usually by intentional self-administration and with the exception of children, rarely accidental. Admissions to hospital in the UK for self-poisoning approach 120 000 annually, and this figure can probably be doubled if the mildly poisoned patients who are sent home from the Accident and Emergency Department, or who are treated at home are included.

Approximately 1 in 5 of all acute medical admissions to hospital are due to poisoning, and about one-fifth of these cases require admission to Intensive Care Units. The national mortality from poisoning is approximately 2 per cent, whereas the hospital inpatient death rate from poisoning is much lower, at approximately 0·6 per cent.

A considerable proportion of the fatal cases have developed hypoxic damage or cardiac arrest either during the journey to hospital or within minutes of arrival at the Accident and Emergency Department. This would indicate a need for meticulous care with the management of the patient with impaired consciousness to prevent needless loss of life or serious brain damage during transport.

The common poisons taken have changed over the years, barbiturates becoming less common, whereas the poisonings from tranquillizer drugs, analgesic drugs and antidepressant drugs have all markedly increased.

GENERAL PRINCIPLES OF MANAGEMENT

The majority of poisoned patients will recover with no more than general conservative supportive therapy which will vary in individual cases from simple first aid to full intensive care. This is best discussed under the following four headlines:

TOXICOLOGY AND COMMON POISONING 223

1. Protection and delay of absorption
2. General supportive therapy
3. Elimination and detoxication
4. Antidotes.

1. **Protection and delay of absorption**
The simplest form of protection is to remove the patient from the environment of the poison, e.g. in carbon monoxide poisoning. The alternative approach is to remove the poison from the patient by promoting vomiting or gastric washout, but these methods should be undertaken with caution. For instance, under no circumstances, should vomiting be induced or gastric washout be attempted if the patient has ingested any corrosive acid or alkali material. To do so would be to encourage dangerous complications of oesophageal or gastric damage. Similarly, if kerosene or petroleum products have been taken, attempts to produce vomiting should be avoided because of the risk of aspiration with inhalational fume damage to the lungs.

Equally important is the complete avoidance of any attempt outside hospital to promote vomiting or to perform gastric washout in any unconscious, or even semiconscious patient, because of the risk of uncontrolled aspiration of stomach contents and contamination of the lungs.

In appropriate circumstances, however, induced vomiting or gastric washout, by removing the poison before it is absorbed, can reduce the severity of poisoning. Gastric washout is only practical in hospital, but induced vomiting can be practised by emergency medical technicians. The usual methods of inducing emesis are:
   a. Pharyngeal stimulation, with fingers. This is fairly safe, but not very effective.
   b. Syrup of Ipecacuanha is more effective, especially in children (*see* Chapter 20).
   c. Strong salt solution is not very effective and runs the risk of danger from hypernatraemia. It should be no longer used, and the practice should be actively discouraged.
   d. Apomorphine—given subcutaneously or intramuscularly is always very effective, but promotes repetitive vomiting. *This is unpleasant and dangerous, and the use of apomorphine should be only very rarely considered, and then only in association with the appropriate antidote (naloxone).*

Oral adsorbent agents
It is possible in cases where induced vomiting or gastric washout is not practical, or where complete removal of poison cannot be achieved, to complement the protection by adding an oral adsorbent drug, which will encourage the poison to cling to it, thus preventing its ultimate

absorption into the bloodstream. Many substances have been recommended as suitable adsorbent agents, such as milk, egg white and olive oil, but only activated charcoal is really worthy of consideration. The adsorbent capacity of activated charcoal (Medicoal) makes it very efficient, safe and cheap. Medicoal is a pleasant, effervescent activated charcoal presentation which is very easy to administer. It must be remembered however, that it complements induced vomiting but does not replace it, and can be used after gastric lavage. Activated charcoal adsorbs barbiturates, tranquillizers, paracetamol, tricyclic antidepressants, phenothiazines and many other drugs.

2. General supportive therapy
Symptoms of poisoning
The general symptoms of poisoning are illustrated in *Table* 21.1. They do not occur in all cases, and are seen more commonly in the severe poisonings.

Table 21.1. General symptoms of poisoning

1. *Impairment of conscious level*
   Coma
2. *Depression of respiration*
   Hypoxia
3. *Depression of cardiovascular function*
   Cardiac irregularities
4. *Impairment of temperature regulation*
   Hypothermia
   Hyperthermia
5. *Stimulation of central nervous system*
   Convulsions
6. *Impairment of renal function*

Impairment of conscious level
The poisoned patient may be awake, drowsy, semiconscious or unconscious. It is important to remember that the situation can rapidly change and that conscious level may deepen into full unconsciousness. It is necessary to assess conscious level. An objective, reliable, easily performed and repeatable assessment may be obtained using the Glasgow Coma Scale (*Table* 21.2). Continued monitoring of conscious level is necessary to assess progress of the poisoned patient in the response to supportive treatment.

Table 21.2. The Glasgow coma scale

Eye opening	
Spontaneous	4 ⎫
To speech	3 ⎬ E
To pain	2 ⎪
Nil	1 ⎭
Best motor response	
Obeys	6 ⎫
Localizes	5 ⎪
Withdraws (flexion)	4 ⎬ M
Abnormal flexion	3 ⎪
Extensor response	2 ⎪
Nil	1 ⎭
Verbal response	
Orientated	5 ⎫
Confused conversation	4 ⎪
Inappropriate words	3 ⎬ V
Incomprehensible sounds	2 ⎪
Nil	1 ⎭

Coma score (responsiveness sum = 3–15 (E + M + V)

Supportive therapy

Respiratory function

Respiratory function is commonly impaired in poisoning and requires careful and immediate attention, particularly in the semiconscious or unconscious patient.
1. Patency of airway
It is essential to ensure that the patient has a clear airway (*see* p. 72).
2. Adequate ventilation
Most poisons that impair consciousness also depress respiration, and it is important at this stage to assess whether respiration is adequate, and if it is not, to support ventilation.
3. Adequate oxygenation
Oxygen should always be given to all patients with impaired consciousness, especially if poisoning has occured from carbon monoxide or any other inhaled fumes or gas.

Cardiovascular support

In acute poisoning the patient is often hypotensive due to vasodilatation. Such hypotension is not usually dangerous as long as the systolic blood pressure is above 80 mmHg and urine output is maintained. Restoration of the blood pressure should be achieved in the first instance by the head-down position, and cautious use of plasma expanders, or other suitable intravenous fluids, such as 0·9 per cent Saline, Hartmann's solution, Haemaccel or Dextrans.

Convulsions

Convulsions can be due to hypoxia, the poison taken, or both. The first line of treatment should be to oxygenate the patient adequately, as adequate oxygenation will remove the cause for hypoxic convulsions, and will raise the threshold for drug-induced convulsions. If the convulsions persist despite adequate oxygenation, they should be controlled using intravenous diazepam or clonazepam. It is important to note that these drugs may produce an increase in respiratory depression which may necessitate artificial respiration.

Hypothermia and hyperthermia

Poisoning can interfere with the normal regulation of body temperature and result in hypothermia and, rarely, hyperthermia. Hypothermia occurs when there has been delay in discovering the poisoned patient and can become so severe as to simulate death. The treatment of such patients is outlined in Chapter 22. When hyperthermia occurs, active cooling with fans and ice bags is necessary to lower the temperature to near normal.

3. Elimination and detoxication

Elimination of poison from the patient can be undertaken by stomach washout, but this is only effective if performed soon after ingestion of the drug. The amount of drug removed by stomach washout is often disappointing. Stomach washout should never be attempted in any patient who has taken corrosive agents or kerosene products and should only be undertaken in semiconscious or unconscious patients after first protecting the trachea and respiratory tract with a cuffed endotracheal tube. In aspirin poisoning and tricyclic antidepressant poisoning, the stomach should always be washed out, even if a period of longer than 4 hours has elapsed since ingestion.

An important aspect of elimination of the poison from the body is the maintenance of adequate urine output, and this is achieved by intravenous administration of reasonable quantities of fluid to maintain a urine output of at least 0·5 ml/kg/hour.

Forced diuresis

In aspirin poisoning effective removal of the drug can be achieved by forced diuresis. In its simplest form this involves encouraging the patient to drink large quantities of fluid, or in its more elaborate form the intravenous infusion of fluid, in moderately large quantities accompanied by the forced production of a diuresis by drugs such as frusemide or mannitol. The aim would be to produce a urine flow of 7 ml/kg/hour.

The method is not without dangerous complications, notably pulmonary oedema from over-infusion, hypokalaemia and hypoglycaemia from uncontrolled diuresis. Very careful hour to hour fluid balance is essential.

Dialysis

Peritoneal dialysis and full haemodialysis have been used for severe cases, but the more recent advent of charcoal column haemoperfusion has to some extent replaced these two methods. Charcoal column haemoperfusion involves passing the blood through devices containing adsorbent particles of activated charcoal, exchange resins and anion resins which remove the poison by adsorption. This method has been shown to be effective in poisoning from barbiturates, salicylates, tricyclic antidepressant drugs, methaqualone and many other drugs.

4. Antidotes

There are only a few specific antidotes available and unfortunately, these are not relevant to the more common poisons taken. However, on the occasions when an antidote can be used, the effect can be dramatic and life saving. The known antidotes available are:

Iron.—Desferrioxamine is a suitable antidote which chelates iron, rendering it ineffective. It can be given orally or intravenously.

Narcotic Analgesic Drugs—A specific antidote naloxone (Narcan) is available, which rapidly reverses the respiratory depressant effect of the narcotic analgesic drugs. More than one dose may be necessary. It is only partially effective against buprenorphine (Temgesic).

Cyanide—the chelating agent Kelacyanor is very effective if given within minutes of taking cyanide, Hydroxycobalamin (Vitamin K) is also useful.

Heavy Metals—such as lead, can be suitably treated with d-penicillamine or dimercaprol as an antidote. Calcium disodium edetate is also very effective.

Nerve Gas Poisons (Pesticides)—the cholinesterase rejuvenating drug pralidoxime is a true antidote when given intravenously.

Paracetamol—Methionine and cysteamine, while not true antidotes, are protective against the hepatic damage from paracetamol. N-acetylcysteine (Parvolex) is an alternative in this situation.

Specific common poisons and their characteristics
Barbiturates

The classic problems of barbiturate poisoning are impairment of consciousness, depression of respiration, hypotension from vasodilatation and hypothermia. The severity of all the above presenting symptoms is increased if the drug is taken in association with alcohol. The greatest life-threatening danger is respiratory obstruction and respiratory depression, hypoxia and cardiac arrest. Blister-like bullous lesions are often seen on fingers, knees and ankles, but these are not specific to barbiturate poisoning. Treatment should be directed at airway and ventilatory support, adequate oxygenation and maintenance of urine output. Forced diuresis is only useful in phenobarbitone poisoning, and charcoal haemoperfusion may be needed in the very severe cases.

Tranquillizer drugs

The commonest group are the benzodiazepines.

The effect of these drugs in overdose is usually mild, showing mainly as impairment of consciousness, with only mild depression of respiration, but this depression can assume serious levels if alcohol has also been taken. Simple airway support is usually all that is necessary, but occasionally artificial respiratory support is needed.

Phenothiazine drugs

These drugs are used as anti-emetics or antipsychotics. The signs of poisoning are usually impairment of consciousness, hypotension and convulsions.

Respiratory depression is less common, other than in very severe cases. Cardiac irregularities are often seen and hypothermia may be present and can sometimes be profound, simulating death. Treatment is entirely supportive. Convulsions should be controlled with diazepam.

Tricyclic antidepressant drugs

The tricyclic antidepressant drugs are the most common drugs used in the treatment of depression. They include such drugs as amitriptyline and imipramine and many others which act similarly. These drugs block the re-uptake of noradrenaline into intracerebral neurones. Symptoms of poisoning can vary from drowsiness, tachycardia and dry mouth, to unconsciousness, convulsions, gross cardiac irregularities and cardiac arrest. Mortality in severe poisoning is usually due to hypoxia and cardiac arrest, which can occur without prior loss of consciousness. Treatment is supportive, with emphasis on adequate oxygenation, control of convulsions and close monitoring and control of cardiac irregularity. Hypoxia, if allowed to occur, will increase the potential incidence of convulsions and cardiac irregularities. Symptoms can occur within 1 hour of taking the overdose, so particular care during transport to hospital is necessary. Antidepressant drugs taken in combination with other drugs such as alcohol or barbiturates increase severity of all potential symptoms. Charcoal column haemoperfusion is useful in severe cases, especially if cardiotoxicity is a main presenting feature.

Monoamine oxidase inhibitor drugs

These drugs are also used in the treatment of depression. They inhibit the action of monoamine oxidase so that pressor substances in food are absorbed unchanged, causing headaches and convulsions ('the cheese reaction'). Poisoning symptoms are coma, convulsions, hypertension and tachycardia. Treatment is entirely supportive, diazepam being administered to control the convulsions.

Salicylate poisoning

Aspirin poisoning remains relatively common, mainly because of easy access to the drug. Accidental aspirin poisoning is commonly seen in children. Early signs of poisoning are sweating, high temperature, buzzing in the ears and vomiting. Drowsiness and clouding of consciousness is a late development, unless some other drug such as a hypnotic or alcohol has also been taken.

Initial alkalosis is replaced by increasing acidosis and central nervous system irritability. Central respiratory and cardiovascular depression only occur in very severe cases. Hypoglycaemia may be a feature. Bleeding from hypoprothrombinaemia and inhibition of platelet aggregation may occur. The severity of poisoning is related to the blood level of salicylate, and the higher the blood level the more severe the effects. Every effort must be made to reduce and control the blood level of salicylate as soon as possible and this may involve oral forced diuresis, forced intravenous diuresis, peritoneal dialysis, haemodialysis or charcoal column haemoperfusion. Good effective forced alkaline diuresis can halve a blood salicylate level in 6 hours, but care must be taken that the therapy does not produce complications of pulmonary oedema. Stomach washout is essential in salicylate poisoning, as the tablets aggregate in the stomach and can erode gastric mucosa leading to perforation.

Paracetamol poisoning

The main problem with paracetamol poisoning is the tendency for delayed liver damage. This is caused by the breakdown products of paracetamol directly affecting liver cells. Drugs such as methionine, cysteamine and N-acetylcysteine (Parvolex) have been shown to protect the liver against damage by paracetamol breakdown products, and are directly indicated if the blood level of paracetamol approaches hepatotoxic levels. The liver damage occurs 2 or 3 days after ingestion of the toxic dose.

Symptoms of acute poisoning are very few, although most patients attend hospital stating the fact they have taken paracetamol. If other drugs have been taken with paracetamol, then drowsiness or coma may present. Distalgesic (a combination of paracetamol and dextropropoxyphene) produces coma and respiratory depression early, due to the dextropropoxyphene, which is a narcotic analgesic drug with direct respiratory depressant effects. These effects can be very quickly neutralized using the narcotic antagonist drug naloxone (Narcan). Once it is known that paracetamol has been taken, stomach washout should be performed and activated charcoal administered. In this context activated charcoal is very effective as it will reduce absorption of any remaining paracetamol by about 70 per cent. Similar results can be achieved using cholestyramine.

Narcotic analgesic drugs

The 'narcotic analgesic drugs', share the quality in overdose of producing marked respiratory depression characterized by very slow deep breathing until breathing ceases altogether. Other classic features are 'pinpoint' pupils, unconsciousness and convulsions. The cause of death is respiratory depression. These drugs can be antagonized by naloxone (Narcan) which has completely revolutionized the treatment of narcotic analgesic poisoning (*see* Vol. 1, Chapter 24). The dose of naloxone may need to be repeated. All other treatment in narcotic overdose is supportive.

Paraquat poisoning

Paraquat is used as a weedkiller. When taken by humans, its absorption into the bloodstream produces lesions in the lungs and other organs, and is almost always fatal. The lung is particularly sensitive to paraquat toxic effects. Paraquat also affects the renal tubules, causing oliguria. Pulmonary oedema, cardiac failure and renal failure are features. The severity of involvement is dependent on the amount of paraquat taken. Treatment involves the administration of Fuller's Earth by mouth. Charcoal haemoperfusion has been tried, but has proved disappointing. At present, there is no antidote for paraquat, and no definitive treatment is available. Patients who have taken only small quantities may survive.

Organophosphorous pesticides

These are the nerve gas poisons that are available on the market as greenfly garden pesticides. The substances inhibit the enzyme cholinesterase in the body and cause toxic cholinergic effects. The substances can be inhaled, absorbed through skin or from the gut. Symptoms include excessive salivation, respiratory paralysis, convulsions from hypoxia and coma.

Treatment is supportive, large doses of atropine to dry the secretions, and the administration of the specific antidote pralidoxime (Protopam). The usual source of poisonings of this variety are children who have accidentally drunk greenfly pesticide and occasional intentional self-poisoning by adults.

TOXICOLOGY AND COMMON POISONING

Cyanide poisoning

Hydrocyanic acid is a constituent of certain pesticides, metal polishes and electroplating solutions. Cyanide, when ingested, poisons the respiratory enzyme systems of the body, and is rapidly fatal. Symptoms appear within seconds and include dizziness, dyspnoea, confusion, coma, and collapse. Cyanosis is not usually present, the skin showing a pink colour, and there is sometimes a smell of bitter almonds on the breath. The antidote for cyanide poisoning is Kelocyanor (dicobalt edetate), or sodium nitrite with sodium thiosulphate. Hydroxycobalamin (vitamin K) is sometimes useful. Supportive treatment is also necessary.

Iron poisoning

This type of poisoning occurs usually in children, who mistake the coloured iron tablets for sweets. Symptoms are epigastric pain, nausea and haematemesis, leading to circulatory collapse. Treatment is prompt administration of the specific antidote desferrioxamine (Desferal) accompanied by gastric lavage.

Carbon monoxide poisoning

Although the replacement of coal gas by natural gas should have resulted in the reduction of carbon monoxide poisonings, this has not been so. Partial combustion of natural gas in faulty appliances produces carbon monoxide as does the internal combustion engine. Carbon monoxide combines with haemoglobin in blood to produce carboxyhaemoglobin, which prevents the combination of oxygen with haemoglobin, leading to increasing hypoxaemia and tissue hypoxia. Symptoms are unconsciousness, with classic 'cherry red' skin appearance, progressing to cardiovascular collapse and pulmonary oedema. Treatment involves removing the patient from the source of carbon monoxide and administration of 100 per cent oxygen, with progression in the more severe cases to hyperbaric oxygen at a pressure of two or three atmospheres.

Poisoning by plants

Many plants are poisonous, such as black bryony, broom, lupins, laburnum, monkshood, hemlock, holly, mistletoe and laurel. There is no specific antidote to any, and as a rule only small quantities are taken. Treatment is mainly supportive.

Deadly nightshade and black nightshade produce berries which cause atropine poisoning, the antidote to which is pilocarpine or physostigmine. Mushrooms and toadstools produce muscarine poisoning, the antidote to which is atropine, along with other general measures of supportive therapy (for further information on poisoning in children, *see* Chapter 19).

Poisons information services

The range and variety of toxic substances that can be ingested is so vast that no presentation could hope to be comprehensive. Poisonings can involve different tablets taken at the same time, and this is becoming more common. The majority of common poisonings can be managed by supportive conservative therapy, plus the occasional use of antidotes when indicated. For other rarer and more exotic cases of poisoning, the guidance available from the National Poisons Information Services should be sought. These centres provide information on toxicity, symptoms and treatment for all known poisons, and the telephone numbers are:
  Belfast (0232) 40503
  Cardiff (0222) 492233
  Dublin (0001) 745588
  Edinburgh (031) 229 2477
  London (01) 407 7600

Further reading

Matthew H. and Lawson A. A. H. (1979) *Treatment of Common Acute Poisons*, 4th ed. Edinburgh, Churchill Livingstone.

Chapter 22

The Trauma of Civil Disturbance

D. G. Ferguson

'If you want a picture of the future, imagine a boot stamping on a human face forever'

George Orwell *'1984'*

The problem of civil disturbance is here now; paramedical personnel may find themselves having to cope with it in its many facets. The terrible thing about civil disorder is the fact that in a civilized society, one person, or group of people, sets out to intentionally injure or kill others.

The key to the conduct of the paramedic in the civil disturbance situation is that he should never get involved, he must never take a side and above all he must ensure his own safety within the bounds of common sense and reason. The temptation for bravado can be very great, but the injured paramedic is of no value to other victims of a riot situation and may only prove a hindrance to his colleagues.

A riot situation may result from an organized march or protest, or it may occur spontaneously, perhaps being initiated by a street fight or the arrest of an individual in an area where he has many sympathizers. Initially, as tempers fray and bystanders become involved, the riot situation can appeal in particular to the teenager. The riot may appear as good fun, as the rioter can break out from the constraints of law and order, and there is the potential to loot and so receive material gain from the situation. The atmosphere is electrifying until such time as the individual becomes involved to such an extent that he is either injured or he is put into a situation in which injury is very likely.

The injuries from a riot may initially be limited to blows from fists or feet. These should never be underestimated, in particular when an individual who has been knocked to the ground is attacked and kicked. It is quite possible to kill somebody in this situation and severe facial, head, chest and abdominal injuries can result. If sticks, metal bars, etc. are being used, again severe head injuries can be inflicted. Stoning is a common activity in rioting and one has only to look at the pictures of a riot to see the very large numbers of stones, half bricks and other missiles laying around the forces of law and order. Stones can cause very considerable injuries and certainly unless the police are wearing riot gear, they will not be protected. The missiles come in various sizes, but it is not uncommon to have bricks and half bricks thrown. Another unpleasant missile is a steel ball-bearing fired from a catapult. This is potentially very dangerous and the injuries can be quite severe, particularly if the face or head is struck.

In this type of situation, the paramedic may be tempted to underestimate the severity of injuries and as with all riot situations he should remove the victims from the riot zone when it is safe to do so, and take them well behind the lines of the rioting factions where they can have treatment rendered to them. Where injuries are more severe, then resuscitation must be initiated.

In hand to hand fighting, the possibility of stab wounds must be considered. These can be easily missed unless there is marked bleeding, or unless the victim is aware of the fact that he has been stabbed. In a stabbing, there will only be a small wound where the knife has entered. The size of the wound gives no indication as to the direction the wounding instrument has taken, nor as to the depth it has reached. From the anatomical position of the wound, that is if it is in the chest or abdomen, a guess can be made as to which organs may be injured. All knife wounds require hospital treatment and many of them will require exploratory operations. The paramedic should ensure that patients are evacuated to hospital with the minimum of delay. Heavy bleeding from a wound can be controlled by local pressure, but there may be massive internal bleeding in the presence of only minor external bleeding.

RIOT CONTROL

'Snatch squads' have been used. The principle is that a team of specially trained soldiers or police with protective equipment and batons, would rush into the riot situation and hopefully arrest the ring leaders and bring them out of the riot. CS gas has been used in Ulster as well as elsewhere in the UK. It can be launched by various methods, and when the grenade explodes amongst the rioters, the gas is released. CS gas causes stinging of the eyes which then water heavily and the nose runs. The victims cough and the whole effect is very unpleasant. It is claimed that no harmful affects result from CS gas unless released in an enclosed space, although there are those who would debate this point. A method of coping with it in the streets is to soak a handkerchief in a solution of vinegar and water, this is then used to cover the mouth and nose. The army and police obviously have gas masks, but one of the problems associated with CS gas is that it is dependent on the direction that the wind is blowing and so in many situations it would not be feasible to use it.

Water cannons were used at the beginning of the 'troubles' in Ulster, but they proved to be unsuccessful. The water cannon works by virtue of spraying the rioters with water and by so doing, hopefully deters them. One of the disadvantages is the noise generated during pressurization of the device giving the rioters an opportunity to get out of the way of the water jets. An attempt was made to put dye in the water, to facilitate the identification of the rioters, but this idea was also abandoned.

Rubber bullets or baton rounds have been used in great numbers in Ulster. They are about 5 in (12·5 cm) long and are fired from a baton gun. The idea behind them was that they would strike the rioters a sharp blow and so deter them. Rubber bullets proved to be very inaccurate and they resulted in a considerable number of facial and chest injuries. They have been superseded by plastic bullets, which are ballistically more stable and although they cause fewer chest and facial wounds, they have been responsible for a number of fatal head injuries.

WEAPONS USED IN CIVIL DISTURBANCES

Petrol bombs

Petrol bombs commonly consist of a milk bottle containing petrol and a piece of rag stuffed in the neck of the bottle. Such a weapon may appear harmless enough, but they are potentially lethal to both victim and aggressor! The rag is lit and the bottle is thrown. When the glass shatters, the petrol is spread over a considerable area. If an individual is close enough, he can be sprayed with petrol and set on fire. The potential danger from a petrol bomb should not be underestimated, as they can cause very severe burns.

Shotgun

Shotguns are readily available to many people and so there is always a possibility that they may be used in a riot situation. The injuries will depend to some extent upon the size of the shot in the cartridges, but generally speaking, at longer range, individuals are just peppered with small pieces of shot. These tend to just penetrate the skin and although extremely uncomfortable do not create any danger to life. However, even at long range, they can cause severe eye injuries. At close quarters, a shotgun is lethal and the injury caused by it may be so massive that the victim will die before medical assistance can be sought. In such situations treatment should be simple first aid measures, with control of obvious haemorrhage and rapid evacuation to hospital.

Low-velocity missiles

A low-velocity missile is one which is travelling at less than the speed of sound which is approximately 1100 ft/sec. These missiles are generally fired from hand guns and this type of weapon causes the majority of gunshot wounds that are seen in an urban setting. Low-velocity missiles cause laceration and crushing of tissues. The injury is restricted to the track along which the missile passes and the missile will often remain within the victim. Low-velocity missiles have a tendency to follow tissue planes within the body. Thus, from the point of view of the surgeon, the bullets can sometimes be difficult to locate, as they have not travelled in a straight line.

High-velocity missiles

High-velocity missiles have been available since the middle of the 19th century and they are missiles which are travelling at a speed greater than that of sound. Modern weapons generally have a muzzle velocity in the region of 3000 ft/sec. The injuries caused by these missiles, which are fired from rifles, are very much greater than that caused by a low-velocity missile. This is related to the energy expended by the missile when it strikes the biological target.
The formula:

$$\frac{M(V_1^2 - V_2^2)}{2} = \text{Energy expended}$$

defines the problem. M represents the mass of the missile, V_1 is the initial velocity of the missile and V_2 is the velocity of the missile after it has struck its target. From this it can be seen that the problem is related to the decrease in velocity of the missile upon impact. The trend with modern weapons is to make a small missile, which travels at a very high speed. The self-loading rifle (SLR), used by the British Army, fires a 7·62 mm bullet, which weighs 9·4 g. This missile has a muzzle velocity of 2800 ft/sec approximately. The Armalite rifle which is often used by terrorists in Northern Ireland, has a 5·56 mm bullet which weighs 3·6 g and has a muzzle velocity of 3200 ft/sec. It is a more unstable missile than the SLR bullet and so it tends to 'tumble' when it hits its target. High-velocity missiles have totally different characteristics from low-velocity missiles. They create shock waves within the victim. These shock waves travel at a very high speed of almost 5000 ft/sec and they create pressures of anything up to 1500 lb/in^2. The shock wave remains within the victim for a very short time, about 0·000001 sec. A feature of high-velocity wounds is the fact that they create a temporary cavity. This is a cavity which will be some 30–40 times the diameter of the missile itself. This cavity is created within the victim; it has a negative pressure and so it sucks bacteria and debris into the wound track. The overall effect of a

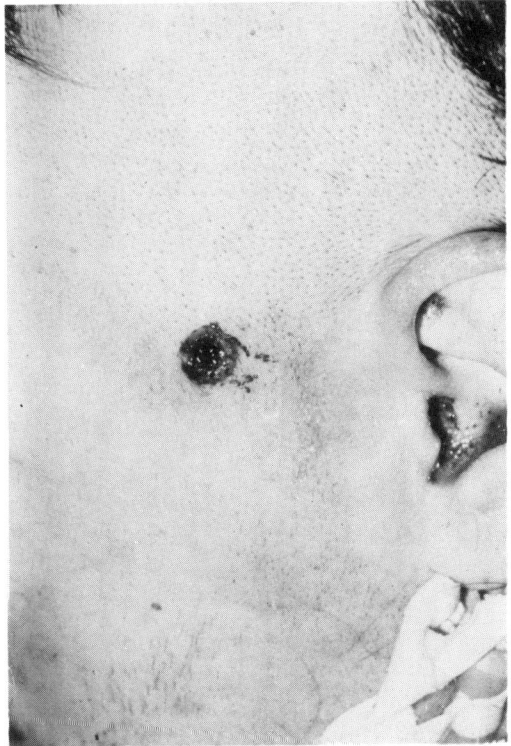

Fig. 22.1. Entrance wound made by a high-velocity missile. It is impossible from the appearance of this wound to determine whether the missile was high velocity rather than low velocity.

high-velocity wound is that the damage to the tissue extends far beyond the wound track itself (*Fig.* 22.3) and vessels and bones can be damaged which are not directly in the line of the missile. The features of a gunshot wound may be fairly unremarkable. Usually the entrance wound is small (*Fig.* 22.1), depending upon the weapon. If the weapon was fired at close range, there may be burns and carbon particles surrounding the wound. High-velocity injuries sometimes have large exit wounds (*Fig.* 22.2), particularly if a bone has been struck by the missile. This is not a constant finding and because the exit and entrance wounds may both be small, it does not preclude the possibility that the missile was a high-velocity one.

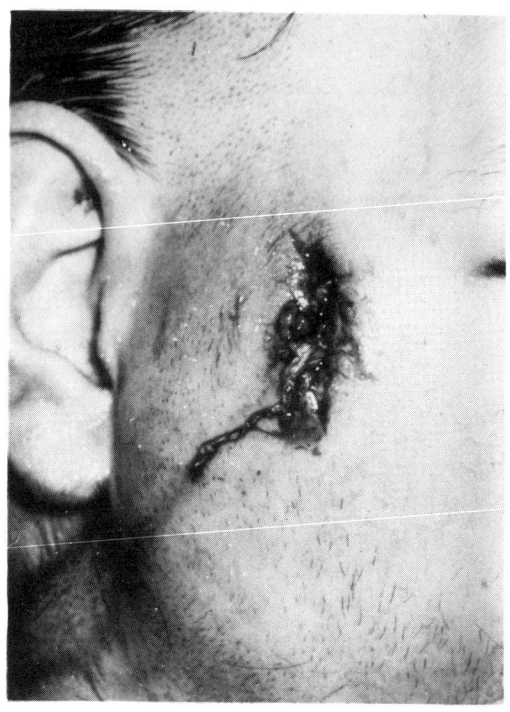

Fig. 22.2. Exit wound from the missile which caused the wound in *Fig.* 22.1. This is a large wound and as such it has the features of a high-velocity exit wound.

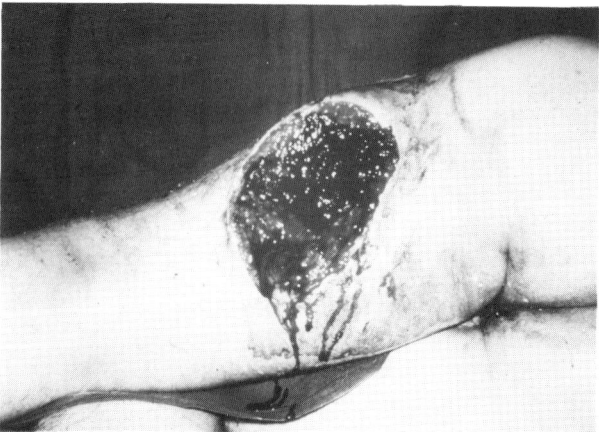

Fig. 22.3. A high-velocity wound to the thigh which has been surgically laid open; there is extensive muscle damage within the thigh.

THE TRAUMA OF CIVIL DISTURBANCE

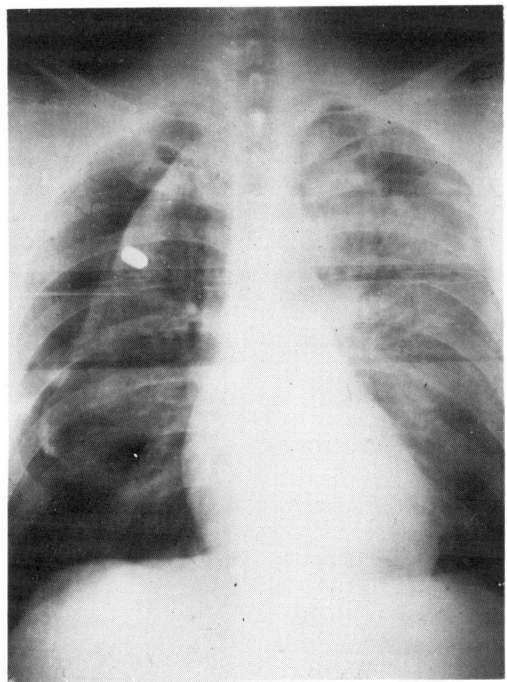

Fig. 22.4. This is a bilateral gunshot wound to the chest, caused by a low-velocity missile. The bullet entered through the left side of the chest, it passed through the upper lobe of the left lung and then it slipped between the oesophagus and the vertebral column without damaging either. This demonstrates the ability of a low-velocity missile to follow its tissue plane. The bullet then came to rest in the right upper lung and was readily visible on X-ray.

At the scene of a shooting, treatment can be rendered to the individual, but generally speaking if the airway is maintained and obvious haemorrhage is controlled by pressure, then the the patient should be rapidly evacuated to hospital. The patient may have been shot a number of times, but this will not be obvious at the scene of the incident and it is only when the patient is fully stripped and a careful examination made, that the various wounds can be found. X-rays are helpful in locating bullets and in determining bony injury (*Fig.* 22.4). It must be remembered that the entrance and exit wounds may not necessarily bear an exact relationship to each other when a patient is lying flat on a trolley, as the individual may have been running or crouching when they were shot, thus the position of his body was very different at the time of the shooting, compared to that when he is being examined in hospital. If

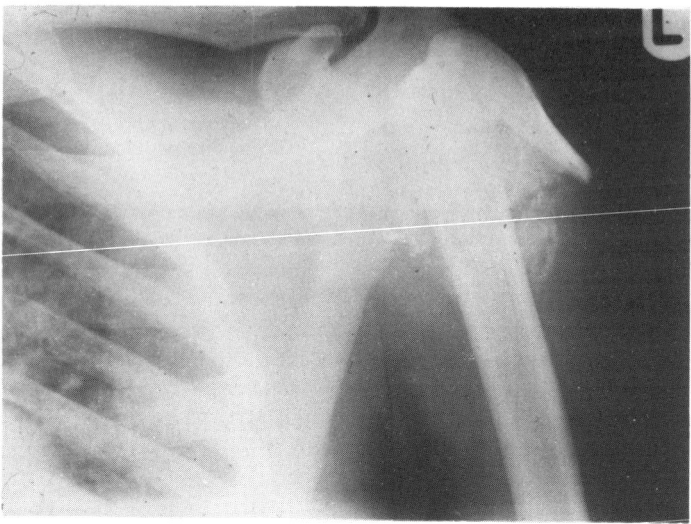

Fig. 22.5. This demonstrates a fracture through the neck of the humerus and it has been caused by a bullet; fragments of metal can be noted around the fracture.

this fact is remembered, then it may be possible to work out the direction from which the bullet was travelling.

The number of holes caused by the bullet or bullets in a patient is important, in that they may all be entry wounds, or there may be an even number of entry and exit wounds. If the number is uneven, then it is reasonable to assume that there is still a bullet within the patient.

All bullet wounds require surgical exploration. The treatment of gunshot wounds is to remove all the dead tissue. This is particularly important in high-velocity wounds. This may result in very large wounds being left, but no attempt must be made to close them as they tend to become infected. Delayed primary suture is carried out on the fourth or fifth day, that is, the wounds are closed at this time. This has proven to be the safest way of treating gunshot wounds. Wounds to the brain, pleura and peritoneum require primary closure, that is closure at the first operation, as these contained structures are at greater risk of infection if left exposed, and the chest must be sealed for normal respiration.

Explosives

Explosive substances have been used in many forms by terrorists. They may be commercial explosives, or home-made explosives, which utilize chemicals found in fertilizers. The explosives can be presented in many forms, extending from parcel bombs and letter bombs, to larger bombs

THE TRAUMA OF CIVIL DISTURBANCE

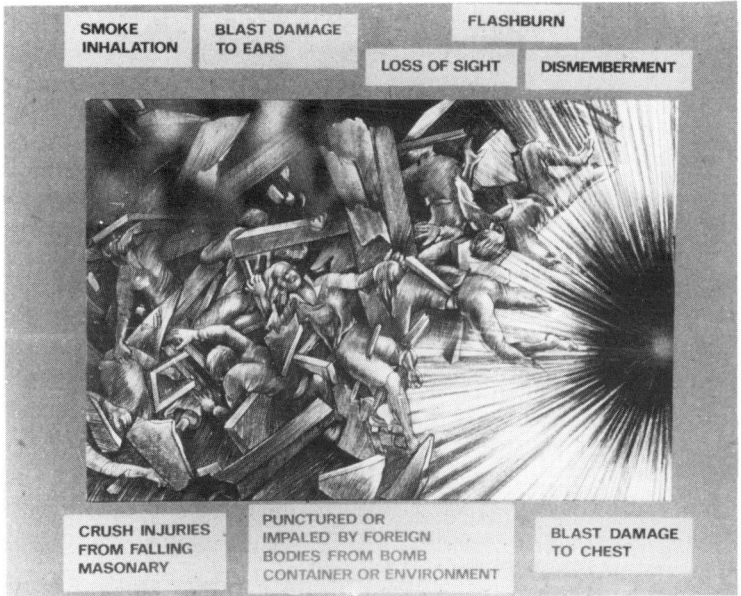

Fig. 22.6. This is an artist's impression of a bomb explosion and it demonstrates many of the features of an explosion.

with complicated anti-handling devices on them. Many of the bombs are utilized in booby-traps. Sometimes a bomb will be packed with nails, thus producing an anti-personnel device which scatters its lethal shrapnel over a wide area. Fairly large bombs are often placed in culverts beside the road, in the hope of blowing up army or police vehicles.

When an explosive substance is detonated, it is rapidly converted into a large mass of gas, which is initially a small volume at a very high pressure; this rapidly expands (*Fig.* 22.6). The result is a positive pressure wave with a thin layer of compressed air just in front of it. This is less than 0·001 in thick. It travels out in a spherical fashion from the point of detonation, at supersonic speed. The speed of the pressure wave rapidly reduces to the speed of sound. The pressure within the wave front is extremely high close to the explosion centre and then decreases according to the third power of the distance from the explosion centre. By virtue of the rapid progress of the shock wave through the atmosphere, it creates a dynamic pressure, which is the blast wind. Following on this, there is a negative pressure wave which lasts about ten times as long as the positive pressure wave. The negative pressure wave can never be more than minus 15 lb/in^2, which is a perfect vacuum. A problem which can occur with a blast wave is seen when it is reflected off a flat surface. The reflected wave may have a pressure 2–9 times as great as the original wave.

As far as the unfortunate individual in the area of an explosion is concerned, the important factors are the maximum pressure of the shock wave, the rate at which it reaches its maximum pressure and the duration of that maximum pressure. The effects of blast are divided into three types. The *primary effect* of a blast is the damage caused to the individual by the variation in the environmental pressure. It mainly affects air-containing structures, such as the lung, gastrointestinal tract, ears and the paranasal sinuses. The *secondary effect* of a blast is the result of missiles which are energized by the blast wave, i.e. shrapnel from the bomb casing, or bits of brickwork, or furniture for example. The *tertiary effect* is the physical displacement of the individual by the blast wind and can either be an accelerating injury or a decelerating injury. The decelerating injury is generally caused by the individual striking a wall.

Experimental work has shown that one of the causes of death from an explosion is the fact that in the lung, the air-containing structures are pulled away from the blood vessels; this results in a breakdown of the fluid–air barrier, and air can leak into the blood vessels and result in air emboli in the coronary arteries, which effectively causes an acute heart attack.

One of the possible effects from a blast is lung injury. 'Blast lung' is not a common problem, but when it does occur, it is very difficult to treat. In the case of people who have received lung damage from a blast, changes occur within the cells of the alveoli and finally there is marked fibrosis of the lungs which makes it impossible for the patients to maintain an adequate level of oxygen in their blood. It was described in the Second World War, that when exposure to a blast had occurred there may initially be no evidence of lung problems, but that these problems could develop after a period of time which could extend from hours to several days. It is always worthwhile bearing in mind, that any victim exposed to blast may develop late pulmonary problems.

The treatment of blast injuries at the site of the explosion is of necessity limited and must be restricted to basic life support.

General principles of coping with the medical problems of civil disturbances are:

1. Ensure that it is reasonably safe for the individual to go into the field of activity.
2. Basic first-aid principles should be applied.
3. It is important to reassure and give confidence to the patients in these situations, as they are often extremely frightened and perhaps are panicking.
4. Rapid evacuation of all serious injuries to a hospital is absolutely

mandatory, in order that specialist advice can be sought and if necessary surgery can be undertaken.

Acknowledgements

May we express our thanks to the Department of Medical Photography at the Royal Victoria Hospital, Belfast, for the use of their photographs, and to Helen Macklehinney, Medical Artist, for the use of her drawing of a bomb explosion.

Further reading

Kirby N. G. and Blackburn G. (ed.) (1981) *Field Surgery Pocket Book.* London, HMSO.

Owen-Smith M. S. (ed.) (1981) *High Velocity Missile Wounds.* London, Arnold.

Chapter 23

Sports Injuries

M. J. Allen

INTRODUCTION

It is impossible to cover all aspects of sports injuries in one chapter. An attempt has been made to cover the general aspects of how injuries are classified, the types of injuries sustained, general aspects of treatment and a note on the prevention of injuries.

In recent years with more and more emphasis being put on physical fitness and the fact that people have more leisure time, more attention is being focused on sport. The number of people taking up sport at all ages and all degrees of physical fitness is increasing so it follows that the number of injuries occurring whilst participating in their chosen sport is also increasing.

However, it should be remembered that the physical nature of a sports injury is exactly the same as other types of injury. The difference lies in the requirements of the athlete who expects a speedy safe return to competition. To achieve this the athlete, often against his wishes, has to be stopped from competing and undergo a period of enforced rest. Sometimes competitions and representative calls make this impossible and the treatment has to be adjusted accordingly but this conflict of ideals only affects the top class athlete.

The aim of treatment is to ensure that the injured athlete returns to his chosen sport as quickly and as safely as is possible and that due consideration has been given to the prevention of long-term effects from his injury.

CLASSIFICATION OF INJURIES

A number of classifications exist, none of which is ideal. The one the author uses is according to the aetiology (cause) of the injury.

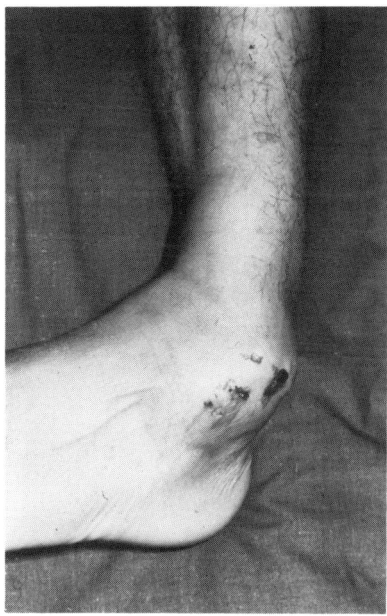

Fig. 23.1. Fracture–dislocation of the ankle.

Direct injuries — caused by direct contact.
Indirect injuries — self inflicted, occur as a result of twisting, turning or sudden bursts of energy. No other player, implement or contact with the ground is present when the injury occurs.
Over-use injuries — caused by repeated over-use of part of the anatomy until it fails.
Iatrogenic (treatment induced) injuries — occur as a result of treatment.
Late-presentation injuries — injuries in which the players purposely present late for treatment.

Direct injuries

Such injuries are caused by direct contact with another player, by an implement such as a squash racket or the ground itself. They usually present acutely and are common in body contact sports such as rugby and soccer.

Examples include lacerations, fractures, dislocations, severe ligament injuries and head injuries. *Fig.* 23.1 shows a severe fracture–dislocation of the ankle.

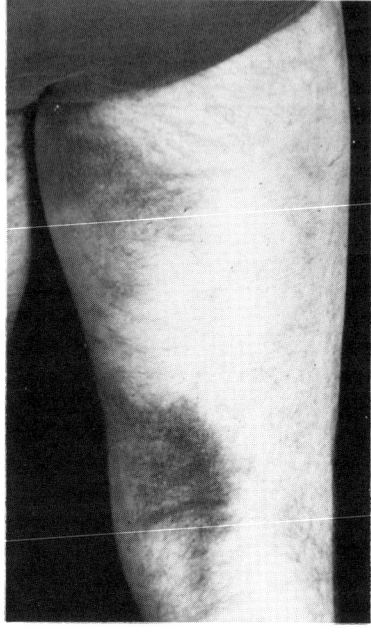

Fig. 23.2. Typical appearance of a torn hamstring. Note the excessive bruising.

Indirect injuries

These are self-inflicted and may present as acute or chronic injuries. Acute injuries can be found in all forms of sports, whereas the chronic type usually falls into the over-use group and tends to occur in marathon runners and track athletes.

Examples of acute injuries include ruptured tendons, such as the Achilles, pulled muscles such as the hamstring (found at the back of the thigh) (*Fig.* 23.2) and torn cartilages in the knee joints.

Examples of the chronic type are to be found in the over-use group.

Over-use injuries

Such injuries are usually chronic examples of indirect injuries.

Examples include stress fractures, chronic tenosynovitis (inflammation of tendon sheaths such as the Achilles), shin splints and chronic ligament sprains.

Stress fractures are fractures that occur in the leg bones as a result of repeated trauma due to excessive running on hard surfaces. Shin splints

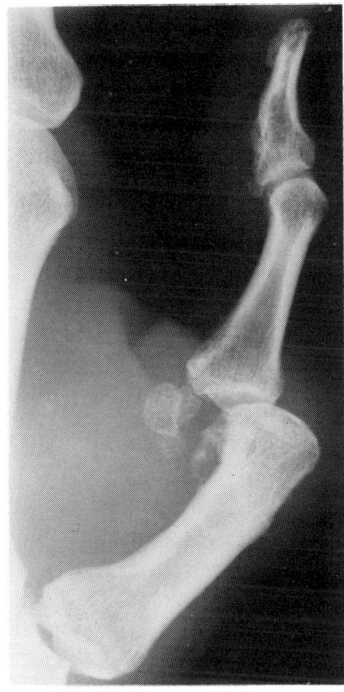
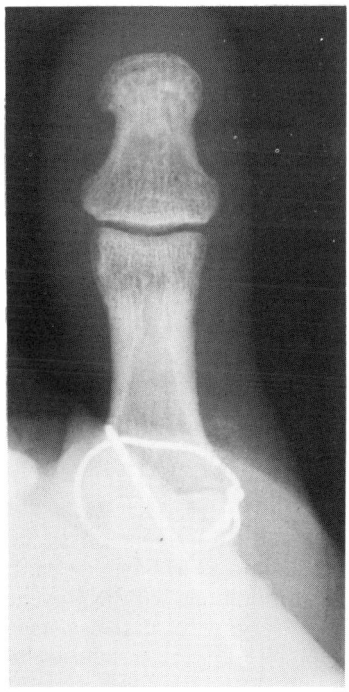

Fig. 23.3. Late-presentation injury—dislocated thumb.

Fig. 23.4. Arthrodesis of the thumb.

almost exclusively occurs in athletes and presents as pain in one or both legs brought on by exercise and relieved by rest. Chronic ligament sprains present as a result of badly managed acute ligament injuries.

Iatrogenic injuries

Such injuries occur as a result of treatment.

Examples include ruptured tendons due to steroid injections and chronic injuries resulting from an acute injury being inadequately treated; the player being brought back to full competitive activity before his acute injury has fully recovered.

Late-presentation injuries

In such injuries the players purposely present late for treatment. Nowadays at the higher levels of sport, competition is so severe that players tend to ignore injuries in the fear that they may lose their team place or miss out on an international call.

Such an example is shown in *Figs.* 23.3, 23.4 in which a player purposely continued to play with a dislocated thumb in fear of losing his place and the possibility of an international call. He presented at the end of the season with a chronic dislocation which required surgery and the joint permanently stiffened (arthrodesis) but had he presented at the time of injury all that would have been required would have been a simple manipulation to realign the digit.

ASSESSMENT AND TREATMENT OF ACUTE SEVERE INJURIES

Assessment of acute injuries

Questions that need to be answered are:
1. Is immediate treatment on the field of play required?
2. Should the player continue?
3. Is immediate hospital treatment required?

Treatment on the field of play

A quick assessment of the injury and a decision as to whether any treatment has to be given on the field of play is required. Treatment in these situations will be preventive to ensure that the injury is not made more severe by careless handling and disregard. The following are examples of those injuries which require immediate attention and treatment on the field of play.

Spinal injuries

Assessment

Findings suggestive of a spinal injury are:
1. Pain in the neck or lower spinal region.
2. Inability to move limbs.
3. Feeling of numbness in the extremities or possible pins and needles.

Treatment

See Chapter 13.

Severe head injuries

Assessment

If knocked out the patient will not respond to questions or commands.

Treatment

A gum shield, if worn, should be removed, together with other objects in the mouth such as dentures or chewing gum. *See* Chapter 14.

Note: There is a high incidence of neck injuries related to unconscious patients so in these situations one should assume that a possible spinal injury has occurred and take the appropriate steps.

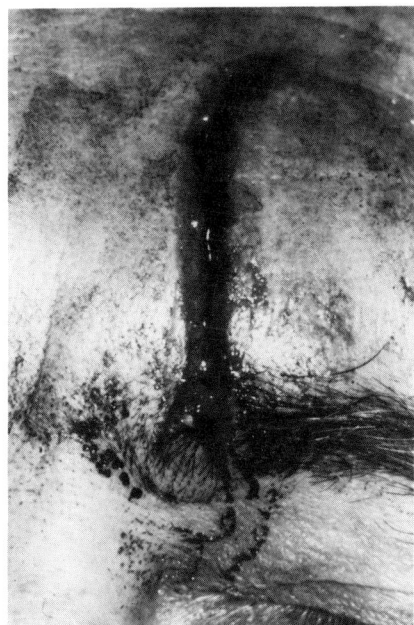

Fig. 23.5. Deep laceration to the forehead just above the eye.

Fractures

Assessment

Signs suggestive of a fracture are:
1. A visible or palpable deformity (*see* Fig. 23.1).
2. Pain at the site of the fracture.
3. Possible bruising (ecchymosis).
4. Loss of function.

Treatment
See Chapter 13.

Complete ligament tears

Assessment
Often it is impossible to differentiate these from a fracture.
Treatment
Is along similar lines to that of a fracture.

Lacerations

Assessment
Profuse bleeding and/or marked parting of the wound edges suggests a fairly severe laceration in need of suturing (*Fig.* 23.5).

Treatment
A clean pressure dressing should be applied to the area.

Should the player continue?
If there is any doubt then the answer is 'no'. If there is any possibility that the player may sustain further more severe damage, then he should be removed from the field of play.

Is immediate hospital treatment required?
If in any doubt the answer is 'yes'.

TREATMENT OF MINOR ACUTE SOFT-TISSUE INJURIES
These so-called minor injuries if not treated properly can lead to chronic problems and subsequent difficulties in management. Such injuries should be treated by an experienced physiotherapist and/or doctor, preferably one with an interest in sports injuries.

Treatment may be split into three phases:
1. Immediate (rest phase)
2. Intermediate (mobilization phase)
3. Long term

Pathology of soft-tissue healing
Soft tissues do not regenerate. They heal by scar formation. Injury to the soft tissues results in pain, swelling (oedema) and haemorrhage with resultant scar tissue formation. Firstly it is important to minimize the scar tissue formation and, secondly, to ensure that it is laid down in the plane of joint movement. To ensure this, early mobilization with reduction in swelling and haemorrhage is required.

Immediate treatment
  [I]ce
  [C]ompression
  [E]levation
  Medication

Ice
This should be placed in a towel or bag so as to prevent ice 'burns' from direct contact with the skin. It should be applied to the maximum area of swelling for approximately 20 min. There are commercially available packs but these tend to be expensive. They have the advantage of being re-usable and easy to store, however.

SPORTS INJURIES 251

Compression

A compression strapping should be applied to the injured area to reduce swelling and to prevent the further collection of fluid. The compression should not be too tight so as to embarrass the blood supply to the limb. Signs of embarrassment to the circulation are pain, pallor or engorgement, pins and needles and loss of function.

It is important that the compression bandage is applied correctly. *Figs.* 23.6–23.12 show serial photographs of the application of stirrup strapping for a lateral ligament injury to the ankle. This is one of the commonest types of injury and correct strapping is vital.

Step 1 (Fig. 23.6)
Two 'U' shaped pieces of orthopaedic felt are cut and shaped to fit around the bones of the ankle joint.

Step 2 (Fig. 23.7)
An elastoplast stirrup is applied from the inner aspect of leg to the outer aspect. To avoid rucks and subsequent blister formation small cuts are made in the strapping, as illustrated.

Step 3 (Fig. 23.8)
After the application of the stirrup it is held by a circular bandage applied as shown.

Step 4 (Fig. 23.9)
The final layer of weave strapping is applied starting from the outer aspect of the foot in order to rest the damaged ligament.

Step 5 (Fig. 23.10)
The final appearance after the weave strapping has been applied from the toes to just below the knee joint. It should be noted that the heel has been left free, this is to encourage up and down movement of the ankle. It is sideways movement that has to be avoided. The difference between correct and incorrect forms of treatment is seen in *Fig.* 23.11 and *Fig.* 23.12.

Elevation
The injured parts should be elevated to reduce swelling.

Medication
There are various forms of medication on the market, some of which are in the form of creams and others in the form of tablets or pain-relieving sprays. Generally speaking most have to be prescribed by a medical

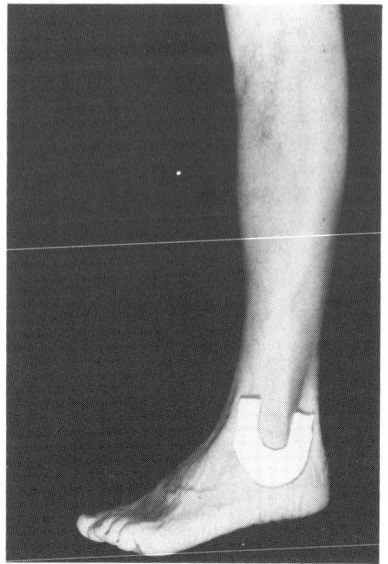
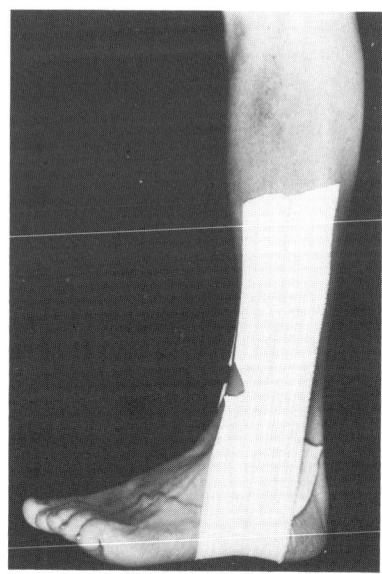

Fig. 23.6. Application of stirrup strapping, Step 1.
Fig. 23.7. Application of stirrup strapping, Step 2.

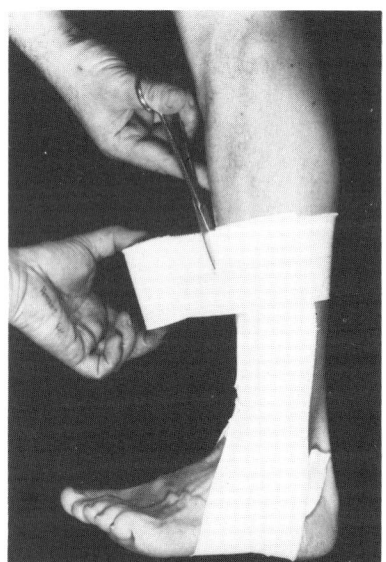
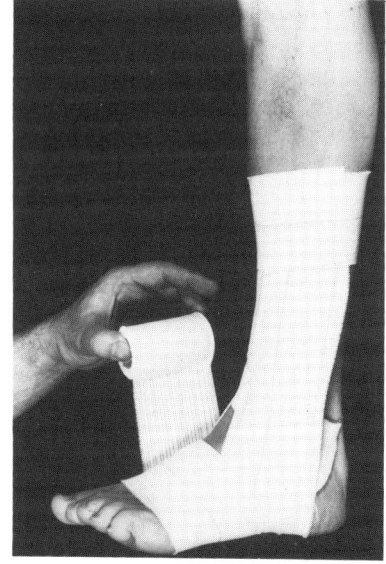

Fig. 23.8. Application of stirrup strapping, Step 3.
Fig. 23.9. Application of stirrup strapping, Step 4.

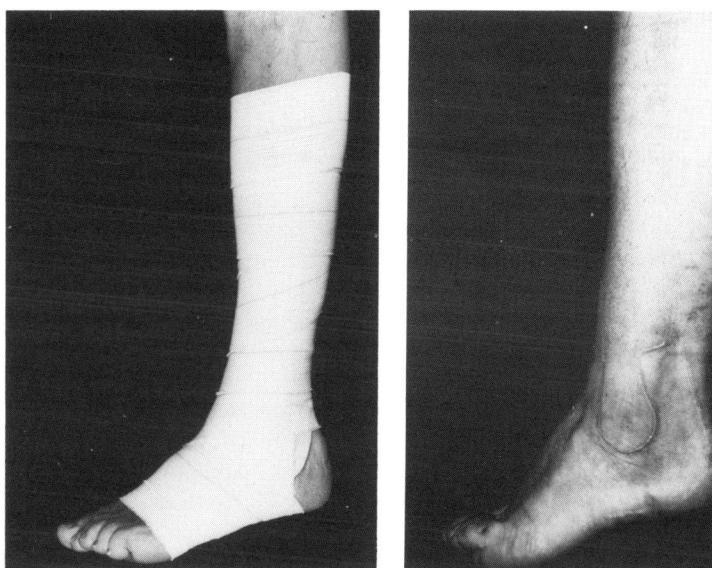

Fig. 23.10. Application of stirrup strapping, Step 5.

Fig. 23.11. Result of stirrup strapping.

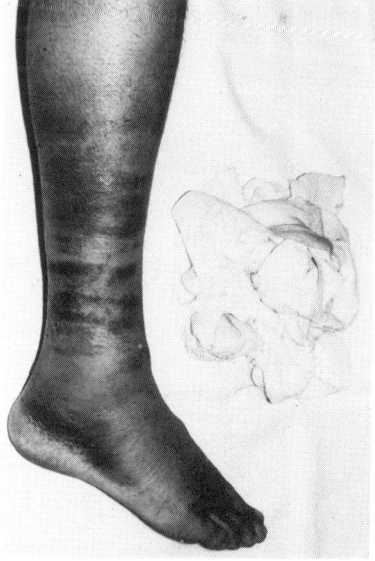

Fig. 23.12. Result after application of crepe bandage.

practitioner. The tablets are known as anti-inflammatory drugs and they relieve pain and swelling. Contrary to the belief of some sportsmen, the tablets and pain-relieving sprays are not to be taken to relieve pain so that they can return to sport immediately. They are to be used so that treatment in the form of mobilization can occur earlier. This phase of the treatment, depending on the severity of the injury, lasts from 48 hours to 10 days.

Intermediate (Mobilization Phase)
Once the initial pain and swelling has subsided early mobilization of the joint can be started. This involves undertaking a controlled exercise programme, an example of which is shown in *Fig.* 23.13. It may be likened to a ladder, an injured sportsman starting at the bottom rung and slowly working himself to the top, back to full activity. If at any stage of his progress up the ladder he suffers adverse reactions then he must go back one step. It must be stressed that this exercise programme should be supervised by a qualified person and great care taken at each step.

The aim of the graduated exercise programme is to reduce adhesions and so help joint movements. It reduces oedema and prevents excessive scar formation. The scar tissue that is laid down is remodelled and muscle power is increased. Finally the athlete returns to his sport fully fit and with little chance of chronic or continued damage to the area.

At this stage it is often beneficial to have various physiotherapy treatments such as shortwave diathermy and ultrasound; however it is beyond the scope of this chapter to discuss these.

Long-term treatment
This involves the prevention of further injury. Having experienced the injury once, protective and preventive measures should be taken to prevent recurrence.

TREATMENT OF CHRONIC AND OVER-USE INJURIES

Often the presenting injury is only a symptom of an underlying abnormality. The abnormality may be in the player's anatomy, type of shoes he wears, the surface on which he performs, or the quality and quantity of his training programme.

Aetiology of the injury
Abnormal anatomy
High arches of the foot (pes cavus) can lead to inflammation of the Achilles tendon as can abnormalities of the heel which can cause

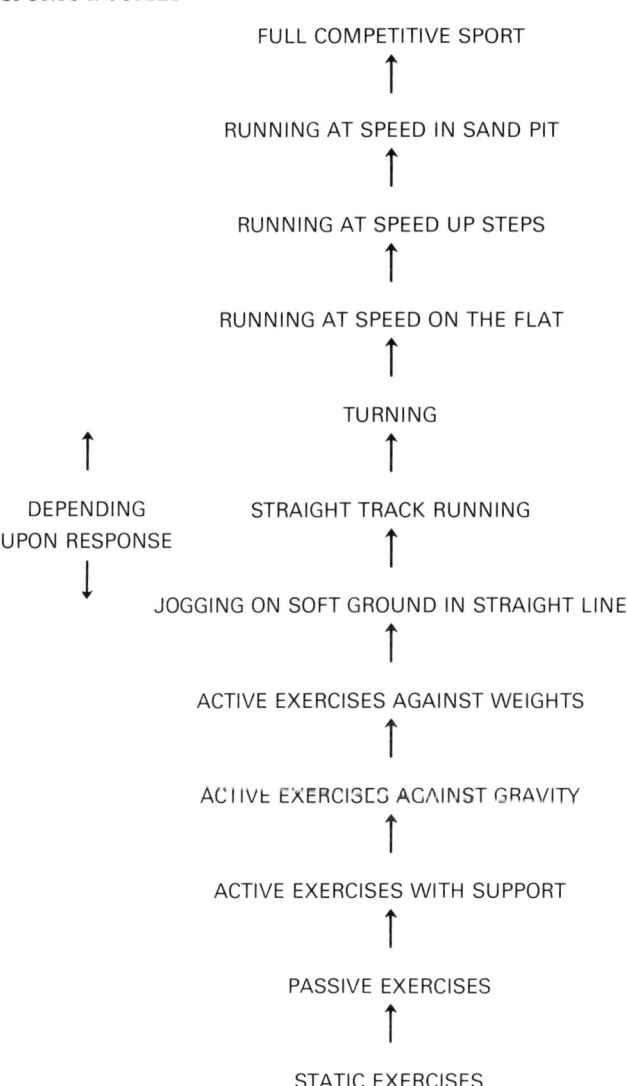

Fig. 23.13. Graduated exercise programme.

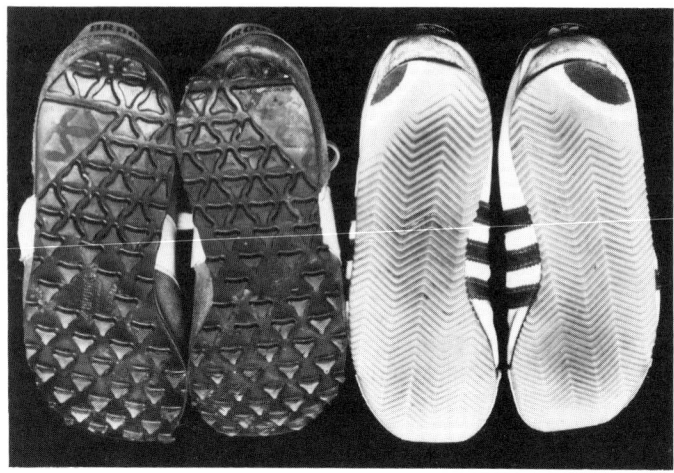

Fig. 23.14. Abnormal wear pattern of shoes.

excessive abnormal wear of the shoes (*Fig.* 23.14) and resultant stresses placed on the Achilles tendon.

Abnormal shoes
Often shoes with so-called Achilles tendon protectors can in fact inflame the tendon.

Surface
Hard surfaces tend to lead to shin splints and if combined with excessive training may lead to stress fractures. The new synthetic surfaces can also cause increase in ligament and cartilage injuries.

Quantity and quality of the training programme
Too much training can do damage as can the wrong type of training. It is important that expert advice is sought.

Treatment of the injury
Most injuries when seen have been present for at least a few months and often years. In the first instance the athlete must stop playing his chosen sport and a full assessment as to the cause of his problem made. It may well be that he might only require a change of shoe or guidance regarding the surface and quality and quantity of his training programme.

COMPLICATIONS OF SOFT-TISSUE INJURIES

These include
1. Adhesions — scar tissue formation.
2. Myositis ossificans — laying down of bone rather than scar tissue.
3. Chronic ligament laxity — the joint becomes unstable
4. Chronic tendon inflammation — the tendons of a joint become inflamed.

Further reading

Clinics in Sports Medicine, March 1982 Vol. 1, No. 1. Ankle and Foot Problems in the Athlete. Philadelphia, Saunders.
Muckle David S. (1982) *Injuries in Sport.* 2nd ed. Bristol, Wright.
Williams J. G. P. (1980) *Colour Atlas of Injury in Sport.* London, Wolfe Medical Publications.
Williams J. G. P. and Sperryn P. N. (1979) *Sports Medicine.* 2nd ed. London, Arnold.
Worth Melvin H. (1982) *Principles and Practice of Trauma Care.* Baltimore, Williams & Wilkins.

Chapter 24

Cave and Mountain Rescue: Some Special Aspects of Prehospital Care

J. C. Frankland

Patients with trauma and with medical emergencies are part of the routine workload of all emergency care personnel. However, the unusual occurs everyday somewhere. The following sections deal with less common problems met in special circumstances. They aim to cover some basic techniques and to mention common pitfalls.

Should you live in suburbia and spend your leisure time in Soho this section may not concern you. However, much of the UK, particularly the North of England and Scotland, is wild terrain, sometimes remote and it can be very hostile.

For those injured off the road in these parts two ambulancemen with a conventional stretcher may be manifestly unable to cope and extra help is mandatory.

All mountain and moorland areas of the UK have their own voluntary Mountain Rescue Teams co-ordinated by the Mountain Rescue Committee and the Mountain Rescue Committee of Scotland. Ninety-two separate teams cover the UK. Call-out in all instances is via the police who hold the statutory responsibility for rescue but are glad to delegate this to their local team with whom they will have an intimate working relationship.

The first requirement of a member of a mountain or cave rescue team is total personal competence in the environment in which he must work even in extreme weather conditions when the demands on his services are most likely. This environment can vary from searching of moors for the lost to the complex technical crag rescues in the extreme weather of Scottish winters; the most remote parts of tough, testing caves presenting perhaps the most challenging problems. All teams have their specialists whether they are controllers, communications experts, first aiders or rock 'tigers' but rescue remains essentially a team effort—the unglamorous jobs like maintaining equipment being as necessary as the actual rescue work.

With increasing leisure time and involvement in outdoor pursuits the collective workload is rising and this is likely to continue. It is encouraging that the rate of accidents is not rising as fast as the increasing number of participants so that modern equipment and safety instruction is saving lives.

For a major mountain search neighbouring teams will be co-opted and a few hundred people may be deployed over a big area. The logistics of supplying and co-ordinating such an operation are complex and senior officers from the statutory services are closely involved. In a few such procedures discreet enquiries may reveal, for example a secret liaison somewhere and the 'victim' is delayed for reasons other than being lost on a mountain! They still have to be sought if there is the possibility that they *are* on the mountain.

If the weather permits, the expertise of the Search and Rescue helicopters of the RAF is frequently sought. The call-out for this procedure is normally made through the senior police officer present. No bills are presented as these marvellous yellow flying machines with their skilled crews are available for civilian rescue if service commitments allow.

Over the past decade the Search and Rescue Dogs' Association (SARDA) has developed and multiplied. Dogs and their handlers receive detailed training to graded levels of skills and are extremely impressive in their effectiveness. They are called at the request of the rescue team leaders and are usually sent into the search area before their human counterparts.

Medical care in remote places is very much a compromise from that available in the intensive care unit. Accurate comprehensive diagnosis cannot be expected as it is usually against a patient's interest to undress him for full examination. The constant fear is of continuing haemorrhage into skull, chest or abdomen which cannot be prevented outside an operating theatre and those victims lost during rescue have often had such problems.

Early evacuation must take priority as far as is practical, with one or two specific exceptions mentioned later representing calculated risks. In English mountains for some years by far the major cause of death has not been the adventurous rock climber or imprudent winter walker but myocardial infarction, up to 70 per cent in some series. The shocked coronary patient on a hillside needs careful handling and, if feasible, on-site care with helicopter evacuation to hospital is generally in his best interest.

Monitoring throughout rescue is essential, preferably by one individual, and in the most difficult circumstances this may be restricted to the level of consciousness, breathing adequacy, pulse rate and temperature readings.

Morale is so important and many fears should be eased when a competent team starts to cope with the job in hand. Experience shows panic and fear to be less of a problem than might be predicted and often the victim's equanimity is inappropriate for his horrific surroundings.

Rescue is never near to hand and particularly in caves a delay of hours is likely before help arrives. This means that some will have died but others will have stabilized, albeit suboptimally.

Resuscitation with intravenous fluids has been less employed by British rescue teams than in the USA or in current military casualty evacuation methods. This may be a deficiency, but a difficult evacuation, particularly from a cave, will not allow simultaneous transfusion of fluids.

PAIN RELIEF

After a fall the second most painful experience for the victim is likely to be when he is picked up, splinted and stretchered. Analgesia before this procedure is generally appreciated, allowing adequate time for its effect. With cold and shock intramuscular injections can be only slowly absorbed so patience helps unless a doctor at the scene can give intravenous analgesia.

Since the early 1950s lay members of teams affiliated to the Mountain Rescue Committees have had access to and been allowed to give morphine to victims. This was initially supplied by Wilson Hey, a Manchester surgeon, who informed the police of his action and was then prosecuted. Shortly afterwards the law was changed and we have had this facility ever since—perhaps one of the earliest pieces of sensible legislation facilitating on-site care for the injured. Over the past decade more teams have enlisted doctors who are experienced climbers or cavers so that the lay use of Mountain Rescue Committee morphine is now minimal. Some cynics have claimed that rescue is the fastest growth sport in the UK!

Many team members have a sensible apprehension about the risks of morphine or pethidine and will instead use pentazocine (Fortral) either orally or parenterally and claim this is an acceptable alternative.

The drowsy patient who has a head injury but remains in pain and shock from limb fractures remains a perennial problem for all. Entonox (a mixture of 50 per cent oxygen and 50 per cent nitrous oxide) seems most appropriate on safety grounds, although bulk and weight are at a premium on the dash up a mountain. It certainly has its uses and with an extended supply tube can be carried in a rucksack alongside the stretcher during evacuation to allow the victim to seek pain relief on demand. At low temperatures an imperfect mixture can be supplied and the cylinder needs adequate insulation (*see* Vol. 1, p. 274).

It is not really feasible to give Entonox throughout evacuation from a cave where the victim usually has to be manhandled through awkward shaped holes in the rock which may be no bigger than his own dimensions. In cave rescue an injured victim who cannot co-operate and give some 'self help' in the predictable frequent awkward sections will have a considerably more prolonged evacuation.

After a normal dose of a strong analgesic drowsiness is likely and for this reason we tend to avoid doses which produce heavy sedation in difficult caves. Each case demands optimal splintage but it is not uncommon to encounter patients who have had just 50 or 75 mg of pethidine initially with major lower limb fractures and who refuse further analgesics during rescues lasting 6 to 8 hours. Their alertness and co-operation makes their passage easier and speedier.

The ideal safe analgesic probably does not yet exist. Teams are currently experimenting with buprenorphine (Temgesic) which can be given sublingually and shows promise. Whatever drug is used, rapport with the patient, careful splintage and as gentle handling as the terrain allows are still mandatory.

IMMOBILIZATION

An essential for rescue splints is that they are practical, withstand rough handling and are easy to apply in difficult situations.

If neck trauma is likely and certainly for the unconscious an adjustable neck splint is essential. It will also help to protect the chin from sagging and threatening the airway.

For mountain rescue bulk is less critical so that leg traction splints are feasible—the Thomas, Hare and Taranga varieties all being used. Pneumatic splints can be appropriate for below-knee injuries if protected from the inevitable sharp rocks. Some European brands made from tough rubberized fabric are more durable than plastic splints. If inflatable splints are used one which can be fitted without removing a boot is a definite advantage, e.g. the 'Athletic Long Leg' splint.

New from the USA and costly but very promising, is a versatile set of interchangeable splints made from strong neoprene with Velcro fasteners and incorporating a semi-flexible metal strip which is bent before application to the required shape (Add-a-splint).

For cave rescue minimal bulk is required and the Heye's splint which stretches from ankle to axilla is ideal for any form of leg fracture. Its absence of working parts which can be fouled by the ubiquitous mud is very much in its favour. In South Wales rescue teams have used the newer plastic cast splinting techniques to impressive effect underground (Baycast).

The ability to improvize is still priceless and notable is the following example. One rescuer lashed a fractured tibia to his own forearm so that he and the victim could crawl together through a constricted convoluted tube in solid rock where nothing else seemed appropriate.

STRETCHERS

Mountain Rescue teams need lightweight stretchers with enough strength to protect the victim during vertical descents from crags and carries over rough ground. Most will split into two so that each half can be carried on the back of a rescuer. The bed of the stretcher is made from netting and not solid fabric so that the man climbing to the victim with half a stretcher on his back does not carry a sail which can cause him to be blown off the rock. Some form of wooden or metal ski runners, head protection frame, extendable carrying poles and haulage attachment points will be incorporated. The Thomas, McInnes or Bell stretchers are generally used by British teams.

On vertical descents the stretcher may be kept horizontal, which is preferable for a shocked victim but may be more difficult technically, or lowered vertically. One rescuer will ride the stretcher attached by a harness and 'walking' down the rockface observing and protecting the victim.

In cave rescue we are denied the luxury of such bulk and most teams still use the Neil Robertson stretcher where stout wrap round flaps will provide all-round protection and add minimally to size. An adjustable metal frame, a protective helmet and extra haulage points need to be added. The canvas and wood fabric of the Neil Robertson stretchers is not durable and can soon suffer from rock friction but the design principle is ideal for the special needs of cave rescue.

Commonly caves will have low 'crawls' or tight vertical fissures, sometimes with a bend midway so that a victim in a rigid stretcher will not pass through. For these he will usually be placed in a nylon whole trunk industrial safety harness and dragged through as delicately as possible inch by inch. Here a co-operative patient will pass through with more ease.

COLD INJURY

Definition

Cold injury describes the damage to tissues produced by exposure to low temperatures. Lesions range from chilblains through to frostbite and from cold damp feet through to immersion foot. The degree of cold and the amount of water coupled with varying exposure times determines the severity of the cold injury. Cold injury can be considered as either freezing or non-freezing injury.

Signs and symptoms

Because cold injuries upset the blood supply to the tissues the signs and symptoms are those associated with restricted blood flow, as seen in other vascular conditions whose pathology is not cold orientated. It is, therefore, essential to record a detailed history either from the casualty or from bystanders. The effects of cold injury can be dramatically reduced by early effective treatment. *Early* signs may well be minimal, just slight tingling followed by stinging, aching or painful sensations. Later the sensation of coldness is followed by numbness with the skin at first red in colour then becoming pale and waxy white.

Late signs after rewarming depend on the severity of the cold injury and range from redness and oedema, vesicle formation to necrosis of the skin. Where the injury is severe enough complete death of the limb may ensue.

Treatment

1. Be gentle with limbs or areas affected. Do not massage affected parts.
2. Remove all constricting clothing from site of injury.
3. *Rapidly rewarm* frozen areas by immersion in warm (35 °C to 40 °C) water, warm air or body heat, e.g. by placing a hand over the injured area.
4. Keep casualties at general body temperature and encourage sleep.
5. Treat all cold injuries as stretcher cases. In high altitude climbing with no rescue facilities and a threat to survival victims should walk to base before rewarming.
6. Do not aspirate intact blisters.
7. Do not apply ointment, petroleum jelly or petroleum jelly gauze to large vesicles (bullae) which should be covered with dry dressings to provide protection and warmth.
8. Analgesics should be given during rewarming as this is painful.

HYPOTHERMIA

Anyone immobilized on a mountain or down a cave is liable to lose heat and deteriorate unless their protective clothing is dry and very adequate. Death within 1 hour from hypothermia down a cave in flood has been documented. When normal clothing becomes soaked its insulation value drops to below 5 per cent of the dry value so that the victim is as if naked from a heat insulation point of view. More threatening than the air temperature level is the wind speed for the 'wind chill factor' rapidly accelerates heat loss. Hypothermia is defined as a drop in 'core' or inner body temperature to below 35 °C—an oesophageal or rectal reading is

264 PREHOSPITAL EMERGENCY CARE

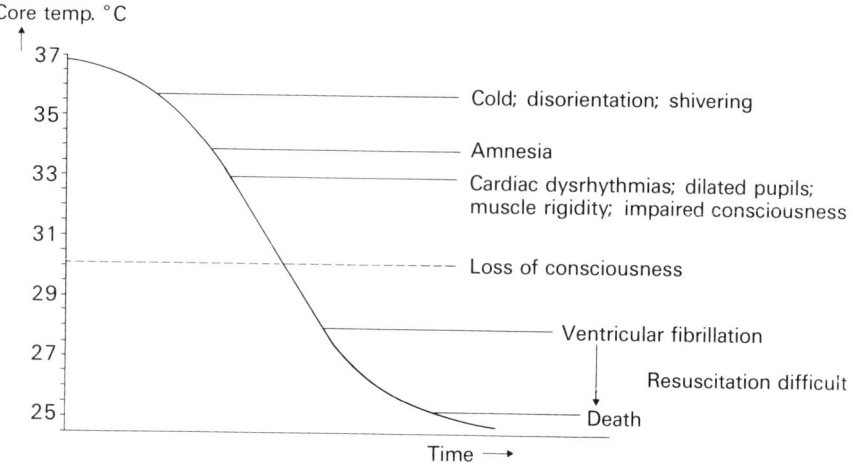

Fig. 24.1. Diagram to show the continuum of deterioration seen with decreasing core temperature.

necessary to measure core temperature. It is most important to appreciate that this is merely an *arbitrary point on a continuum of deterioration* and that those above this limit can rapidly deteriorate and die in adverse conditions (*Fig.* 24.1).

In addition to accidental exposure to low temperatures outdoors other causes of hypothermia are:
1. Accidental hypothermia in the elderly—usually following immobilization from, e.g. a stroke or fall in a poorly heated room.
2. The inability of small babies, especially premature infants, to regulate their temperatures.
3. Some drugs when taken in overdose.
4. Hypothyroidism and hypopituitarism.
5. Collapse due to alcohol or a suicide attempt.

Out of doors, more common than pure hypothermia is the dangerous combination of fatigue and heat loss best described as the 'exposure exhaustion syndrome'. Such victims are apathetic, may well have impaired judgement so that they take inappropriate decisions in a survival situation and will sometimes have a detectable *smell of ketones (acetone) on the breath*. This is an important simple diagnostic observation.

Signs and symptoms
1. Loss of general interest in surroundings.
2. Lack of mental and physical co-ordination.

CAVE AND MOUNTAIN RESCUE

3. Low body temperature.
4. Uncontrollable shivering which stops as severe hypothermia develops.
5. Irrational behaviour
6. Slow heart rate and respirations.
7. Loss of consciousness.
8. Breathing and heart beat become increasingly difficult to detect.

Diagnosis

In extreme cases the casualty is comatose and pale and could be mistaken for dead. Respirations are shallow and infrequent and the pulse is weak or absent. The pupils do not react to light but are *not* dilated.

Never assume that a patient is dead because heart beat and respirations appear absent.

Shivering is the body's automatic reaction to loss of heat and casualties who are in the uncontrollable shivering state are not profoundly cooled (*see Fig.* 24.1). When the shivering ceases with the continued lowering of body temperature, complications may appear which need skilful appraisal of cardiac and respiratory adequacy. Effective resuscitation and attention to the airway are vital.

The significance of a core temperature at or below 35 °C is that such a victim will deteriorate if exertion is forced on him. The peripheral or 'shell' circulation to limb muscles will be shut down to conserve heat loss and opening this up by exercise will divert the cooler shell blood back to the warmer core with likely serious consequences. Such victims need to be carried or rewarmed before they can be walked out.

The first priority in dealing with a cold patient is to supply adequate insulation. The traditional teaching is that wet clothing should be removed and replaced by dry clothing carried in by the rescue team. In practice now many would just remove outer wet clothing and then apply thick *fibre pile* clothing which will 'wick' water away from wet underclothing and still remain an effective insulator if it becomes wet.

Survival bags of polythene or space blankets are on sale in most outdoor pursuits shops and are becoming more widely carried by walkers. The lightweight space blankets afford very little effective insulation to a cooled patient whose radiant heat loss will be minimal and the faith which many first aiders have in space blankets is probably unjustified. They are certainly better than nothing and are very compact and easily carried.

If a cold victim is being treated anywhere a space blanket covering alone is inadequate. It should be covered with a blanket and then a second or third blanket and finally something windproof and waterproof; perhaps another space blanket.

Of more value out of doors is the heavy duty (500 gauge) orange plastic survival bag which gives complete cover and is much more effective than a space blanket. Inside one of these with dry clothing and a sleeping bag and sheltered from the wind, victims will rewarm spontaneously from their ongoing metabolism. If a warm rescuer is put in alongside the cold victim his recovery will be hastened. We all have a fantasy that one day the victim will be a pretty girl and that it will be our turn in the bag, but somehow this never seems to happen! Rescue on big mountains and down caves can be prolonged and can sometimes take over 12 hours. A practical difficulty exists in monitoring body temperature during this time. Ideally, rectal or oesophageal temperatures should be measured but this is impractical. An effective cocoon of insulation round the whole body is necessary to allow spontaneous rewarming and disturbing this to measure rectal temperature would be detrimental and impossible when the victim is strapped in a stretcher.

A thermometer capable of subnormal ($< 35\,°C$) readings kept under the tongue for a measured 3 minutes will give a temperature reading several degrees below core temperature. The value of this information is that if the procedure is repeated the *change* in reading will indicate if the victim is rewarming or cooling.

This information is probably of more value than absolute levels of temperature in circumstances where high technology treatment is not available. Carry at least two such thermometers as breakage through fumbling is likely when your own hands are cold.

In 1972 Lloyd described airway rewarming as the first on-site means of supplying active treatment for hypothermia. Since then compact equipment has become commercially available and many rescue teams now think the method of value. There are many anecdotal stories attributing survival to airway rewarming but less objective laboratory data although a US Coastguard trial in 1977 reported it a significant advantage on cold human volunteers.

The principle is that the victim is given air to breathe which is warmed to around $50\,°C$ and fully saturated with water vapour. This heat is dispersed directly via the large blood flow through the lungs and thence to the body core. The heat supplied is not large being in the order of $5.0\ kJ/m^2/hr$ but perhaps more important the method can totally prevent the body's respiratory heat loss of around $35\,kJ/m^2/hr$. This is usually the body's largest source of further heat loss when there is profound skin cooling and peripheral circulatory stasis.

The method is certainly not a substitute for adequate insulation which must also be carried out assiduously.

Experience has shown much benefit from this technique so that many consider it worth the inconvenience of carrying the equipment down caves which is probably the ultimate test. In practice most victims were not the critically cooled, who are unconscious, but those less cold through being immobilized. Such persons certainly appreciated the subjective benefits of breathing warm air almost to the point of addiction! With insulation and airway rewarming they will improve so that stretcher evacuation is often avoided to the benefit of both parties.

Other methods of rewarming include chemical heat packs used by the US Militia and a 'Thermal Sarong' which is a sleeping bag containing tubes through which ethylene glycol liquid heated by a butane burner circulates. These latter are very expensive and are understandably scarce amongst UK teams.

When a cooled victim must be carried through cold surroundings a new simple piece of equipment can be used to reduce airway heat loss in transit. It is simply a plastic mask over the nose and mouth attached to a short tube which is placed inside the victim's anorak or sleeping bag. Incorporated in the tubing is a cardboard condenser so that the inspired air becomes humidified by the moisture from the expired air. It is also slightly warmed by being drawn from inside the clothing surrounding the body. This simple technique is tolerated and welcomed by victims but will increase respiratory dead space and is probably not appropriate for those with any chest injuries or respiratory embarrassment.

A difficult decision with hypothermia victims can be in determining whether life still exists. This is commonly met after recovery from snow burial. Recovery without brain damage after one hour of proven cardiac arrest has been documented and many victims found apparently drowned with the face elevated by a life jacket are hypothermic and may be resuscitated. Children submerged in cold water for up to 45 min have recovered without cerebral impairment. Within the constraints of common sense the diagnosis of death from hypothermia can only be that of failure to respond to resuscitation.

In a remote mountain area hospital resources may be hours away and immersion in a warm bath at the nearest house may be necessary. This should be organized during, not after, rescue.

The trunk but not the limbs should be placed in a deep bath of water at 41 °C or as hot as the elbow can stand if no thermometer is available. Only outer garments should be removed before immersion to minimize handling. Many victims will show aggressive uncontrollable movements after immersion and the head must be kept as low as is safe and firmly supported.

A cold victim will rapidly cool the surrounding water which should be constantly stirred and its temperature maintained by 'topping up' so that around 40 gallons of water are necessary. This attention to maintaining the water temperature is most important.

The patient should be kept immersed until visible sweating develops on the forehead and then be allowed to stabilize, lying flat in a warmed bed.

The method is lifesaving but potentially hazardous if done indiscriminately. Keeping the victim's trunk and head horizontal and maintaining the water temperature are the most important factors. Food and warm drinks will benefit the exposure exhaustion syndrome patients but most will be apathetic and need encouragement to take sustenance. Lack of judgement and inappropriate decision-making are early features of cold patients who may totally lack both a subjective feeling of cold or an awareness that they are deteriorating. It is common to find walkers collapsed carrying, but not wearing, insulating clothing and ignoring nearby sources of shelter.

Further reading

Frankland J. C. (1975) Medical Aspects of Cave Rescue. *Trans British Cave Research Assoc.* **2**, 53–63.
Frankland J. C. (1981) Hypothermia and exposure. *Br. Med. J.* **282**, 369.
Keighly J. H. (1980) A comparison of mountain rescue bags. *Clothing Res. J.* **8** 46–56.
Lloyd E. Ll. et al. (1972) Accidental hypothermia—an apparatus for central rewarming as a first aid measure. *Scott. Med. J.* **17**, 83–91.
McInnes H. (1972) *International Mountain Rescue Handbook.* London, Constable.

Airway Rewarming Manufacturers

'Reviva'. Peter Bell Engineering, The Slack, Ambleside, Cumbria, UK.
'The Little Dragon'. Mike F. Mitchell, Coppelrigg, Kentmere, Cumbria, UK.

Splint Pack Distributors

'Add-a-splint'. G. & W. Bonser, Vale View, Blackrock, Abergavenny, Gwent, NP1 0LW.

Chapter 25

Aviation and Underwater Medicine

J. E. Butter

AVIATION MEDICINE

Introduction

It is a common enough experience for medical and paramedical personnel to be involved with helicopter evacuation procedures. Such procedures are hazardous both for medical staff and patients unless properly understood and rehearsed. It is the latter which provides the stumbling block for the unprepared, and the purpose of this section is to provide an outline of the theory of aviation medicine as applicable to paramedical, ambulance and nursing responsibilities and to allay some of the fears and folklore surrounding helicopter ambulance duties. The role of the helicopter in today's civil and military medical evacuation of casualties (CASEVAC), or the planned transfer of patients from one hospital to another (MEDIVAC), is a subject which all medical staff *must* be prepared to study in advance.

Detailed considerations
1. The medical need
Helicopters have obvious advantages over other vehicles for the transportation of the injured or sick, indeed, they have revolutionized medical support to major disasters and the battlefront and have come to dominate the rescue services along our coasts and in the mountainous regions of the world. The value of the helicopter is such that it is all too easy to extol its virtues and forget, or ignore, its inherent disadvantages in the disciplines of patient care. It is important to ask the following questions before reaching the point of decision to use a helicopter:
    a. Is the flight in the best interests of the casualty.
    b. Is there any other form of transport available which is adequate?
    c. Is speed essential?

The helicopter is, after all, just a vehicle and as such is about as much use as a well-equipped ambulance or a rickshaw unless it forms an integral part of the patient's overall care. In the CASEVAC mission, the helicopter forms part of the general medical package, the object of which is to deliver the patient from the scene of the accident to a suitable receiving unit in the best possible condition. The aircrew in Search and Rescue aircraft are all trained first aiders whose skills will be able to sustain life and complete suitable treatment measures before landing. For those paramedical personnel working on oil rigs in the oceans of the world, working in inaccessible areas or as part of special medical teams their skills may well mean additional training to act as temporary aircrew with a full understanding of the medical aspects of flying. Flight safety and flight drills must be an integral part of their paramedic training. The decision to fly requires a total knowledge of the risks, dangers and physiological aspects of the patient's condition which will be affected by altitude. There will, of course, be times when flying is not at all appropriate but no other means of rescue or transportation is available and under these circumstances compromise is an essential quality.

2. *The aviation difficulties*

This section highlights some of the aviation difficulties which must be considered by the aircrew before they make the decision to fly or not. Such a decision will be based upon their assessment of the risks to the safety of the aircraft and its occupants. The condition of the patients does have a bearing on the aircrew decision but will not dominate it.

It will be seen that aviation difficulties are equally divided between 'aircraft' and 'medical' but contribute as a whole to the overall package of patient care and safety (*Table 25.1*):

Aircraft	Flight safety checks	Responsibility of aircrew
	Weather conditions	The decision to fly will be made by aircrew
	Altitude limits	Most patients will be flown at the lowest possible altitude compatible with flight safety. The altitude ceiling will be an aircrew/medical compromise
	Number of casualties	Weight within the aircraft limits the amount of fuel that can be carried and consequently the range

AVIATION AND UNDERWATER MEDICINE

Medical
- I.V. infusions — I.V. infusions are best set up before the flight starts because vibration, turbulence and space create difficulties
- Inflatable splints — The air inside an inflatable splint expands as altitude increases and it may burst or cause vascular problems
- Endotracheal tube cuffs — Will also expand. Remedy is to fill with water
- Medical equipment — Check with aircrew before taking gas cylinders or other inflammables into the aircraft
- Patient's condition — Make sure that your patient will withstand the flight. Don't be frightened to cancel

3. CASEVAC and MEDIVAC

There are two kinds of casualty evacuation in helicopter operations:
  a. CASEVAC—Unplanned rescue, immediate care and transportation to a medical reception area.
  b. MEDIVAC—Planned transfer of casualties between hospitals for specialized or urgent treatment.

In the CASEVAC there is a sense of urgency and spontancity of action, whereas the MEDIVAC is carefully planned, carefully executed and wholly premeditated. Remember, helicopters are superb rescue machines but very poor transport for the critically ill.

4. The casualty reception unit

This flow diagram overleaf is designed as a guide for a safe and satisfactory conclusion to the flight.

The helicopter rotor downdraft will whisk away hats and loose items which may well be sucked into the engine intakes. Open coats will be blown up over heads and cause, at the very least, a nuisance.

5. Preparation for in-flight care—and the unexpected

Once the aircraft is in the air only on-board equipment and help can be used. If oxygen is required take a spare cylinder. It will be wise to take spare clothing and washing gear as it is not always possible to get a return flight. Helicopters travel fast and 1 hour's journey out may take upwards of 8 hours to get back. One may be diverted due to bad weather and end

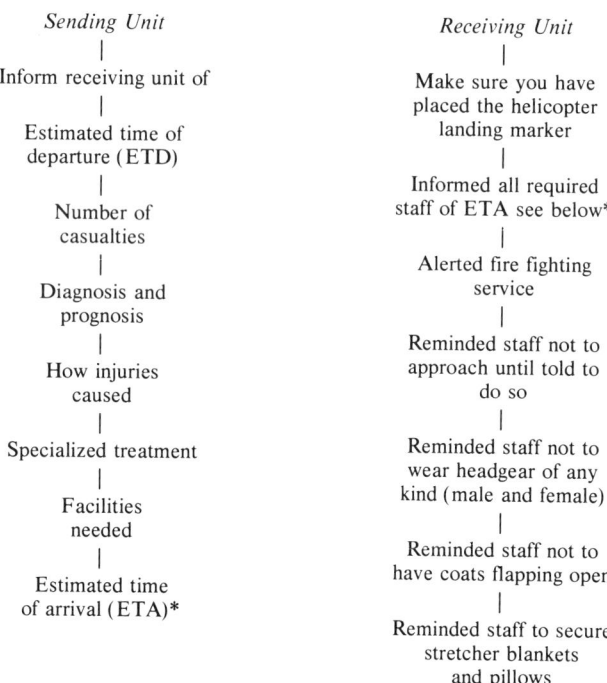

up in totally unusual surrroundings. If the mission is a CASEVAC and the casualty is bleeding heavily extra large dressings may be required to stem the flow. Aircraft vibrate and the vibration frequency may be just the one to negate the pressure between pad and limb. Different parts of the body vibrate at different frequencies (e.g. abdomen at a different frequency from a limb). If a patient has a fracture and the aircraft vibration frequency equals that of the limb extra care will be needed. The pilot may be asked to slow down or to take some other action which may reduce the problem.

Aircrew tend to get used to motion sickness due to regular flying and Experience in dealing with the problem. Casualties and their medical escorts may well find themselves in the uncomfortable situation of feeling sick. Aircrew should be informed and will provide suitable advice and assistance.

6. *Thorough briefing and planning*

Prevention of classic errors and untimely illustrations of lack of knowledge can be prevented by understanding the problem and seeking the best possible advice.

Table 25.1. Care of casualties in helicopters

General stress/ noise	*All patients*—Helicopters are alarming *Psychiatric patients*—violent and suicidal reactions are difficult to cope with in the air *Desperately ill patients*—do not fly well. Get them as stable as possible *before* the flight	A gentle, confident reassuring manner will work miracles. Try to obtain a headset for the patient—it will occupy him and settle his mind
Vibration/ turbulence	*Haemorrhage*—vibration may well encourage wounds or internal bleeding to get worse or restart *Fractures*—unstable fractures may be very painful or become complicated as bone fragments move	Ask the pilot to fly gently rather than gallantly. Make sure that pads and splints are firm
Cold	*Hypothermia*—almost anyone who has been in the sea or on a mountain will be at risk. So will any other patient if he is not properly wrapped up and the aircraft door is left open	Do not undress or handle roughly. Prevent further heat loss. Wrap patients up well with windproof clothing
Pressure changes	*Abdomen*—a wide variety of troubles can cause pain or damage with gas expansion. Operation wounds can burst *Ears*—patients may not be able to 'clear' their ears if they have a common cold as well as other injuries	The greatest pressure changes occur in the first few hundred feet. Avoid rapid altitude changes and fly as low as possible. Beware of inflatable splints and endotracheal tube cuffs
Hypoxia	*Chest*—anyone with breathing difficulty, be it due to disease or lung injury will become hypoxic before healthy aircrew *Haemorrhage*—loss of blood means reduced oxygen carrying capacity *Heart patients*—risk of myocardial infarction is increased *Head injuries*—hypoxia will compound head injury damage	Look for signs of respiratory distress. Fly low and give O_2 or refuse to fly these patients
Decompression sickness	*Divers*—anyone who has been below 30 feet in the last 24 hours *could* have problems. This includes casualties of RTAs on the way home from diving, not just the person who already has decompression sickness	Fly as low as possible. The difference between 100 and 200 feet is enough to matter

7. Altitude

For practical purposes the atmosphere can be considered as 20 per cent oxygen and 80 per cent nitrogen. This proportion never varies. However, as altitude increases the atmospheric pressure falls and the partial pressure of oxygen (Po_2) falls proportionately.

8. Oxygen uptake

In a mixture of gases each gas will exert its own pressure independently of the others and atmospheric pressure is the sum of the partial pressures of its components. From the point of view of the casualty and his respiration one is interested only in the partial pressure of oxygen because this is an important factor in the rate of uptake of oxygen in the lungs. At sea level the atmospheric pressure is 760 mmHg (1000 mb) and we need only 20 per cent of the air to be oxygen. As altitude increases so does the need for greater concentrations of oxygen with each breath the casualty, the medical staff and the aircrew takes.

9. Altitude problems

Hypoxia

This means that the body is short of sufficient oxygen to perform efficiently. In the uninjured and healthy this allows almost normal function up to 10 000 feet, but in the injured or critically ill the 'ceiling height' may well be only several hundred feet. Casualties with reduced ability to maintain normal respiration due to trauma, respiratory depressants, or the effects of various pathological processes are at considerable risk of hypoxia in normal circumstances let alone that compounded by altitude. The body is designed to perform optimally at sea level and the size of the lungs, the power of the heart and the number and size of the blood vessels are adapted to life on the surface. Those who are born at high altitudes adapt from the moment of conception to cope with the lower (Po_2). Mountain climbers and those who move to higher altitudes later in life adapt to a limited extent after a while. Casualties cannot adapt during short flights and so the lower the altitude the pilot can fly safely is the best option for the patient. In helicopters there is no oxygen supply or pressurized cabin, consequently occupants rely upon the available oxygen in the air. As the body is deprived of oxygen it will be the brain which will suffer first and this in turn will affect the body's trauma-compensating responses, thus compounding the difficulties of basic life support.

Barotrauma

As the atmospheric pressure drops the gas within the body expands. The lungs have ready communication with the exterior, so pressure equalization occurs without any difficulty although pulmonary (lung) barotrauma can be a severe problem for divers. In aviation the difficulties arise with the closed or semi-closed air spaces.

a. *Closed air spaces*
1. *Gas in the gut:* Patients who have abdominal problems and who are CASEVAC cases may have problems. The gas expands and may not be able to get out, either up or down. If so it will cause distension of the bowel which is painful. The gas may perforate the bowel at a weak point, e.g. a gangrenous appendix.
2. *A badly filled tooth* may have a gas pocket behind the filling. Pain will be experienced above a certain altitude as the expanding gas presses on the nerve. The pain disappears again on the way down at about the same height. The remedy is to have a new filling put in. In casualties who have a pneumothorax, with increasing altitude this gas will expand and compress the lung, impairing breathing further.

b. *Semi-closed spaces*
So-called because they are open to the atmosphere, but by a communicating channel which is narrow and may be blocked easily.
1. *The middle ear* communicates with the atmosphere via the eustachian tube which opens high up at the back of the throat.
2. *The sinuses*—cavities in the facial bones open by different channels into the side of the nose. All these passages are lined with an epithelium which swells up when inflamed (e.g. by a cold) and can be blocked by mucus. If the passages are obstructed, it is usually not difficult for expanding air to force its way out during ascent, but it commonly fails to re-enter on descent. The eustachian tube, in particular, is so shaped at the outer end as to aggravate this tendency because of a flap valve, preventing air going into the ear during descent if the subject has even a slight cold.

The effect of this blockage or partial blockage will be to prevent or delay repressurization of the ear or sinus on the way down. A pressure differential builds up across the wall of the sinus or across the ear drum.

The result is one or more of the following:
 i. The ear-drum bursts—this is, of course, painful.
 ii. A blood vessel inside the ear or sinus bursts and the compartment repressurizes with blood instead of air. Again this is painful and in contrast to the burst ear-drum, which often heals without permanent damage, there may be long-term consequences as a result of the clot and scar formation inside the ear.
 iii. Finally, the blockage in any tube may give way and release the pressure once sufficient differential has built up. The patient will experience increasing pain and then a violent 'bang' as the equalization takes place.

In all three cases the violence of the equalization will cause a pressure wave to ricochet around the inside of the middle and inner ear and this is likely to result in severe vertigo.

Flying with even a slight cold increases the risk of all these complications.

Note that these problems, in contrast to those of closed air spaces, tend to occur more on descent. It will not be possible to apply the checks to CASEVAC casualties and flying them with respiratory tract infections must be accepted as a reasonable risk.

Decompression sickness

This is caused by a rapid drop in pressure allowing dissolved nitrogen in the bloodstream to come out of solution just as carbon dioxide (CO_2) bubbles out of fizzy drinks when the top is taken off, releasing the pressure. When this happens in a blood vessel, the bubbles cause a gas lock which obstructs the flow, like an air lock in a water pipe. According to where the obstruction occurs, the casualty suffers the bends (joints), the creeps (skin), the chokes (chest), the staggers (spinal cord) or a complete collapse which looks typically like a faint. It does not occur below 18 000 ft and is uncommon until above 26 000 ft. The treatment is recompression, sometimes to slightly greater than atmospheric pressure.

The above altitude limits do not apply to divers, that is, anyone who has been breathing underwater or under increased pressure before the accident. The risk of decompression sickness relates to the depth of the dive and the time interval between surfacing and aircraft take-off time as well as the altitude of the flight. Thus the shallow water diver flying to not more than 1000 feet faces little risk whilst the deep water diver (such as oil rig or clearance diving) may be at risk for up to 48 hours even at low altitudes.

A rather different situation obtains when a diver has got decompression sickness after surfacing from a dive and requires treatment. Helicopters are often called upon to transport such a patient to a recompression chamber since speed is often an important element. There is potential conflict, therefore, between direct flight and staying at low altitudes. Even an extra few hundred feet can have a severe effect on the patient and the aim should be to stay as low as practicable.

UNDERWATER MEDICINE

To survive underwater man needs to breathe gas at a pressure equivalent to the surrounding water pressure. Various gases may be used and pure oxygen can be appropriate up to a depth of 8 m. Compressed air is the most popular and can be used to about 50 m. Diving beyond 50 m calls for great technical skill and special mixes of oxygen and helium are used.

For the recreational diver enjoying the delights of his sport the inherent decompression sickness problems of deeper diving do not present themselves. However, those who go deeper, either deliberately or by accident, create for themselves, and the medical support teams called in to assist them, a series of medical evacuation and treatment problems.

Diving is always potentially dangerous and requires a high degree of fitness and general health. Good equipment, sound instruction and the practise of drills coupled with detailed planning of each and every dive will obviate many of the potentially hazardous and disastrous events under water.

Special effects of breathing gases

Four gases require consideration:
1. Oxygen
2. Carbon dioxide
3. Nitrogen
4. Carbon monoxide

Oxygen

Oxygen is essential to life, consequently, any gas mixture used in diving must, as one of its components, contain oxygen. A diver is put at risk not only by compression but also from oxygen poisoning, the signs and symptoms of which are:

A. *Early Signs* (underwater)
 1. Twitching lips
 2. Twitching face muscles
 3. Vision disturbances

B. *Later Signs* (on the surface)
 Convulsions

The convulsive phase mimics an epileptic fit and the treatment is much the same. The patient must be protected from injuring himself and biting his tongue. The convulsions can last up to 2 min with a return to the conscious state between 4 and 8 min later and from which a full and normal recovery can be expected. The treatment of oxygen poisoning is:
1. Breathing air
2. Prevention of self-injury
3. Supportive measures by symptomatic assessment

Carbon dioxide

For divers a build-up of carbon dioxide is unlikely unless special procedures are being carried out. For example, military divers use a system of rebreathing air, which has had the carbon dioxide removed within a closed breathing apparatus system, the purpose of which is to ensure that a trail of bubbles is not created and the divers' presence not revealed.

The same system is, however, used by clearance divers and, therefore, may present itself to offshore medical personnel. The symptoms of carbon dioxide poisoning are:
1. Increase in respiration rate
2. Skin flushing
3. Severe headaches
4. Unconsciousness

The treatment of carbon dioxide poisoning is to:
1. Remove face mask
2. Allow spontaneous recovery or
3. Symptomatically assess and treat

For divers who reach the surface unconscious one must also consider the possibility of *air embolism*.

Nitrogen

The partial pressure of nitrogen increases as the water pressure increases and this may give rise to the narcotic effect (the 'narks') which reduces awareness of any dangers, produces a euphoric effect and a marked reduction in physical and mental performance. There is no treatment for nitrogen narcosis as it regresses during ascent and cannot occur on the surface.

Carbon monoxide

Carbon monoxide competes with oxygen for uptake by haemoglobin and is some 200 times more effective in doing so. Consequently carbon monoxide poisoning is very dangerous and leads to rapid unconsciousness and death. The diver will be quite unaware of his problem before he loses consciousness and the only sign will be the classic pink to cherry red lips. Carbon monoxide poisoning is usually due to the gas being inadvertently compressed with contaminated air, often from exhaust fumes of internal combustion engines being run nearby. Treatment includes giving 100 per cent oxygen.

Decompression sickness

As a diver descends the pressure exerted increases, causing nitrogen to become dissolved, first in the bloodstream and then in the body tissues. During ascent this gas comes out of solution and provided the ascent is controlled and regulated by diving tables there will normally be no ill effects. Unfortunately this is not always the case and when these nitrogen bubbles form in the bloodstream and the tissues of the body a condition known as decompression sickness results.

Minor decompression sickness is characterized by a feeling of unusual tiredness, itching of the skin and, maybe, a skin rash. Such signs and symptoms are warnings that there may follow a serious condition and divers should be carefully monitored if they make any general complaint about feeling unwell. Divers themselves are readily aware of the problems facing them and will be quick in drawing attention to anything they feel is unusual.

Serious decompression sickness falls into four main areas and affects several parts of the body:

1. Cerebral decompression sickness (CDS)

The neurological signs and symptoms suggestive of brain damage are much the same as those to be expected from head trauma, but the history is the conclusive aid to diagnosis. If a diver has neurological problems after a dive one must assume that he has cerebral decompression sickness and transfer him to a compression chamber as soon as possible.

2. Vestibular decompression sickness (VDS)

Divers who seem to be staggering about after a dive may well be suffering from vestibular decompression sickness which affects the balancing mechanism of the innner ear. The inability to keep his balance, nausea or vomiting and perhaps a 'dizzy' feeling are all indicative of VDS.

3. Spinal decompression sickness (SDS)

Nitrogen bubbles which occur within the spinal cord will cause the signs and symptoms of sensory and motor nerve disturbances. Usually the diver will complain of 'pins and needles' of the limbs and, perhaps, the trunk. He may experience a general weakness if the condition is mild or paralysis if more severe. Such functions as passing urine become difficult or impossible.

4. Lung decompression sickness (LDS)

Chest pain, the inability to breathe freely and, in severe cases, hypovolaemic shock are all signs and symptoms of LDS. A large quantity of nitrogen bubbles in the bloodstream will block the pulmonary circulation manifesting themselves as a 'mild' or 'severe' LDS.

Pulmonary barotrauma

The diver as he descends compresses the air in his lungs. It may be that the ascent is achieved in one continuous expiration as the compressed air slowly expands and only if the diver stops his expiration will damage from barotrauma begin. Once on the surface he will complain of chest pain or difficulty in breathing which may be associated with coughing up blood. With more severe barotrauma he may well present with a pneumothorax or gas embolism, the latter caused by air finding its way into the bloodstream and thence to the brain as a cerebral arterial air (gas) embolism.

Cerebral air embolism
Air blocking the circulation to or within the brain will have the same effect as any other embolism. An air embolus will cause the following signs and symptoms:
1. Visual disturbances
2. Paralysis
3. Weakness
4. Paraesthesiae (tingling and numbness)
5. Behavioural changes
6. Convulsions
7. Coma

Should a diver make a rapid ascent the likelihood of a cerebral air embolism must be considered by medical staff. The convulsions and coma may well present very soon after surfacing and cardiopulmonary resuscitation will dominate treatment in the initial stages.

Treatment of decompression sickness
Speed is essential in the successful treatment of decompression sickness. Delays in securing treatment considerably lower the survival graph. Once the diagnosis of the disease is made immediate transfer to a recompression facility is mandatory. It is essential that before diving takes place the recompression facilities available for use are well known to all concerned. Patients should be transferred in the recovery position inclined to the left side. The use of oxygen will be beneficial if the journey is a long one. A deterioration in the patient's condition may apparently occur soon after the oxygen is administered but this should improve after a short period of time. Transfer of patients in helicopters, which are unpressurized, should be limited to safe flying at as low an altitude as the pilot will permit and under no circumstances should he fly over 1000 feet above sea level.

The immersion victim
Drowning and hypothermia
The two conditions are difficult to separate and must be considered together because in the case of the immersion victim they are interrelated. Immersion casualties can be considered as passing through four distinct stages in which the mechanisms leading to incapacitation or death are slightly different.

a. Initial immersion or cold shock ('hydrocution')
During the first two or three minutes of being in the water (below 15 °C) the casualty may be overcome by *'cold shock'*. If the victim is not well

clothed or used to very cold water the sudden immersion of the skin in cold water produces severe stress. This can lead to reflex effects on the heart and involuntary gasping respirations. Such respirations can lead to uncontrolled inspiration when waves splash over the face so that water is inhaled. These reflexes can incapacitate a fit and healthy competent swimmer while in the unfit or the elderly the stress can cause cardiac arrest. For those persons who try to effect rescues and who are quite unprepared for the 'cold shock' the resultant 'shock' to their bodies can be disastrous with the would-be rescuer also a casualty.

b. Short-term immersion

This is defined as immersion for between 4 and 30 min. Even competent swimmers, if they are unused to the cold, will have considerable difficulty in swimming in cold water. The use of a suitable life-jacket is essential to prevent drowning—regardless of swimming expertise.

c. Long-term immersion

This is defined as immersion lasting over 30 min. The major problem here is lack of thermoregulation which inevitably results in hypothermia. Useful consciousness will be lost when the core temperature drops by 2 or 3°C, and at this stage the casualty will drown unless an adequate airway is maintained, *clear of the water.* As a consequence severe hypothermia will only occur in immersion casualties who are wearing life jackets.

d. Post-immersion collapse

See below under Special Treatment Considerations.

Rescue of immersion victims

The rescue of immersion victims is often very difficult especially if the sea is rough, if oil or other pollutants are in the sea or if suitable means of lifting or recovering survivors or bodies is not available. If possible, arrangements must be made in advance to devise a means of lifting survivors on to the rescue platform. Survivors will have their chances of continued survival greatly increased if they are lifted horizontally and not made to stand after rescue.

Treatment of immersion victims

As soon as the immersion victim is rescued it must be assumed that he will be suffering from hypothermia and drowning and no attempt should be made to differentiate between the two conditions. Initial treatment is therefore aimed at restoration of adequate ventilation, the prevention of hypotension and reduction of further heat loss. Resuscitative efforts must be started as soon as is practical and continued until such time as it is obvious that such efforts are in vain. About 60 per cent of all near-drowning victims vomit during resuscitation and for those who seem alert 100 per cent oxygen administered for about 5 min will be of considerable benefit and continued oxygen therapy should be given as necessary. Conscious patients should be encouraged to cough and take deep breaths which helps to remove water from their lungs and re-expand areas of collapsed lung.

Special treatment considerations

Hypovolaemic collapse

The sudden reduction in cardiac output which occurs on removal from the water—resulting from the fall in central venous pressure due to the removal of the supportive hydrostatic squeeze—may result in sudden loss of consciousness or even death.

As far as is practicable, therefore, efforts should be made to protect the individual from this known hazard during and immediately after rescue.

After rescue the victim should be laid horizontally with the lower limbs slightly elevated, or jet-splints applied to prevent peripheral venous pooling. Such recommendations about posture must be reconciled with the requirement to maintain a clear airway.

The unconscious or semi-conscious patient should be insulated with a blanket or sleeping bag and allowed to rewarm spontaneously. Clothing should not be removed—except for loose outer clothing—to avoid unnecessary manhandling; external sources of heat, e.g. hot water bottles, heat lamps, etc. should not be used as they may precipitate rewarming collapse.

Rewarming collapse

Surface rewarming (except by immersion in a hot bath, *see* p. 267) dilates the blood vessels in the periphery thus causing a hypovolaemic collapse. Thus in the absence of adequate monitoring facilities, rewarming should be slow, i.e. spontaneous, except for those patients who are alert and shivering, and obviously not severely hypothermic. Alert, shivering patients may be permitted to have a hot shower, but it is necessary to observe them while they are doing so because of the danger of fainting.

Hypoxia

Although the patient may be breathing, ventilation may be inadequate because of the presence of small amounts of water in the lung or areas of collapse. This may be manifest at the time of rescue or may develop up to 72 hours later. Consequently, patients who have inhaled moderate amounts of water should be observed for signs of respiratory distress (tachycardia, cyanosis and reduced pulse pressure). If conscious, the patient may be coughing, complaining of chest pain and auscultation will reveal crepitations and other clinical signs.

Such patients may require ventilatory assistance. In conscious patients, this procedure must be explained in order to gain their cooperation. All such patients must be admitted to hospital as soon as possible for observation, chest X-ray, blood gas analysis and other investigations.

Secondary drowning

This is delayed failure of lung function due to an outpouring of secretions caused by the irritant effects of aspirated vomit and other foreign material such as sand and mud. It can occur from 15 min to 4 days after the near drowning incident and requires *urgent* resuscitative measures, including ventilation. High dose steroid therapy, given as soon as possible after the incident probably reduces the risk of this delayed, life-threatening emergency, if transfer to hospital is likely to be prolonged, the patient's condition may also be helped by infusion of 500–1000 ml of a plasma expander such as dextran or gelatin.

Further reading

The Air Attendants' Handbook, published by The St John Ambulance Association and Brigade of the Order of St John.

Aviation Medicine

Read, Keith E. E. (1971) *Aeromedicine for Aviators*. London, Pitman.
Whiteside T. C. D. (1979) *Health and Clinical Factors*, Aviation Medicine, Vol. 2. London, HMSO.

Underwater Medicine

Bennett P. B. and Elliott D. H. (1982) *The Physiology and Medicine of Diving*. Eastbourne, Bailliere Tindall.
Diving and Subaquatic Medicine. Police Diving Manual. (1983) 2nd ed. London, HMSO/Home Office.
Hills B. (1977) *Decompression Sickness*. Vol. 1. *The Biophysical Basis of Prevention and Treatment*. New York, Wiley.

Chapter 26

Nuclear, Biological and Chemical Warfare

J. E. Butter and S. J. Mather

The purpose of this chapter is to provide paramedical personnel with information on the biomedical effects of nuclear weapons, biological and chemical agents, to ensure that personnel understand the protective precautionary measures to avoid contamination themselves when dealing with casualties who have been exposed, and to appreciate the value of *co-ordinated* first aid measures.

Horrific as it is to contemplate, we are living in an age where nuclear explosions may happen, either as a result of an accident or through a deliberate act of war. A comprehensive review of the subject is beyond the scope of this book but we have attempted to outline the major effects of a nuclear explosion, the effects of biological and chemical agents, and the difficulties that would be consequent upon such events, particularly in so far as the provision of medical aid is concerned.

THERMONUCLEAR WEAPONS

Terminology

The yields of thermonuclear weapons at present available to the 'superpowers' are of the order of tens of *kilotons* to about 1·5 *megatons*. The 'tonnage' refers to the equivalent effect of that many tons of TNT. In other words, a 1 megaton warhead produces an explosion equivalent in its destructive power to 1 million tons of TNT. Of course, nuclear weapons produce many other effects, quite apart from the destructive effect of the blast which make them different in almost every way from even millions of tons of TNT. The bomb which devastated Hiroshima was a mere 13 kilotons in size!

NUCLEAR, BIOLOGICAL AND CHEMICAL WARFARE

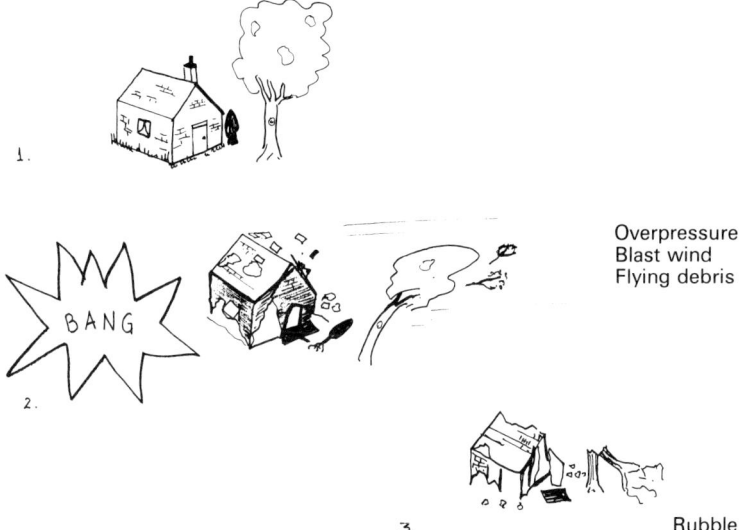

Fig. 26.1. Once the blast wave has passed and the damage sustained, the medical problem is based upon conventional triage and rescue.

Ground burst versus air burst

If a nuclear weapon is exploded on the ground, a so-called ground burst, the effect differs from that of one exploded at altitude (an air burst). The ground immediately beneath such an explosion is known as 'ground zero'.

An air burst increases the area over which the force of the explosion has its effect but, relative to the ground burst, has less effect at ground zero. There would also be less local radiation but more extensive thermal effects.

It is realistic to assume, with multi-warhead missiles that an effective nuclear exchange would be of the order of 20 megatons, spread out over several targets. The possibility of 'limited' nuclear warfare with tactical nuclear weapons being used only on the battlefield and avoiding escalation into strategic, intercontinental exchanges seems naive. Any planning for defence or the provision of medical services must assume that the natural consequences of the first transgression to the use of nuclear weapons will be all-out nuclear war which neither side could win.

Conventional explosions

The destructive action of conventional explosions is due to the transmission of energy in the form of a blast wave with resultant mechanical damage to persons or property (*Fig.* 26.1).

Nuclear explosions

The energy of a nuclear explosion is transferred to the surrounding area in three distinct forms:
Blast
Thermal radiation
Nuclear radiation
For a low-altitude atmospheric detonation of a moderate-sized weapon the energy is roughly distributed as:
50 per cent blast.
35 per cent as thermal radiation (made up of a wide range of the electromagnetic spectrum including infrared, visible and ultraviolet light and some soft X-ray).
15 per cent nuclear radiation (including 5 per cent as initial ionizing radiation consisting of neutrons, and gamma rays emitted within the first minute of detonation and 10 per cent residual radiation in the fallout (*see below*).

Considerable variation from this distribution will occur depending on the size of the weapon, location and whether ground or air burst. Much of the energy of the explosion would be in the form of intense visible light and electromagnetic radiation both above and below the visible spectrum. The flash would cause permanent damage to the retina many miles from the explosion. Transient 'flash blindness' could occur at greater distances but 'transient' in this context might imply many days of blindness which, given the adverse circumstances, might prove fatal.

The temperature in the immediate vicinity of the explosion would be millions of degrees Celsius. As the 'mushroom' cloud rises upward, the temperature at ground zero falls rapidly but re-radiation from the expanding hot gas cloud would still produce a surface temperature of many thousands of degrees. Any flammable material, such as clothing, fuel stores, cereal crops and forests would be likely to ignite spontaneously. Forest fires and burning buildings would perpetuate the fire. The intense winds created by the explosion and the heat would blow at anything from 100 to 1000 miles per hour, creating a 'firestorm' and consuming all the available oxygen so that even survivors of the blast might be killed by suffocation.

Electromagnetic pulse

The gamma radiation emitted by the bomb, when absorbed by the atmosphere, would result in a high-voltage electromagnetic 'pulse', mainly in the radio frequency band. Radiocommunications, computers, telex and telephone equipment could be rendered completely ineffective. Air bursts, particularly those in the atmosphere, could be expected to disrupt radio communications over hundreds of miles. Missile guidance systems and radar would also be affected.

Blast

The explosion would initially create a shock wave moving at supersonic speed; 5-10 psi overpressure would lead to ruptured ear drums, air embolus, pulmonary contusion and damage to the bony thoracic cage. Such effects might be expected to occur several miles from ground zero. Those who were not killed in this way might be fatally injured by flying debris.

Radiation

The exact nature and intensity of the radiation emitted depends upon the construction characteristics of the bomb and whether the explosion was a ground or air burst. Ground-burst weapons suck up millions of tons of dust into the cloud, which then becomes radioactive. This radioactive cloud gives rise to many different isotopes, with differing half lives. It is this radioactive material which returns to earth as 'fall out'. It is estimated that plutonium from such a blast could persist in the environment for half a million years!

The medical effects of nuclear explosions

The numbers killed and injured following an 'average' hypothetical explosion of 20 megatons over a populated area could be expected to be 9·5 million people killed outright and 5 million injured. Most of those injured would then succumb to the effects of disease, hunger, radiation sickness or further injury. There would be no buildings in the city standing, no uncontaminated water or food for those without the benefit of a hardened nuclear shelter. Communications would be devastated and in all-out nuclear war, no neighbouring area is likely to be able to offer aid.

Medical services, which rely for their operation on sophisticated electronic, mechanical and technical services would be completely overwhelmed. The entire resources of the peacetime National Health Service in the UK could not cope with the medical effects of even one nuclear attack on a major British city. In such a situation medical personnel would be little more use than trained first aiders. Epidemics of disease such as typhoid, cholera, hepatitis and dysentery would be rife and uncontrollable.

Thermal injuries

In nuclear warfare burn injuries will dominate the problems of medical personnel where radioactive contamination is not a consideration.

Diagnosis

The area of the burn will, as is already accepted, be the critical determining factor in treatment regimes.

Head and neck burns

Burns of the head frequently are complicated by oedema which can result in respiratory obstruction. Burns of the face present a psychological as well as a surgical problem and if the hot gases have been inhaled damage to the trachea may well indicate tracheostomy.

Burns of the respiratory tract

Such burns are very serious and have a high mortality rate if they extend deep into the alveoli. These patients are critically ill and do not tolerate movement or transportation well. Pulmonary oedema may well develop abruptly and without warning and is extremely difficult to manage.

Radiation injury

Radiation injury alone or in conjunction with other injuries will be common in nuclear warfare. Radiation injury can result from a single exposure to prompt radiation at the time of detonation, or from high levels of fallout radiation, or from repeated exposures to both with complex patterns of recovery, or from an accumulation of radiation damage.

There are three phases in the clinical course of radiation sickness:
Phase 1 Transient incapacitation
Phase 2 Latent period
Phase 3 Clinical illness

The diagnosis of radiation sickness is based primarily upon the picture presented by the patient. A detailed history may well be difficult to obtain since many of the patients will not know that they have been exposed, especially if it is due to fallout.

There are three syndromes worthy of limited discussion to explain the clinical process and the biological effects of radiation:
Haematopoietic syndrome
Gastrointestinal syndrome
Central nervous system syndrome

The haematopoietic syndrome

Doses of radiation in the low to midlethal range will produce depression of bone marrow function with cessation of blood cell production. The time of onset of the depression of cell production in the marrow will vary considerably, and the concomitant clinical problems toward uncontrolled haemorrhage, decreased resistance to infection and anaemia will vary considerably from as early as 10 days to as much as 6–8 weeks after exposure. Therefore, the signs that a patient may present with are:
Haemorrhagic disease
Susceptibility to infection

Loss of weight
Loss of hair
If bone marrow depression reaches a critical level below which it is unable to restore sufficient numbers of granulocytes and thrombocytes to the circulating blood, death from overwhelming infection and haemorrhage will occur.

The gastrointestinal syndrome

The doses of radiation which will result in the gastrointestinal syndrome are higher than those causing the haematopoietic syndrome and the clinical phase occurs earlier. After a short latent period of a few days to a week or so, the characteristic severe fluid losses, haemorrhage and diarrhoea begin. The pathological basis for this syndrome is a combination of severe loss of gastric mucosa and injury to the fine vasculature of the submucosa. A problem in diagnosis will arise in patients with sublethal haematopoietic depression due to radiation and with symptoms due to some other cause such as infection. It would, for example, be difficult to differentiate between patients with lethal radiation sickness and those with potentially nonlethal radiation sickness complicated by dysentery.

The central nervous system syndrome

This syndrome is associated with very high doses of radiation. The latent period is very short, ranging from several hours to 1–2 days. The clinical picture is that of a steadily deteriorating state of consciousness with eventual coma and death. Convulsions may or may not occur and because of the very high doses of radiation required to cause this syndrome, personnel close enough to the nuclear explosion to receive such high doses would generally be well within the range of lethality due to blast or thermal effects.

In any event there would be 100 per cent mortality from the cerebral effects and hypotension. A great dilemma exists for those attempting to identify potential survivors in the first hours after a nuclear attack since many other mechanisms may produce similar symptoms.

Treatment would only be feasible for isolated incidents which were the result of an accident. Full intensive care facilities with the back up of a major hospital would be required. In the context of nuclear war it would be unrealistic to expect to offer anything but the simplest treatment to mass casualties. This would involve making them as comfortable as possible. Skilled triage would be necessary to ensure that scarce resources were not wasted on those with no chance of survival. Those who had received total body irradiation would not present any radiation hazard to others.

Treatment

The haematopoietic syndrome
Antibiotics
Whole blood or fresh platelet transfusion
Bone marrow transfusion

The gastrointestinal syndrome
Transfusion of fluids
Antibiotics
Bone marrow transfusion

The central nervous system syndrome
Symptomatic treatments

External contamination from radioactive material

The danger here is of penetration of the skin by radioactive particles or absorption of radiation through the skin. The exact effect would depend upon the type of radiation being emitted (alpha, beta or gamma) and the amount and the length of time for which the individual had been exposed. Such a person does present a risk to others because transfer of radiaoactive particles to another individual is a possibility. Decontamination after an isolated accident is feasible but it is doubtful whether effective decontamination could be achieved for the numbers of casualties who would be affected following a nuclear attack.

Internal contamination

Ingestion of radioactive particles is likely to occur together with external contamination. Again, the effects would be dose-dependent. In isolated cases, emergency iodine prophylaxis may be employed.

Iodine prophylaxis

Fallout, as mentioned above, would contain many radioactive isotopes with varying half-lives. Iodine 131 could be expected to occur in large quantities following both nuclear power-station accidents and nuclear warfare. The theory behind the treatment relies upon the administration of potassium iodide which is taken up by the thyroid gland. If enough potassium iodide is given, the gland would be saturated with iodide, inhibiting the uptake of radioactive iodine 131.

Local burns

Local burns may occur from the absorption of high doses of gamma rays. These may be difficult to elucidate in the presence of other, traumatic, injuries, classic burns and whole body irradiation.

Ecological effects and the 'nuclear winter'

a. Consequences due to fallout

Lethal levels of fallout could be expected for weeks or months at least and even years in some areas. Agricultural land and water supplies could remain radioactive for hundreds of years. It is doubtful whether many people could be sheltered from the fallout for long enough to provide a viable and disciplined work force to rebuild towns and cities and cultivate what would be a terribly hostile landscape. Deaths from radiation sickness and infection would continue to occur for months. Later, there would be an increase in deaths from cancer.

b. Consequences due to the destruction of modern society

The use of nuclear weapons, with their potential for massive destruction, would produce situations in which epidemic outbreaks of disease amongst the population would become highly probable, and if large heavily populated areas are devastated the social organization which is required to support effectively a modern medical care system will be severely compromised. If the ravages of war are beyond the capabilities of either the society itself or the armies in the area to repair then decimation of the population by the classic diseases such as dysentery, typhus, cholera, etc. will ensue.

The fires would continue to rage for weeks, converting atmospheric oxygen into oxides of nitrogen and ultimately depleting the ozone layer high in the atmosphere. The results of this would be catastrophic because the resulting thin ozone layer would allow intense ultraviolet radiation to penetrate to the earth's surface.

Such intense ultraviolet radiation could cause full-thickness skin burns in unprotected individuals within a few hours. Agriculture as we know it today would cease as the crop yield, in the face of this radiation, without modern fertilizers and harvesting equipment, would be very poor. Fuel supplies would soon be exhausted, cultivation of the land returning to at best a medieval level.

Depletion of the ozone layer and other atmospheric changes would also produce a marked diminution in the earth's surface temperature.

c. 'The nuclear winter'

A nuclear conflict, as we have already mentioned, could be expected to carry millions of tons of the earth's surface high into the atmosphere. This dust would block out up to 99 per cent of the sunlight falling upon that area. Natural disasters, such as the Mount St Helens eruption are known to have produced significant changes in the world's weather systems and there is good evidence that other, similar, events in history have also done so. Such a phenomenon might account for the disappearance of the dinosaurs on earth.

A combination of changes in the weather systems, changes in surface temperature and almost perpetual dark would render an area barren in the extreme. No crops could be grown under such circumstances and animals without shelter would quickly die in the subzero temperatures which would certainly occur in Europe, Canada, the USA and the Soviet Union.

Isolated nuclear accidents

Isolated incidents, such as radiation leaks at power stations or nuclear fuel-processing plants, might be serious enough to cause death or serious injury to whole communities, but in the global context the consequences would be much less severe than a nuclear explosion in so far as the emission is likely to be in the form of radioactive gas, without a dust cloud or fires and on a much smaller geographical scale. The mainstay of population defence would be evacuation or shelter for those in the path of the gas cloud, together with iodine prophylaxis (since a large proportion of the emission would predictably be in the form of iodine 131).

In such an incident, the affected population would have the benefit of support facilities and sophisticated medical care in adjacent communities. All the trappings of modern civilization would be intact, giving exposed persons who had not received a lethal dose of radiation a good chance of survival.

Medical planning for nuclear war

The success of medical support operations will depend to a great extent on the adequacy of planning, training and preparation. The main points are listed below:
1. Organization of the medical support system
2. Mobility of medical support
3. Casualty assessment
4. Stores support and re-supply
5. Personnel replacements
6. Handling large numbers of casualties
7. Patient decontamination
8. Suitable shelters for patients and staff
9. Personal protection against radiation

CHEMICAL AGENTS

Chemicals can affect the body in a variety of modes. The use of chemical agents as a deliberate attempt to incapacitate populations cannot be ruled out in times of conflict between nations, nor can the accidental chemical disaster be ruled out in the form of chemical factory explosions or a workforce's accidental exposure to toxicants within the factory. The chemicals can be grouped into the following:

NUCLEAR, BIOLOGICAL AND CHEMICAL WARFARE

Nerve agents
Blister agents (vesicants)
Choking agents (lung damage)
Blood agents (cyanogen)
Incapacitants

Nerve agents

Nerve agents are all organophosphorus esters related to insecticides such as parathion. They are liquids varying in volatility similar to that between petrol and heavy lubricating oil. Colour ranges from pale yellow to colourless and they have very little smell. They are rapidly destroyed by strong alkalis and chlorinating compounds. Nerve agents very strongly inhibit the enzyme cholinesterase which catalyses the hydrolysis of acetylcholine into choline and acetic acid. This action prevents impulses travelling along the nerves thus creating symptoms ranging from minor nasal mucosal irritation to respiratory arrest. The time course will vary between minutes to hours depending upon the dose.

Pathology

The damaging effects of nerve agents are predominantly on *function* rather than structure.

Treatment

Restoration of vital body functions
Atropine by injection
Decontamination
Oxime therapy (to restore cholinesterase function)
Supportive care

Blister agents

Blister agents are known more commonly as mustards and are able to penetrate rubber, wood, leather and skin.

Pathology

Once the skin is contaminated there is a latent period where no effects are experienced. This is followed by erythema and the formation of blisters if the dose has been high enough. Some discomfort will be noticed in the eyes. Patients may also present with throat and gastrointestinal symptoms.

Treatment

Skin—Erythema and itching can be reduced by the topical application of local anaesthetic creams or other soothing preparations. Blisters are covered with sterile petroleum jelly gauze and topical antibiotics may be of use.

Eyes—Application of analgesic drops or ointments. Antibacterial preparations where appropriate.
Throat—Gargles and symptomatic therapy.
Gastrointestinal tract—Give 0·5 mg atropine sulphate and sedatives. Make every effort to replace fluids and electrolytes.

Choking agents
Chemical agents which attack the lungs, primarily causing pulmonary oedema are classed as lung-damaging agents. Of these phosgene is the most dangerous and the only one likely to be used.

Pathology
A mild irritation of the eyes and upper respiratory tract are minor distractions which are secondary to the noxious effect phosgene has on the lungs. Primary effects are damage of the bronchiolar epithelium, development of local emphysema and partial collapse of alveoli.

Treatment
  Rest
  Warmth
  Sedation
  Oxygen
  Antibiotics

Blood agents
Blood agents attempt to inhibit cellular respiration, consequently oxygen carried by the haemoglobin is not consumed and this explains the bright colour of venous blood of casualties exposed to hydrocyanic acid (cyanide) intoxication.

Treatment
Artificial ventilation with 100 per cent oxygen, specific antidotes.

Incapacitants
Incapacitating agents are chemicals which produce temporary disabling conditions which persist for hours or days after exposure. Medical treatment is not required but does assist recovery at a more rapid rate. Examples are 'CS' and 'tear' gas.

Medical support in chemical accidents
All site medical personnel must be prepared to receive casualties injured or contaminated with chemical agents. If a person is injured and unable

to decontaminate himself then this process must be performed by other personnel, including the medical staff.

Rescuers must be able to:
Manage casualties so that injuries resulting from chemical agents are minimized and the other injuries not aggravated.
Protect personnel handling contaminated casualties or working in contaminated areas.
Avoid the spread of contamination in ambulances or other evacuation facilities.

BIOLOGICAL WARFARE

The possibility of contamination by bacteriological or viral agents by an aggressor is a horrific, but real, threat.

The choice of agent will depend upon the particular military strategic aims and the surrounding environment. Contamination may be airborne (aerosols), through the water or food supply, or through any other commodities in widespread use by the target population or military forces.

Agents with a high mortality, e.g. *Bacillus anthracis* or *Clostridium botulinum*, may be used if it is required to inflict rapid losses but these agents are unusual contaminants and a suspicion of bacteriological warfare may be aroused early once the first cases are identified.

A more subtle and insidious approach would be to use an agent more commonly found in normal circumstances, such as a variety of the influenza virus, or dysentery, which may not lead to a suspicion of biological warfare until a large number of the target population have been incapacitated.

The use of biological agents is not without its risks for the aggressor, however.

Requirements for suitable agents

The agent must be available in large quantities, be able to maintain its virulence (infectivity) and survive storage in this state for long periods. Some viruses may be freeze-dried and 'reconstituted' at a later date.

Agents which are to be introduced into the water supply of the target population must be very potent in order to be effective once dilution has occurred.

There must be no natural or acquired immunity in the target population which would reduce the effectiveness of the attack.

The incubation period of the agent should be as short as possible in order to minimize delay between the initial contamination and the clinical effect.

Factors influencing the development of infection or effect upon the target population

Dose—the number of organisms required to produce the disease
Viability of the organism
Ease of contamination
Incubation period
Immunity of the target population

Organisms which might be considered for use in biological warfare

Anthrax
Botulinus
Cholera
Dysentery (shigella)
Plague
Typhoid
Q-fever
Rocky mountain spotted fever
Typhus
Dengue
Encephalitis viruses
Smallpox
Yellow fever
Influenza
Fungi (coccidioidomycosis; histoplasmosis)

Detection of contamination

This may be very difficult at the time of contamination, which may be from an aircraft, shell or by the hand of saboteurs. Cultures may take up to 48 hours to produce a reliable identification from any one individual. Identification of viruses may be especially difficult.

Clinical signs of disease are likely to be the only available means of detection initially.

Protection against biological agents

A high index of suspicion that the enemy may be using biological agents is a prerequisite for early detetion. Low-flying aircraft especially should arouse concern, especially if the weather conditions would favour contamination.

Personal protection depends upon the following:
1. Any clothing will help prevent direct contamination but special suits (NBC suits) are available to protect the armed forces. Used with a respirator, these give a high level of protection. Civilian populations, however, are very much at risk from inhalation of aerosols.
2. A high standard of personal and public hygiene is essential; pest control measures must be ruthless.
3. Decontamination of food and water.
4. Immunization.
5. Shelter from aerosols and insect vectors. This is only likely to succeed if effective air filtration plants are available and working.

Decontamination

Most of the agents which are likely to be used will rapidly lose their virulence and are unlikely to pose a continuing threat. Persistent, very virulent organisms would prevent rapid occupation of territory by an invading army.

Decontamination can be achieved by thorough washing in hot soapy water. Cleansing of the hair and nails and any cuts or abrasions is particularly important.

Clothing should be changed and burned if possible. Failing this, garments should be boiled or soaked in bleach.

Vehicles, buildings and utensils should be washed with hypochlorite solution (bleach).

All water supplies should be boiled or treated with 'purification' tablets.

Treatment

Treatment will consist of the normal medical management of the infection, isolation of patients and appropriate decontamination of contacts, investigation and control of the source and protection of the population at risk as far as is practicable in the prevailing conditions.

Further reading

Ervin F. R. et al. (1962) The medical consequences of nuclear war. *N. Engl. J. Med.* **266**, 1126–1145.

Hubner K. F. and Fry S. A. (ed.) (1980) *The Medical Basis for Radiation Accident Preparedness.* New York, Elsevier.

Lapp R. E. and Andrews H. L. (1972) *Nuclear Radiation Physics.* 4th ed. Englewood Cliffs N J, Prentice-Hall.

Lewis K. N. (1979) The prompt and delayed effects of nuclear war. *Scientific Am.* **241**, 35–47.

The Medical Effects of Nuclear War (1983) London, BMA.

Index

Abdomen, 9–10, 18, (*Figs.* 12.1, 12.2) 123–131
Abdominal trauma, 128
Acetone, smell of, on breath, 264
Acidosis, 40
Addison's disease, 185
Adsorbent agents, 223
Air embolism, 278
Airway, 54–61, 72, 154, 205, 211
  oropharyngeal, (*Fig.* 6.8) 58
Altitude hypoxia, 48, 274
Amnesia, 148
Amniotic cavity, 190
Analgesia, postoperative, 46
Analgesics, 43–45, 85, 208
  local, 45
  'mild', 47
Aneurysm, aortic, (*Fig.* 11.1) 105
Antenatal care, 191
Antigravity Suit, (*Fig.* 19.1) 203
Antihypertensive drugs, (*Table* 11.1) 108
Apex beat, 6
Appendicitis, 128
Arterial thrombosis, cerebral, 159
Aspirin poisoning, *see* Salicylate poisoning
Asthma, 9, 95
Asystole, 77
Atrial fibrillation, 115, 116
Atrial flutter, 116
Apomorphine, in treatment of poisoning, 223
Auscultation, (*Fig.* 2.2) 7, 8, 9, 72, 127
Aviation medicine, 269–76

Barbiturate poisoning, 227
Barotrauma, 274, 279
Bigeminy, 120
Biological warfare, 295–7
BIPP (bismuth iodoform paraffin paste), 175
Blast injuries, 87–88
Blast lung, 242
Blastocyst, 190
Bleeding, *see* Haemorrhage

Blood, artificial, 39
pH, 21
Blood, coughing up, 17, 85, 95
Blood loss, (*Table* 10.1) 99
  assessment, 29–30
Blood pressure, 16
Blood transfusion, hazards, 39–41
Blood sugar, measurement in the field, 19
Blue lips, 4
Blunt trauma, 102
Body fluid compartments, (*Fig.* 4.1) 26
  (*Fig.* 4.2) 33
Bones, examination, 10
Bowel sounds, 9, 18
Brainstem reflexes, 155
Bronchial breathing, 8
Bronchitis, 9, 93
Bulbar paralysis, 158
Buminate, 38
Burn injury, assessment, 206
  of the eye, 167
  immediate care, 204
  pathophysiology, 204
  transport, 208
  in childhood, 220–221

Capillary refill time, 27
Carbon dioxide, partial pressure, 20
  poisoning, 278
  treatment, 278
Carbon monoxide poisoning, 49, 87, 231, 278
Cardiac arrest, 70–74
Cardiac contusion, 102
Cardiac cycle, 15
Cardiac failure, *see* Heart failure.
Cardiac massage, 72, 201, 212
Cardiogenic shock, 49, 79, 199
Cardiopulmonary resuscitation, 70–81, 210–12
  children, 210
  complications of, 79
Cardiovascular system, 6–7, 12–17

299

CASEVAC, 269
Central nervous system, 18
Central Nervous System syndrome (radiation injury), 289
Cerebral abscess, 157
Cerebral embolus, 159, 280
Cerebral haemorrhage, 160
Cerebrospinal fluid, leaking, 4
Chemical measurement in the field, 19
Chemical warfare agents, 292–5
Child abuse, 221
Cholecystitis, 129
Closed chest cardiac massage, (*Fig.* 7.2) 72
Coagulation problems, 40
Cold injury, 262
Cold shock, 280
Colloids, 37–39, 102
Colour of patient, 17
Coma, 153–154
  diabetic, management of, 154
Compression strapping, (*Figs.* 23.6–23.12) 251
Consciousness, level of, 18
Convulsions, 226, 228, 230, 277
  in children, (*Table* 20.1) 219
Corrosive agents, immediate care, 204
Crepitation, 9, 32, 283
Crepitus, 142
Cricoid pressure, 65
Critical care, 1, 2
Crystalloids, 35–36
CS gas, 234
Cushing's disease, 185
Cyanide poisoning, 49, 231
Cyanosis, 4, 17

Decompression sickness, 276, 278–9
  treatment, 280
Decontamination, 297
Defibrillators, 80
Dextrans, 37, 102, 226
Dextrose, 5% solution, 36
Dextrose–saline solution, 36
Diabetes insipidus, 177
Diabetes mellitus, 178–84
Dialysis, 227
Dislocations, 142
Distalgesic poisoning, 229
Drowning, 218, 280
  secondary, 283
Drowsy child, 218–19

Eclampsia, 196
Ectopic beats, 6, 115, 117
Electrocardiogram (ECG), 13
Electroencephalogram (EEG), 162
Electromagnetic pulse, 286
Electromechanical dissociation, 78
Emergency medical technician, 2
'Emergency Position' for transport of patients (*Figs.* 6.6, 6.7) 56–57
Emphysema, 7, 93
Encephalitis, 157
Endocrine system, 177
Endotracheal intubation, (*Fig.* 6.11) 61–67, 134, 212, 217
Entonox, 43, 208, 221
Epididymo-orchitis, 131
Epiglottitis, 215
Epilepsy, 161–2
Epistaxis, 174
Exercise programme, controlled, (*Fig.* 23.13) 254
Explosions, conventional, 285
  injuries caused by, (*Fig.* 8.5) 87
  nuclear, 286
  medical effects, 287
Explosives, 240
External fixation, 143
Extravascular compartment, 30
Eyeball tension, 31

Fat embolus, 144
Fetal distress, 197
Flail chest, 17, 85
'Flail' segment, (*Fig.* 8.4) 85
Flotation catheter, 29
Fluid balance, 25
Fluids, intravenous, 25
Fluid replacement, in trauma, 101, 205
Fluid therapy, 32
Follicle stimulating hormone (FSH), 190
Foreign body, in eye, 165
  inhaled, 88, 216
  in nose, 175
  removal, 54–55
  in thorax, 88
Forced diuresis, 217, 226, 229
Fractures, blow out, of orbit, 167
  closed, 141
  open, 141
  of ribs, 85
  skull, 149
  spiral, (*Fig.* 13.8) 140

INDEX

Fracture-dislocation of ankle, (*Fig.* 23.1) 245
Fresh Frozen Plasma (FFP), 38

'G' suit, (*Fig.* 19.1) 106, 203
Gangrene, 139
Gastric lavage, *see* Stomach washout,
Gastroenteritis, 130
Gastrointestinal syndrome (of radiation injury), 289
Genitalia examination, 10
Glasgow coma scale, 10, 18, 147, (*Table* 15.1) 153
Graafian follicle, 190
Great vessels, trauma to, 104
Ground burst, 285
Ground zero, 285
Gunshot wound, 237

Haemaccel (polygeline), 37, 102, 226
Haematemesis, 129
Haematocrit, 28
Haematopoietic syndrome of radiation injury, 268
Haemoglobin measurement, 19, 28
Haemoptysis, 85, 95
Haemorrhage, antepartum, 194
 cerebral, 160
 control of, 100
 extradural, 148
 postpartum, 195
 subarachnoid, 148, 160
 subdural, 148
 traumatic, 98–99
Haemorrhagic shock, 98–102
Haemothorax, (*Fig.* 8.3) 85, 103
Hartmann's solution (Ringer lactate), 36, 206, 226
Head injury, 147–50, 153, 177
 in children, 214
Heart block, 78, 113
Heart failure, 28, 94, 121
Heart, penetrating injuries, 103
Heart sounds, 7, 71
Heimlich manoeuvre, 54 (*Fig.* 6.3) 89
Hernia, 130
History taking, scheme for, (*Fig.* 2.1) 5
Human Albumin Solution (HAS), 38
Hydroxyethyl starch, 39
Hypercarbia, 51
Hyperglycaemia, 184

Hyperkalaemia, 40, 71
Hypertension, 106–8, 120, 160, 191, 196
Hyperthermia, 226
Hyperthyroidism, 188
Hypoglycaemia, 79, 183, 199, 227, 229
Hypothermia, 177, 226, 228, 263, 280
Hypothyroidism, 187
Hypovolaemia, 4
Hypovolaemic shock, 71, 198, 215, 282
Hypoxia, 48–50
 altitude, 48, 274
 and immersion, 282
'Hypoxic drive', 51

Immediate care, 1
Immobilization in rescue work, 261
Incapacitants, 294
Infarction, pulmonary, 95
 myocardial, 108
Infection, ear, 173
 eye, 168
Injuries, abdomen, 150
 chest, 150
 facial, 150
 head, in sport, (*Fig.* 23.5) 248
 musculoskeletal, 132–46
 neck, 150
 soft tissue, in sport, 250
 spinal, 134
 in sport, 248
 peripheral nerves, 151
Insulin, 178, 182
Internal fixation of fractures, (*Fig.* 13.10) 144
Intestinal obstruction, 126
Intracellular compartment, 32
Intravenous fluid therapy, (*Figs.* 4.3, 4.4) 34, 129, 130, 138
Iodine prophylaxis, 290
Iron poisoning, 227, 231

Joint(s), 10
 examination, 10–11
 facet, (*Fig.* 13.2) 134

Kernig's sign, 156
Ketamine, 45
Ketoacidosis, treatment of, 184

INDEX

Labour, 192
Laryngotracheobronchitis, 215
Larynx, (Fig. 9.1) 92
Lead poisoning, 227
Liquid debris, removal of, (Fig. 6.4) 55
Localizing signs, monitoring, 18
Locomotor system, 10–11
Lucid interval, 149
Lymphadenitis, 130

Major disaster, 3
'Mast' suit (Fig. 19.1) 203
Maxillofacial injuries, (Fig. 13.1) 133
MEDIVAC, 269
Melaena, 129
Meningitis, 155–6
Mesenteric infarction, 130
Mismatch transfusions, 40
Missile injuries, (Figs. 22.1–22.5) 236
Mobile Coronary Care Unit, 110
Mobitz (Type II) heart block, 114
Monitoring,
 abdomen, 18
 cardiovascular, 12–17
 respiratory, 17
 temperature, 18
 urinary, 18
Monoamine oxidase inhibitors, poisoning, 229
Morula, 190
Mountain rescue teams, 258
Mouth-to-mouth resuscitation, (Fig. 7.1) 72
Myocardial infarction, 49, 71, 108, 259
Myxoedema, see Hypothyroidism

Narcotic analgesics, poisoning, 230
Nasal cannulae, (Fig. 6.2) 53
Nasopharyngeal airway, (Fig. 6.9) 60
Neck rigidity, 156, 160
Neck veins, engorged, 28
Nervous system, 10
Neurogenic shock, 199
Newborn, resuscitation, 213
Nitrogen narcosis, 278
Non-accidental injury, 221
'Normal' saline, 36
Nose bleed, see Epistaxis
Nuclear accident, 292
 explosions, medical effects, 287
 thermal injuries, 287

Nuclear war, medical, planning for, 292
Nuclear winter, 291
Nursing process, 22

Obturator airway, oesophageal, 58
Oedema, 28, 31, 205, 250
 cerebral, 149
 pulmonary, 94
On-site care, 2–3
Oxygen, apparatus, portable (Fig. 6.12) 66
Oxygen, partial, pressure, 20
 poisoning, 277
 treatment, 277
 tent, 53
 therapy, 48–69, 217, 282, 294
 masks, (Fig. 6.1) 52
 uptake, 274

Packed cell volume, see Haematocrit
Pain, in abdomen, 124
 assessment, 12
Pain relief, in cave rescue, 261
Palpation, 6, 9, 11
Pancreatitis, 129
Paracetamol poisoning, 227, 229
Paramedical personnel, 2
Paraquat poisoning, 230
Pelvic fracture (Fig. 13.6) 138
Peptic ulcer, 129
Percussion, in examination of the patient, 7
Perforating eye injury, 166
Peritoneal fluid administration, 35
Peritonitis, 126
Pesticides, poisoning, 227, 230
Phenothiazine poisoning, 228
Plants, poisoning by, 231
Plasma proteins, 228
 in fluid therapy, 38
Plaster-of-Paris, 143
Plastic bullets, 235
Platelet count, 20
Pneumonia, 92–93
Pneumothorax, (Fig. 8.3) 84, 85, 89
 spontaneous, 96
 tension, 89, 96, 103
Poisons Information Service, 232
Poisoning
 in children, 216
 management, 217, 222

INDEX

Poliomyelitis, 158
Polyurethane foam, hazards of, 87
Potassium, plasma, 20
Pre-eclampsia, 196
Pregnancy, 190, 191
   diagnosis of, 190
Pre-hospital care, 1, 2
Prolapsed cord, 196
Pulmonary embolus, 71, 144
Pulmonary oedema, 9, 94, 151, 227, 231
   due to left ventricular failure, 79
Pulse monitor, 12
Pupils, 10, 18, 71
Pyelonephritis, 130
Pyrogens, 39

Quinsy, 91

Radiation, 287
   injury, 288
   treatment, 290
Radioactive material, external
   contamination, 290
   internal contamination, 290
Records, 23
Recovery position, (*Fig.* 6.5) 56, 133, 154
Renal colic, 130
Respiratory distress syndrome, adult
   (ARDS), 96
   children, 213
Respiratory system, 7–9, 17
Retina, detached, 170
Rhonchus(i), *see* Wheezes
Rifle, Armalite, 236
   selfloading (SLR), 236
Ringer lactate solution (Hartmann's
   solution), 36, 206, 226
Riot control, 234
Rubber bullets, 235
Rugby football injuries, 245
'Rule of Nines', 206, 207

SAGM blood, 38
Salicylate poisoning, 229
Seatbelt, injuries, 9
Septic shock, 71, 199
Shock state, features, 199
   treatment, 201

Sinus bradycardia, 113
Sinus rhythm, 111
Sinus tachycardia, 112
'Site medical officer', 3
Skin elasticity, 31
Skin, examination of, 4
Smoke inhalation, 86–87
Soccer injuries, 245
Sodium, serum, 20
Spinal injuries, 248
Spine, damage to, (*Fig.* 8.2) 82–83, 134 151
Splints, 261
Squash injuries, 245
Status epilepticus, 162
Stomach washout (lavage), 229
Stretchers, in mountain rescue, 262
Stridor, 91, 215
Sudden Infant Death Syndrome (SIDS), 213
Supraventricular tachycardia, 74, 112
Survival bags, 265
Sweating, 12, 71, 74, 229
Syphilis, 156

Temperature, peripheral, measurement, 11–12, 27
Testis, torsion of, 131
Tetanus, 158
Tetraplegia, 151
Thermonuclear weapons, 284, 292
Thyroid disease, 187
Thyroxine, 188
Tongue, 31
Tourniquets, 100–1
Trachea, palpation, 7
Tracheostomy, 67–69 (*Figs.* 6.13, 6.14) 89, 134
Traction, (*Figs.* 13.11, 13.12) 144
Trauma, to great vessels, 104
   to respiratory system, 82
   to thoracic contents, 85–86
Tranquillizers, poisoning by, 228
Transfusion hazards, 39–41
   reactions, 39
Traumatic haemorrhage, 98–99
Tricyclic antidepressants, poisoning by, 228
Trismus, 158

Umbilical cord, 190
Underwater medicine, 276

Ureteric colic, 130
Urinary system, 18
Urine, blood in, 4, 18
  examination, 10
  output, 27, 29, 31
  retention, 131

Vascular compartment, assessment of, 25–30
Vasoconstriction, selective, 26
Vasodilators, (*Table* 11.2) 109, 202
Ventricular, trigeminy, 120
  ectopic beats, 117, 118
  fibrillation, 76, 119
  standstill, 119, 120
  tachycardia, 75, 118
Venous return, 26

Vocal resonance, 8
Venous pressure, 6
Vertebrae, crush fracture of, (*Figs.* 13.2, 13.3) 134

Warfare,
  biological, 295
  chemical, 292–5
  nuclear, 284–92
Water cannon, 235
'Wedge' pressure, 29
Wenckebach (Type I) heart block, 113, 114
Wheezes, 9
Wound, gunshot, 235
  scalp, 150